Toward Replacement Parts for the Brain

Toward Replacement Parts for the Brain

Implantable Biomimetic Electronics as Neural Prostheses

edited by Theodore W. Berger and Dennis L. Glanzman

A Bradford Book
The MIT Press
Cambridge, Massachusetts
London, England

MIT Press books may be purchased at special quantity discounts for business or sales promotional use. For information, please email special_sales@mitpress.mit.edu or write to Special Sales Department, The MIT Press, 55 Hayward Street, Cambridge, MA 02142.

This book was set in Times New Roman on 3B2 by Asco Typesetters, Hong Kong, and was printed and bound in the United States of America.

Library of Congress Cataloging-in-Publication Data

Toward replacement parts for the brain : implantable biomimetic electronics as neural prostheses / edited by Theodore W. Berger and Dennis L. Glanzman.
    p.   cm.
"A Bradford book."
"This book has its origins in a meeting, entitled "Toward replacement parts for the brain: intracranial implantations of hardware models of neural circuitry" that took place in Washington, D.C. in August 1999."
Includes bibliographical references and index.
ISBN 0-262-02577-9
1. Neural circuitry. 2. Neural networks (Neurobiology) 3. Brain–Computer simulation. 4. Biomimetics. 5. Computational neuroscience. I. Berger, Theodore W. II. Glanzman, Dennis., L.
QP363.3.T695   2005
612.8′2′011—dc22   2004051171

10   9   8   7   6   5   4   3   2   1

Contents

Preface

This book has its origins in a meeting entitled "Toward Replacement Parts for the Brain: Intracranial Implantation of Hardware Models of Neural Circuitry," that took place in Washington, D.C., in August 1999. The meeting was sponsored by the National Institute of Mental Health (NIMH), the University of Southern California (USC) Alfred E. Mann Institute for Biomedical Engineering, and the USC Center for Neural Engineering. The motivation for the meeting was a growing realization among neuroscientists, engineers, and medical researchers that our society was on the threshold of a new era in the field of neural prosthetics; namely, that in the near future it would be possible to mathematically model the functional properties of different regions or subregions of the brain, design and fabricate microchips incorporating those models, and create neuron/silicon interfaces to integrate microchips and brain functions. In this manner, our rapidly increasing understanding of the computational and cognitive properties of the brain could work synergistically with the continuing scientific and technological revolutions in biomedical, computer, and electrical engineering to realize a new generation of implantable devices that could bidirectionally communicate with the brain to restore sensory, motor, or cognitive functions lost through damage or disease.

Recognizing the ambitious nature of such a vision, the goal of the meeting and thus of this book, was to explore various dimensions of the problem of using biomimetic devices as neural prostheses to replace the loss of central brain regions. The first two chapters focus on advances in developing sensory system prostheses. The remarkable success in development and clinical application of the cochlear implant, and the rapid progress being made in developing retinal and visual prostheses, provide the best foundation for considering the extension of neural prostheses to central brain regions.

Cortical brain areas in particular present their own set of challenges. Beyond the issues of designing multisite electrode arrays for the complex geometry and cytoarchitecture of cortical brain (chapters 3 and 12) it is clear that neural representations of sensory receptive fields are not static, but in fact are dynamic, changing over time and with experience (chapter 4). The limitations of using static, multisite electrode arrays to extract information from a dynamically changing population of neurons must be taken into account when designing neural prosthetic systems triggered by sensory ensemble codes. Sophisticated analyses of multielectrode recordings from the hippocampus in behaving animals (chapters 5 and 6) emphasize the complexity of neural representations typical of memory systems in the brain. Hippocampal neurons respond to multiple dimensions (modalities) of a given learning and memory task, with key, higher-level features distributed across populations of spatially disparate cells. How to extract information from systems with such complex functional properties in real time, process that information, and then transmit the processed output back to other parts of the brain to influence cognitive function and behavior constitutes a considerable challenge.

Given the multiple levels of function that characterize the nervous system (i.e., molecular, cellular, network, or system), chapter 7 provides one of the few existing theoretical frameworks for modeling the hierarchical organization of neural systems. Chapter 8 offers some practical approaches for how to organize multidimensional time series data to achieve representational schemes for sensorimotor coupling.

Despite these complexities, considerable progress is being made in implementing biologically realistic neural system models in hardware. The importance of this step is that, to design and construct a neural prosthetic system that can interact with the brain, the mathematical models required to capture the nonlinear dynamics and non-stationarity of neural functions need to be miniaturized for implantation in the brain or on the skull, and need to take advantage of the parallel processing and high-speed computation offered by microelectronic and optoelectronic technologies. Examples of such first steps in very large-scale integration (VLSI) are described here for the hippocampus (chapter 12) and thalamocortical systems (chapter 13). In addition, the use of photonics and holographic technologies for achieving high-density connectivity between neural processors (chapter 14) and multiple-pattern storage for context-dependent connectivities and functions (chapter 15) offer novel and exciting possibilities for achieving the complexity of neural system functions in hardware. Chapter 16 offers a series of intriguing insights on the potential synergy between neuroscience and computer engineering; that is, how the capabilities of current VLSI and photonic technologies can facilitate the implementation of biologically based models of neural systems, and how our increasing understanding of neural organization and function can inspire next-generation computational engines.

Finally, designing and controlling the interface between neurons and silicon is a critical consideration in the development of central brain neural prostheses. Communication between biotic and abiotic systems must be bidirectional, so that the "state" of a neural system "upstream" from a damaged brain region can be sampled (e.g., electrophysiologically recorded) and processed by a biomimetic computational device, with the processed output then used to "drive" or alter (e.g., electrophysiologically stimulate) the state of a neural system "downstream" from the damaged region. Moreover, the "sampling" and "driving" functions must be achieved through an interface having sufficient density of interconnection with the target tissues, and correspondance with their cytoarchitecture (see chapter 12), to maintain the requisite input-output neural representations required to support a given level of cognitive function.

Perhaps most important, the neuron/silicon contacts must be target specific and maintained for multiyear durations to justify the surgical procedures required for implantation. Three chapters (9, 10, and 11) describe some of the latest updates in designing neuron/silicon interfaces and offer insights into the state-of-the-art problems and solutions for this aspect of implantable biomimetic systems.

There were other aspects of the global problem of how to achieve the collective vision of implantable biomimetic neural prostheses that were covered at the original meeting but, unfortunately, they are not readily compatible with a written volume. For example, we considered the need for new graduate education programs to provide next-generation neuroscientists and engineers with the expertise required to address in the scientific, technological, and medical issues involved, and discussed the technology transfer and commercialization obstacles to realizing a viable medical device based on an interdisciplinary science and technology foundation for implantable neural prostheses.

I SENSORY SYSTEMS

1 We Made the Deaf Hear. Now What?

Gerald E. Loeb

Neurons and modern digital electronic devices both process information in the form of all-or-none impulses of electricity, respectively called action potentials and logical states (bits). Over the past 50 years, electrophysiological techniques have been developed to provide sophisticated, safe, and reliable interfaces between electricity carried as ion fluxes in water and electricity carried as electron motion in metal conductors. Neural prostheses consist of the use of such interfaces to replace or repair dysfunction in the human nervous system. This chapter reviews the promises and the reality of what has been and might be achieved in the areas of sensory and motor prostheses, in the hope of providing some useful lessons and strategies for undertaking even more ambitious projects to repair higher neural functions such as cognition, memory, and affect.

Some years ago, the *New Yorker* printed a cartoon showing a bookstore patron gazing balefully at three aisles of books labeled, respectively, "nonfiction," "fiction," and "lies." That is a useful, if somewhat harsh and labile, way to categorize the status of a given scientific proposal to do something "difficult." Using an electronic device to fix a broken nervous system is certainly difficult. The first two *New Yorker* categories are akin to the distinction sometimes drawn between problems of "engineering" and those of "science," which raises the delicate question of what falls into the third category. Let us start with some examples drawn from other fields and then try to relate this categorization to actual or potential neural prostheses in order to understand their technical feasibility, clinical potential, and strategic risk.

The cliché question from the layperson is, "If we can put a man on the moon, why can't we cure cancer?" Putting a man on the moon is in the category of engineering because all the laws of physics required to demonstrate its feasibility are known, and calculations based on those laws can demonstrate that it is feasible. In fact, theoretical feasibility has been demonstrable for over a century, but practical achievement required a lot of technology, time, and money.

At some point between Jules Verne and the Apollo missions, putting a man on the moon shifted from fiction to nonfiction. I submit that the point occurred when someone, probably early in the history of modern rocketry, actually performed the myriad calculations related to gravity fields, rocket acceleration, fuel efficiency, life-support systems, etc. and couldn't find any reason why it would not work.

In contrast, curing most cancers remains in the category of scientific research rather than engineering or clinical practice because we still do not know enough about what causes cancer or how cells control their reproduction to even identify a particular strategy for curing cancer in general. One can construct plausible scenarios for how it might be possible to cure cancer, but they must be based on suppositions or hypotheses about how cells work that are as yet unproven. Thus, such scenarios are a credible form of science fiction, permitting even scientists knowledgeable in those fields to indulge in a "willing suspension of disbelief."

Stories based on time travel, perpetual motion machines, or extrasensory perception, for example, represent a different form of science fiction. One can only suspend disbelief if one doesn't know enough about physics, thermodynamics, or neurophysiology to realize that the bedrock theory upon which those sciences are based makes those ideas fundamentally impossible, not just temporarily impractical. I submit that such stories become "lies" when they are offered up to the lay public with the promise that if they spend enough money on a particular fiction, it can be made real. They are particularly pernicious lies if one tells such stories to patients and their families, who would like to believe and use them as a basis for important personal decisions on alternative methods of treatment and rehabilitation.

This is not to say that scientific theory cannot be overturned; an eighteenth-century physicist would have dismissed a story about atomic energy and transmutations of the elements as such a lie. Nevertheless, it would have been prudent even then to recognize that the scenario could never be realized by alchemy and to wait for the eventual development of quantum mechanics. With the benefit of hindsight, we can look at the prior criticisms of research on neural prostheses to see if this categorization might have provided guidance in selecting projects that turned out to be useful.

Cochlear Implants

In the early days of cochlear implants (circa 1975), many knowledgeable auditory neurophysiologists believed (and some forcefully stated) that a functionally useful auditory prosthesis could not be built. Their arguments were not based on theoretical limits on the electrical excitability of the auditory nervous system. The biophysics of neurons in general had been well worked out 50 years earlier, and experiments in humans had already demonstrated that perceptions of sound could be produced by reasonable and safe electrical stimulation. Their objection was based on their personal hypotheses regarding how the central nervous system might process and perceive various temporospatial patterns of electrical activity in the ensemble of auditory neurons.

Even as practiced today with multichannel intracochlear electrodes and sophisticated digital signal processors, cochlear stimulation creates temporospatial patterns
of neural activity that are greatly distorted from what would have occurred if those
sounds had been presented acoustically to a normally functioning ear. It turns out
that the brain is much more tolerant of some types of distortion than others and
that it is possible to present this relatively crude electrical stimulation in ways that
the brain accepts as quite natural sound. In fact, recent psychophysical tests in cochlear implant patients suggest that the intelligibility of speech as a function of number
of information channels follows essentially the same curve in cochlear implant users
as it does in normal hearing individuals. It levels off at about four to six channels regardless of how many stimulation channels the implant can provide (Wilson, 2000,
1997).

On the other hand, there are a lot of ways to present the same number of information channels that are not intelligible at all. In fact, a substantial minority (about
20%) of cochlear implant recipients never acquire high levels of speech recognition,
for reasons that remain mysterious (Kessler et al., 1995; Loeb and Kessler, 1995).
Thus, it was plausible but not provable to assert in 1975 that functional hearing
would not be produced by multichannel cochlear implants. Fortunately for tens of
thousands of deaf people and for the field of neural prosthetics in general, this asser-
tion turned out to be wrong. Cochlear implants progressed from plausible science
fiction to engineering and clinical fact, although it took 20 years to complete this
transition.

There are still reasons for trying to increase the number of useful channels actually
provided, but they fall into the category of incremental improvements rather than enabling technology. Such improvements might be expected to enhance performance in
cluttered acoustic environments with background noise. They might also address the
problematic minority who have difficulty using implants, but this is less certain. The
underlying problem that limits the number of effective channels is related to the ten-
dency for electrical stimulation currents to spread longitudinally in the fluid-filled
scala tympani before passing through the subjacent bony walls into the spiral ganglion, where the auditory neurons are stimulated. Addressing this problem requires
substantial changes to the design of the electrode arrays (for example, see figure
1.1), which raises various challenges for manufacturing techniques, surgical insertion
strategies, and biocompatibility.

Alternatively, it may be more useful to address the temporal distortions produced
by the present electrical stimulation waveforms. There are various speech encoding
and stimulus waveforms in use (recently reviewed by Wilson, 2000), but they all introduce an unphysiological degree of synchronicity in the firing of the auditory neurons. The auditory nervous system is exquisitely tuned to decode temporal patterns
(Loeb et al., 1983), so this may be more important than the simple rate coding that

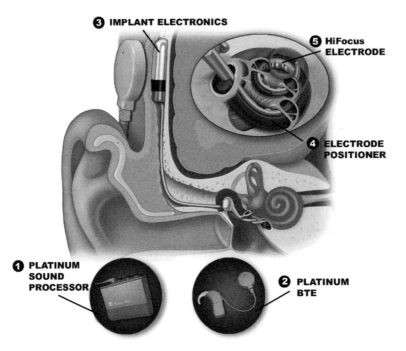

Figure 1.1
A cochlear prosthesis consists of an external sound processor (optional configurations shown in inserts 1 and 2) that transmits power and data to an implant (3) that generates complex patterns of stimulation pulses delivered to the cochlea by a multichannel electrode system. Insert 5 shows a new cochlear electrode array that attempts to improve the localization of each stimulation channel by pushing the array (4) against the medial wall of the scala tympani (closer to the spiral ganglion cells to be stimulated) and by incorporating silicone bumps between contacts to block the longitudinal spread of stimulus currents. (Illustration of the CLARION^{TM} system with HiFocus^{TM} electrode provided courtesy of the manufacturer, Advanced Bionics Corp., Valencia, Calif.)

appears to dominate most sensory encoding systems. By applying very high stimulus pulse frequencies, the auditory neurons can be desynchronized to fire on random sub-harmonics of the stimulation frequencies, reducing this unnatural synchronization (Rubinstein et al., 1999). Unfortunately, such stimulation is less efficient in terms of the mean power consumption needed to produce a given level of perceived loudness. This would conflict with the emphasis on smaller, lighter prostheses that can be worn on the ear (see Figure 1.1, insert 2) or even fully implanted in the body. Given steady improvements in the power efficiency of digital signal processing, the power budget for cochlear implants is increasingly dominated by the power dissipated by pushing stimulation currents through electrodes and cochlear tissues. The combination of more channels and higher stimulus pulse rates would require substantially larger, heavier batteries or more frequent recharge cycles.

It is not clear whether either the temporal or spatial enhancement strategies will be useful in any particular patient, much less in all. There are some suggestions that cochlear implant patients and perhaps even normal hearing individuals vary considerably in their relative dependence on the wide range of partially redundant acoustic cues that distinguish speech. Conventional cochlear implants are based on replicating the Helmholtzian place-pitch encoding, but some listeners may depend more on decoding of the high-frequency temporal cues that arise from phase-locked transduction of complex acoustic waveforms (Loeb et al., 1983). For example, some subjects prefer interleaved patterns of biphasic pulses that avoid electrotonic summation between channels. Other subjects prefer and perform just as well with simultaneous multichannel stimuli consisting of complex analog waveforms obtained by bandpass filtering and compressing the dynamic range of the raw acoustic signal.

Despite the wealth of electrophysiological and psychophysical data that can be collected from patients with multichannel cochlear implants, no correlations have yet emerged that account for their often striking differences in performance and preference. Thus, it is not surprising that there are essentially no preoperative predictors to decide which patients should receive which cochlear electrode or which speech-processing system. This forces engineering teams to try to design into the implants a very wide range of signal-processing and stimulus generation and delivery schemes, greatly complicating what is already perhaps the most complex biomedical device ever built. That complexity, in turn, demands a high level of sophistication from the clinicians, who must decide how to program each implant in each patient, and a high level of design for the supporting software that allows those clinicians to navigate and manage all those options.

Despite (or perhaps because of) all these emergent complexities and competing strategies, cochlear implants remain the visible proof that sophisticated neural functions can be successfully replaced by well-designed neural prosthetic systems. They succeeded clinically and commercially because even the relatively primitive single-channel and multichannel devices that emerged in the late 1970s provided useful benefits for the large majority of patients in whom they were implanted (Bilger, 1983). This provided the impetus for much further research and development that vastly improved both the basic performance and general usability of cochlear implants. It also provided a wide range of improved general design and manufacturing tools and techniques that should be applicable to other neural prosthetic devices, provided that we understand their underlying basic science.

Visual Prostheses

Research on visual prostheses has been going on for even longer than cochlear implant development, but it is still stuck in the category of science fiction. In 1965, when the scientific community got wind of Giles Brindley's plan to implant an array of cortical surface electrodes in a blind volunteer patient, a secret conference was convened largely to vilify the attempt (notes from that conference can be found as an appendix to the proceedings of a later meeting edited by Sterling et al., 1971). As with cochlear implants, it was well known from biophysical theory and prior experimentation that electrical stimulation of the striate cortex (Brodmann's area 17, now known as V1) could produce sensations of light (Penfield and Perot, 1963). Contemporary hypotheses about visual perception suggested, however, that it would not be possible to create useful, stable percepts from such stimulation. In the event (a few months later), the patient reported seeing "phosphenes" that were much more stable and well defined than had been predicted (Brindley and Lewin, 1968). This led to about 10 years of aggressively pursued research to build a practical visual prosthesis based on this approach. It turned out that the surprisingly punctate phosphenes produced by relatively high levels of poorly focused stimulation were the product of the surround-inhibitory neural circuitry of cortical columns, which were discovered about this time. These same circuits, however, also produced uncontrollable nonlinear interactions between adjacent sites of surface stimulation when an attempt was made to combine them into images (reviewed by Girvin, 1988). In the end, this plausible attempt to convert science fiction into engineering fact had to be abandoned.

In order to overcome the problem of the interaction of stimulus channels, some researchers turned next to developing intracortical microstimulation. Very fine microelectrodes can be inserted about 2 mm into the cortex so that they stimulate just a few neurons within a cortical column, using microamperes of current rather than milliamperes (Ranck, 1975). Given the concurrent advances in the neurophysiology of vision, this approach is now primarily an engineering rather than a science problem. Unfortunately, it is a very large problem. Small arrays with a few microelectrodes have been used successfully to produce stable and apparently combinable phosphenes in patients (Schmidt et al., 1996; Bak et al., 1990). Scaling this up to hundreds or thousands of separately controlled channels to produce useful (but still crude) images poses daunting problems for fabrication, surgical implantation, biocompatibility, protective packaging, interconnections, power consumption, psychophysical fitting and programming, image acquisition, and real-time data processing. There are promising technologies under development for each of these requirements, but their combination into a clinically safe, effective, and practical system remains only plausible, not certain.

Over the past decade, attention has shifted toward the very different strategy of electrically stimulating the retina. Obviously this is not a viable strategy for blindness caused by damage to the retinal ganglion cells whose axons make up the optic nerve (e.g., glaucoma, retinal detachment, optic nerve compression), but it might work for patients with primary degenerative diseases of the photoreceptors (e.g., retinitis pigmentosa and macular degeneration). The problem is that the retinal cells are very small; biophysical theory predicts that they should be difficult to stimulate electrically. Initial experiments in patients with intact retinas (who were undergoing removal of the eye because of malignant tumors) appeared to confound this prediction because microampere currents produced sensations of light. In fact, this is an unsurprising consequence of introducing small biases in a system of photoreceptors and intraretinal circuitry that employs spontaneous activity to create very high sensitivity to weak but coherent incident energy, such as light reflected from dimly illuminated objects. The transduction systems of both the intact retina and the intact cochlea are built in this way. It has long been known that the first sensations induced by weak electromagnetic fields are visual and auditory auras. In the absence of this background activity from the receptors, however, the postsynaptic neurons that generate all-or-none action potentials to convey sensory information to the brain revert to their type-specific and predictable biophysical properties.

When electrical stimulation is applied to the vitreous surface of a retina without photoreceptors, the lowest threshold neural elements are the long, myelinated output axons of retinal ganglion cells coursing horizontally over the retinal surface on their way into the optic nerve. Any local subset of these axons would map into a wedge-shaped sector of the retina. The resulting "phosphene" would not be a promising primitive from which to create complex visual images. One clever alternative is to take advantage of the different membrane time constants of the myelinated retinal ganglion axons and the unmyelinated bipolar cells, which are local interneurons oriented perpendicularly to the retinal surface (Greenberg et al., 1999). Electrical stimulation becomes more efficient when pulse duration approximates this time constant (Ranck, 1975), so it is possible to selectively stimulate bipolar cells with much longer pulses ($\sim$2 ms) than normal ($\sim$0.2 ms). Long pulses may cause problems, however, if they also require high stimulus currents and repetition rates to produce stable phosphenes. A retinal prosthesis is likely to need large numbers of closely spaced, relatively small electrodes to achieve useful image resolution. The individual stimulus pulses may exceed the charge density limits of the electrode materials (Loeb et al., 1982) and the aggregate power dissipation may cause excessive heating of the retina. Initial experiments with relatively crude electrode arrays have been encouraging (Humayun et al., 2003).

Epiretinal stimulation is likely to lead to the same problems of subliminal channel interaction that were encountered with cortical surface stimulation. It is possible that the same fix will be feasible—using penetrating microelectrodes to inject current much closer to the target bipolar neurons, thereby reducing power requirements and channel interactions. However, the bipolar cells are biophysically much less excitable than cortical pyramidal cells, and the retina is a much more delicate place in which to implant such electrode arrays. Thus, for the time being, this strategy is plausible science fiction in need of well-focused experiments to determine theoretical feasibility. If it is theoretically feasible, then the effort can shift to the formidable technical obstacles inherent in transmitting large amounts of data and power to dense electrode arrays that have to function for many years in the presence of saltwater and constant motion.

An alternative approach to retinal stimulation seeks to avoid the enormous complexity of external image acquisition and transmission of power and data to multichannel electrode arrays. The idea is to use integrated silicon arrays of photocells and electrodes implanted into the retina itself, between the superficial photoreceptor layer on the scleral side and the rest of the retinal ganglion circuitry on the vitreous side (Chow, 1991). It is a relatively simple matter to compute the maximal electrical current that can be derived from converting incident photons to electrons, assuming any reasonable photoelectric efficiency. Unfortunately, the answer is in the nanoampere range. There is no biophysical reason to expect such tiny stimulus currents to evoke action potentials in retinal cells deprived of background depolarization from photoreceptors.

Neuromuscular Reanimation

For the past 30 years, much of the technology developed for stimulating peripheral nerves and muscles has been predicated on the notion of getting paraplegics to walk. Despite substantial research efforts, there are no commercially available systems for locomotion; most research on functional electrical stimulation (FES) of the legs has retreated to the goal of providing FES-assisted standing. Paradoxically, the feasibility of electrically stimulating muscles to contract and move the limbs has been known since Luigi Galvani's discovery of bioelectricity in 1790. Is this an example of poor execution or unreasonable expectations?

The main challenge to the creation of clinically viable FES comes neither from science nor engineering but largely from selecting realistic objectives and tactics. There are many useful and practical clinical problems that can be addressed, given our present understanding of neurophysiology and currently available technologies, but getting paraplegics to walk is not one of them. Paraplegia presents a heterogeneous set of conditions in a relatively small population of patients. Moving around by wheelchair is readily available, relatively cheap, safe, and actually more energy efficient than normal walking or running. Equal-access laws have removed most mobility barriers in public places. Conversely, moving the legs with electrical stimulation of the muscles is highly invasive, cumbersome to program and to use, and inefficient and slow, even in a laboratory environment. In an uncontrolled field environment, it is likely to be quite dangerous as a consequence of inadequate strategies for coping with unpredictable footing and obstacles, the inability to control and minimize injury from falls, and the inability to get up after a fall. The kinematics and kinetics of unperturbed gait are easily measured in normal subjects, but the central neural strategies for achieving stability in the face of a wide range of perturbations and long delays in actuator response are not understood at all. Given these limitations, the resulting product would be unlikely to reduce health care costs or to improve the employability of paraplegics, in which case there would be no motivation for insurers to pay for it.

We have chosen instead to focus initially on the myriad secondary problems of muscle paralysis and paresis (Loeb and Richmond, 1999). Many of these result in substantial morbidity and large health care costs, but may be treatable with a modest number of stimulation channels and little or no real-time control. We have developed a modular, generic technology consisting of wireless intramuscular stimulators that can be injected nonsurgically into a wide range of sites (Cameron et al., 1997; figure 1.2). Each of these BION (*bio*nic *n*euron) implants receives power and digital command signals by inductive coupling from an external coil that creates an amplitude-modulated radio-frequency magnetic field in the vicinity of the implants (Troyk and

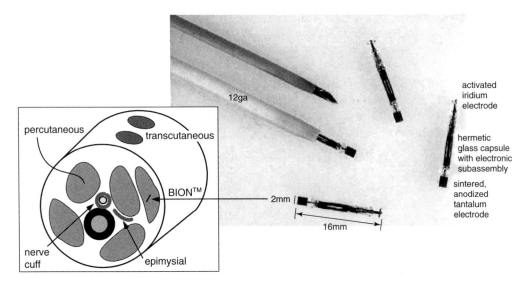

Figure 1.2
Various approaches to stimulating muscles include transcutaneous and percutaneous electrodes and surgically implanted multichannel stimulators with electrodes attached to nerves and muscles. BION implants are shown as they would be injected into muscles through a 12-gauge hypodermic needle. Each implant receives power and digitally addressed and encoded commands from an external controller and transmission coil. This system is in clinical trials to prevent disuse atrophy and related complications of upper motor paralysis, such as stroke and spinal cord injury. In principle, coordinated stimulation of many muscles could reanimate a paralyzed limb, but this will require substantial advances in sensing command and feedback signals from the patient and in emulating the complex and poorly understood control circuitry of the brain and spinal cord.

Schwan, 1992). The patient is provided with a portable controller (Personal Trainer) that creates preprogrammed sequences of stimulation to exercise the muscles.

The first clinical applications of this technology have aimed to prevent or reverse disuse atrophy of paretic muscles (Dupont et al., 2004). One clinical trial now under way involves stimulation of the middle deltoid and supraspinatus muscles of stroke patients to prevent chronically painful subluxation of the flaccid shoulder. Another involves strengthening the quadriceps muscles to protect an osteoarthritic knee from further stress and deterioration. Other applications in the planning phase include prevention of venous stasis and osteoporosis in patients with spinal cord injuries, reversal of equinus contractures of the ankle in cerebral palsy patients, and correction of footdrop in stroke patients. Still other clinical problems that may be candidates for such intramuscular stimulation include sleep apnea, disorders of gastrointestinal motility, and fecal and urinary incontinence. For most of these applications, clinical utility is as yet uncertain, morbidity would be unacceptable, and cost will be paramount. The generic, modular, minimally invasive and unobtrusive nature of BIONs makes them feasible to apply first to relatively simple clinical problems that might not justify the expense and morbidity of surgically implanted multichannel systems.

The BION technology is suitable for more ambitious FES to reanimate paralyzed limbs, but first the present microstimulator technology must be enhanced to include sensing and outgoing telemetry of the signals required for command and control. Work is under way to accommodate bioelectrical signals such as electromyography (EMG), motion and inclination as sensed by microelectromechanical system (MEMS) accelerometers, and relative position between implants, which can be used as a form of electronic muscle spindle to compute joint angles. These will be combined in progressively more ambitious ways to address various deficits of grasping and reaching in quadruplegic patients who have partial control of their arms. Such applications are less likely than locomotion to run afoul of our still-primitive understanding of sensorimotor control because speed, energy efficiency, and safety are much less critical.

Conclusions

The clinical and commercial success of cochlear implants has greatly increased the credibility of the field of neural prosthetics in general and the levels of technology and funding available to pursue new applications. That this success was achieved despite knowledgeable naysayers should not be cause for hubris. The laws of physics apply equally to bioelectricity and to conventional electronics, so they cannot be ignored. They represent the first and most easily predictable of many scientific, medical, and logistical hurdles that must be overcome to produce any useful neural prosthesis.

References

Bak, M., Girvin, J. P., Hambrecht, F. T., Kufta, C. V., Loeb, G. E., and Schmidt, E. M. (1990) Visual sensations produced by intracortical microstimulation of the human occipital cortex. *Med. Biol. Eng. Comput.* 28: 257–259.

Bilger, R. C. (1983) Auditory results with single-channel implants. *Ann. N. Y. Acad. Sci.* 405: 337–342.

Brindley, G. S., and Lewin, W. S. (1968) The sensations produced by electrical stimulation of the visual cortex. *J. Physiol. (London)* 196: 479–493.

Cameron, T., Loeb, G. E., Peck, R. A., Schulman, J. H., Strojnik, P., and Troyk, P. R. (1997) Micromodular implants to provide electrical stimulation of paralyzed muscles and limbs. *IEEE Trans. Biomed. Eng.* 44: 781–790.

Chow, A. Y. (1991) Artificial Retina Device. U.S. Patent 5,024,223.

Dupont, A. C., Bagg, S. D., Creasy, J. L., Romano, C. Romano, D., Richmond, F. J. R., and Loeb, G. E. (2004) First patients with BION® implants for therapeutic electrical stimulation. *Neuromodulation* 7: 38–47.

Girvin, J. P. (1988) Current status of artificial vision by electrocortical stimulation. *Neuroscience* 15: 58–62.

Greenberg, R. J., Velte, T. J., Humayun, M. S., Scarlatis, G. N., and de Juan, E., Jr. (1999) A computational model of electrical stimulation of the retinal ganglion cell. *IEEE Trans. Biomed. Eng.* 46: 505–514.

Humayun, M. S., Weiland, J. D., Fujii, G. Y., Greenberg, R., Williamson, R., Little, J., Mech, B., Cimmarusti, V., Van Boemel, G., Dagnelie, G., and de Juan, E. (2003) Visual perception in a blind subject with a chronic microelectronic retinal prosthesis. *Vision Res.* 43: 2573–2581.

Kessler, D. K., Loeb, G. E., and Barker, M. S. (1995) Distribution of speech recognition results with the Clarion cochlear prosthesis. *Otol. Rhinol. Laryngol.* Suppl. 166: 283–285.

Loeb, G. E., and Kessler, D. K. (1995) Speech recognition performance over time with the Clarion cochlear prosthesis. *Ann. Otol. Rhinol. Laryngol.* Suppl. 166: 290–292.

Loeb, G. E., and Richmond, F. J. R. (1999) FES or TES: How to start an industry? In *Proceedings of the 4th Annual Conference of the International Functional Electrical Stimulation Society*, pp. 169–172.

Loeb, G. E., McHardy, J., Kelliher, E. M., and Brummer, S. B. (1982) Neural prosthesis. In D. F. Williams, ed., *Biocompatibility in Clinical Practice*, vol. 2. Boca Raton, Fla.: CRC Press, pp. 123–149.

Loeb, G. E., White, M. W., and Merzenich, M. M. (1983) Spatial cross-correlation: A proposed mechanism for acoustic pitch perception. *Biol. Cybern.* 47: 149–163.

Penfield, W., and Perot, P. (1963) The brain's record of auditory and visual experience. *Brain* 86: 595–696.

Ranck, J. B., Jr. (1975) Which elements are excited in electrical stimulation of mammalian central nervous system? A review. *Brain Res.* 98: 417–440.

Rubinstein, J. T., Wilson, B. S., Finley, C. C., and Abbas, P. J. (1999) Pseudospontaneous activity: Stochastic independence of auditory nerve fibers with electrical stimulation. *Hear. Res.* 127: 108–118.

Schmidt, E. M., Bak, M. J., Hambrecht, F. T., Kufta, C. V., and O'Rourke, D. K. V. P. (1996) Feasibility of a visual prosthesis for the blind based on intracortical microstimulation of the visual cortex. *Brain* 119: 507–522.

Sterling, T. D., Bering, E. A., Pollack, S. V., and Vaughan, H. G., eds. (1971) *Visual Prosthesis: The Interdisciplinary Dialogue*. New York: Academic Press.

Troyk, P. R., Schwan, M. A. K. (1992) Closed-loop class E transcutaneous power and data link for microimplants. *IEEE Trans. Biomed. Eng* 39: 589–599.

Wilson, B. S. (1997) The future of cochlear implants. *Br. J. Audiol.* 31: 205–225.

Wilson, B. S. (2000) New directions in implant design. In S. B. Waltzman and N. L. Cohen, eds., *Cochlear Implants*. New York: Theme Medical Publishers, pp. 43–56.

2 Microelectronic Array for Stimulation of Large Retinal Tissue Areas

Dean Scribner, M. Humayun, Brian Justus, Charles Merritt, R. Klein, J. G. Howard, M. Peckerar, F. K. Perkins, E. Margalit, Kah-Guan Au Eong, J. Weiland, E. de Juan, Jr., J. Finch, R. Graham, C. Trautfield, and S. Taylor

During the 1990s a number of research groups began exploring the feasibility of an intraocular retinal prosthesis (IRP). The hope of providing vision for the blind has attracted a great deal of attention in the scientific and technological world. Recent advances in the fields of microelectronics, neurophysiology, and retinal surgery have advanced to the point where an implantable visual prosthetic system, based on electrical stimulation, is considered feasible.

Another type of neural prosthesis, the cochlear prosthesis for deaf patients, has been successfully developed and commercialized (Agnew and McCreery, 1990; Heiduschka and Thanos, 1998). Development of a retinal prosthesis is generally following in the footsteps of the cochlear prosthesis, but is a number of years behind at this point. Although there are other approaches to a visual prosthesis, this chapter focuses primarily on the development of an intraocular electronic stimulator array. Many issues need to be resolved before successful implants become practical for long-term human use. This chapter describes the scientific and technical issues related to development of an intraocular retinal prosthetic device.

It is important to note that the retina is a true extension of the brain, and in that regard, there are many similarities between the design of an IRP and a device for direct stimulation of the brain or other sensory areas of the central nervous system (CNS).

The first section of this chapter gives a brief description of the retina and some background on work in visual prosthetics. The second section gives an overview of the concept for an IRP. Electrical stimulation of the retina is discussed in the third section. The fourth section discusses the development of a curved-surface electrode array fabricated using channel glass. Efforts to design and fabricate a microelectronic stimulator array for an advanced IRP are described in the fifth section.

The Retina and Prosthetic Devices

The retina is the innermost layer of the eye. It is basically composed of two layers, the outer retinal pigment epithelium (RPE) and the inner neural (sensory) retina

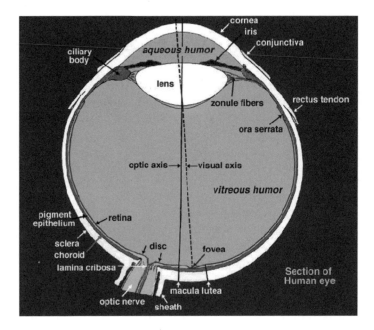

Figure 2.1
Sagittal section of an adult human eye (from Ogden, 1989; modified by Kolb, 2001).

(figure 2.1). The sensory retina is a delicate sheet of transparent tissue varying in thickness from 0.4 to 0.15 mm. The anatomical site for detailed fine vision, called the fovea, is in the center of the macula. The outermost layer of the sensory retina consists of photoreceptors (figure 2.2); in the macular region, the photoreceptors are mostly cones (color-sensitive). Other more inner layers of the sensory retina are the inner nuclear layer with bipolar, amacrine, and horizontal cells; and the ganglion cell layer. The axons of the ganglion cells form the optic nerve after traversing the nerve fiber layer.

Photoreceptor loss from diseases such as retinitis pigmentosa (RP) and age-related macular degeneration (AMD) are the leading cause of legal blindness. Despite near-total loss of photoreceptors in these diseases, there is relative preservation of the other retinal neurons. By stimulating the remaining functional retinal layers, it may be possible to restore visual perception. In other diseases, this approach may not be practical. For example, in glaucoma (high intraocular pressure with optic nerve damage), the ganglion cells are primarily damaged. In diseases such as retinopathy of prematurity, diabetic retinopathy, and vascular diseases of the retina, all the layers are affected. In these diseases, it is highly unlikely that electrical stimulation of the retina can restore visual function, and other approaches such as retinal transplantation or electrical stimulation of the visual cortex should be investigated.

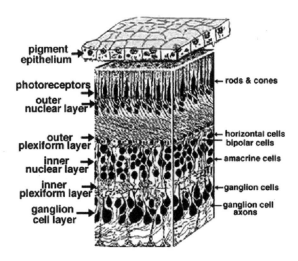

pigment
epithelium

photoreceptors

outer
nuclear layer

outer
plexiform layer

inner
nuclear layer

inner
plexiform layer

ganglion
cell layer

← rods & cones

← horizontal cells
bipolar cells

← amacrine cells

← ganglion cells

ganglion cell
axons

Figure 2.2
Three-dimensional section of human retina (from Polyak, 1941; modified by Kolb, 2001).

Background of Visual Prosthetics

During the eighteenth century, scientists began to understand that electricity could stimulate biological tissues. Galvani showed that electrical stimulation could cause contraction in muscle preparations (Galvani, 1791). Fritsch and Hitzig (1870) demonstrated the electrical excitability of the cerebral cortex in a dog. They were able to use this finding to localize electrophysiological functions of the brain. Glenn and colleagues (1959) developed a totally implanted heart pacemaker using radiofrequency waves to transfer information. This technological breakthrough overcame the problem of stimulating deep neural structures without the danger of infection that can accompany percutaneous leads. Djourno and Eyries (1957) reported electrical stimulation of the acoustic nerve in a totally deaf human by direct application of an electrode in the inner ear.

Today, a number of research projects around the world are aimed at developing prosthetic vision systems. The approaches can be categorized most simply by where the actual stimulation occurs. The device discussed in this chapter addresses the technical problem of positioning a high-density electrode array against the retina to achieve very high-resolution imagery. Other efforts in the United States, Germany, and Japan are building on the basic idea of stimulating retinal cells with a small number of electrodes on a microelectronic chip.

In the past, another approach has been to bypass the retina altogether and stimulate the visual cortex of the brain. In this approach, an array with penetrating microelectrodes is positioned against the visual cortex. This involves invasive brain surgery through the cranium. Both of these approaches are discussed in the sections that follow.

There are two major advantages of the cortical stimulation approach (Normann, 1999). First, the skull is a stable stimulation site and will protect the electronics and the electrode array. Second, the approach bypasses all distal visual pathway pathologies. However, it has a number of disadvantages. The retinotopic mapping on the cortical surface is poorly understood, so patterned stimulation may not produce patterned perception. Furthermore, it is unclear what visual perceptions will be evoked by stimulation of cortical neurons. Also, the complex topography of the cortical anatomy makes it a difficult site for implantation. Finally, surgical complications can lead to severe consequences.

Other groups are attempting to develop retinal prostheses that will cause visual perception by electrical stimulation of the healthy inner layers of the retina in patients who suffer from diseases such as retinitis pigmentosa and age-related macular degeneration. Progress in the field of neural prosthetics has converged with advances in retinal surgery to enable the development of an implantable retinal prosthesis. Initial experiments with intraocular stimulation were performed by de Juan and Humayun several years ago (Humayun et al., 1994). Since that time, several research groups have begun the development of retinal prostheses (Zrenner et al., 1999; Humayun et al., 1999; Chow and Peachey, 1998; Eckmiller, 1997; Wyatt and Rizzo, 1996; Veraart et al., 1998; Yagi and Hayashida, 1999). Their approaches can be classified according to where their device will be positioned—on the retinal surface (epiretinal) or in the subretinal space (subretinal).

Epiretinal implantation has the advantage of leaving the retina intact by placing the implant in the vitreous cavity, a naturally existing and fluid-filled space. Studies at John Hopkins University Hospital have demonstrated that this position for an array is biocompatible (Majji et al., 1999). Other groups are examining this approach as well (Eckmiller, 1997; Rizzo and Wyatt, 1997). The basic concept that has been described in the past is to mount a miniature video camera (e.g., a charge-coupled device, CCD) on a pair of glasses. The video signal and power of the output would be processed by a data processor, and the information transferred to intraocular electronics by either an 820-nm wavelength laser (Rizzo and Wyatt, 1997) or radiofrequency transmission from an external metal coil to an intraocular coil (Troyk and Schwan, 1992; Heetderks, 1988). The power and data transmitted from the laser or the coil would be converted to electrical current on a stimulating chip that would then control the distribution of current to the epiretinal electrode array. A later section of this chapter discusses a means of naturally imaging light onto an epiretinal prosthesis.

Subretinal implantation of a retinal prosthesis is being developed by Zrenner (Zrenner et al., 1999; Guenther et al., 1999) and Chow (Chow and Peachey, 1998;

Chow and Chow, 1997; Peyman et al., 1998). This approach essentially replaces the diseased photoreceptors with a microelectronic stimulator device. However, the surgical implantation requires detaching the retina, and the location of the device may be disruptive to the health of the retina (Zrenner et al., 1999). The histology of the retina after long-term implantation of a device showed a decline in the densities of inner nuclear and ganglion cell layers (Peyman, et al., 1998). The outer layers of the retina are nourished by the choroid. For this reason, Zrenner's group included nutrition openings in each unit of their device. These issues are being examined in recently announced phase I clinical trials of a subretinal implantation by Chow and colleagues in Chicago. A disadvantage of this approach is that it is not applicable to patients with AMD because the retina is no longer transparent.

Another approach to a retinal prosthesis was proposed by Yagi at the Kyushu Institute of Technology, Japan (Yagi and Hayashida, 1999; Yagi and Watanabe, 1998). He proposed to develop a device called the hybrid retinal implant. This device would be an integrated circuit and include both electronic and cellular components. The neurons on the device would extend their axons to the central nervous system and thus create a natural device/CNS interface.

The epiretinal and subretinal approaches have several advantages over the cortical approach. They both have the ability to use existing physiological optics of the eye, less severe consequences in case of infection, obvious spatial mapping or retinotopic organization, and natural processing of the electrically stimulated images along the proximal visual pathways. However, the retina encodes many properties of the image that are passed on to the higher visual centers (color, intensity, motion, etc.). Therefore it may be necessary to integrate some image-processing functions into a retinal prosthesis. This issue is the subject of the next section.

Overview of an Intraocular Retinal Prosthetic Device

The basic concept of an IRP is straightforward: Visual images can be produced in the brain by electrical stimulation of retinal cells. A layer of retinal cells, such as a ganglion cell layer, can be stimulated by using an adjacent microelectronic array that inputs electrical impulses to create the perception of an image. The axons of the stimulated ganglion cells then transmit the image through the optic nerve to cells in the visual cortex. This is in place of the normal phototransduction process that occurs in a healthy retina. In a large percentage of blind patients, the photoreceptors are diseased but the other retinal layers are still responsive to electrical stimulation (de Juan et al., 1989).

One concept for a high-resolution retinal prosthesis is shown in figure 2.3. A ray trace of photons incident on a retina without a prosthesis is shown in the top half of figure 2.3. Note that the incoming photons pass through several layers of transparent

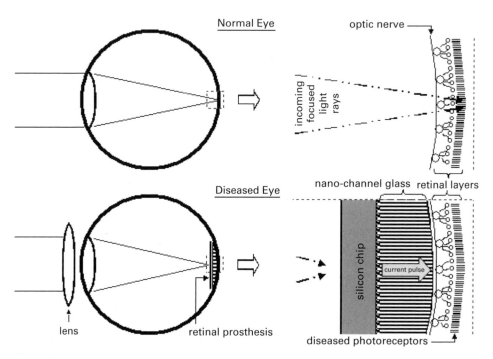

Figure 2.3
Basic concept for a retinal prosthesis. A ray trace of photons incident on a retina without a prosthesis is shown in the top half of the figure. Incoming photons pass through several layers of clear retinal cells before being absorbed by the photoreceptors. In the bottom half of the figure, a retinal prosthesis is shown positioned against the retina.

retinal cells before being absorbed by the photoreceptors. In the bottom half of figure 2.3, a retinal prosthesis is shown positioned against the retina. In this case, the photons are absorbed by a microelectronic imaging array that is hybridized to a glass disk containing an imbedded array of microwires. The glass disk has one flat side, while the other side has a curved surface that conforms to the inner radius of the retina. The microelectronic imaging array is made of thin silicon containing very large-scale integrated (VLSI) circuitry and photon detectors that convert the incident photons to an electronic charge. The charge is then converted to a proportional amount of electronic current that is input into the retinal cells. The cells fire and a signal is transmitted through the optic nerve.

A number of technical issues must be addressed in designing and fabricating a retinal prosthetic device that will generate a high-resolution image. First, there is the problem of creating an electrical interface between the high-density electrode array and the curved surface of the retina. The electrode array must have a spherical, convex shape to conform to the spherical, concave surface of the retina. The electrode array must be biocompatible and safe for permanent implantation. Second, the electrical stimulation pulse shapes and repetition rates need to be determined in general and may need to be optimized for each patient. Third, direct electrical stimulation of the ganglion cells precludes certain image-processing functions that normally would have occurred in earlier layers of the retina. Therefore, preprocessing operations may need to be performed on the image before stimulation of the retina. Fourth, the power supply to a permanent implant will need to be engineered so there are no wires or cables through the eye wall. Fifth, because a normal retina processes image information created by the photoreceptors in a simultaneous manner, it is assumed that a prosthesis should similarly excite retinal cells in a simultaneous manner (as opposed to a sequential raster scan like that used in video displays).

A microelectronic stimulator array is described here that addresses many of these technical issues. The current joint effort between the U.S. Naval Research Laboratory and Johns Hopkins University Hospital is aimed at developing a microelectronic IRP stimulator array that will be used in preliminary short-term tests in an operating room environment. The test device will receive input images from an external camera connected via a microcable. These tests will determine the requirements for a permanent IRP implant that images incident photons, as shown in the bottom half of figure 2.3.

The test device will allow short-term human experiments (less than an hour) to study basic issues involved with interfacing a massively parallel electrode array to retinal tissue. The design combines two technologies: (1) electrode arrays fabricated from nanochannel glass (NCG) (Tonucci et al., 1992), and (2) infrared focal plane array (IRFPA) multiplexers (Scribner et al., 1991).

Nanochannel glass is a technology that uses fiber optic fabrication techniques to produce thin wafers of glass with very small channels perpendicular to the plane of the wafer (Tonucci and Justus, 1993a,b). Typical NCG wafers that will be required for retinal prostheses are several millimeters in diameter and contain millions of channels, with channel diameters on the order of 1 μm. The channels are filled with a good electrical conductor, and one surface of the glass is ground to a spherical shape consistent with the radius of curvature of the inside of the retina. The electrical conductors on the curved surface should protrude slightly to form efficient electrodes. NCG technology is discussed in a later section.

For the test IRP, a microelectronic multiplexer is required. The IRFPA community has been developing a similar multiplexer technology over the past decade. These arrays use microelectronic multiplexers that are fabricated at silicon foundries. The multiplexer is a two-dimensional array that reads out the infrared images captured by a complementary detector array that converts photons into an electrical charge. The charge is integrated and stored in each pixel (sometimes referred to as a unit cell) for a few milliseconds. The full image is then multiplexed off the array at

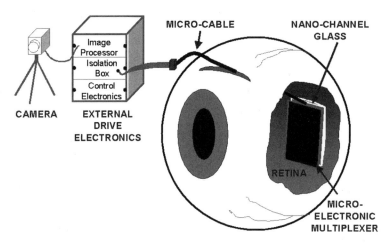

Figure 2.4
An intraocular retinal prosthetic test device positioned against the retina as it would be in a short-term human experiment performed by an ophthalmologist. External-drive electronics are needed to control the device and interface it with a standard video camera.

frame rates compatible with commercial video. For a test IRP, the process is essentially reversed, and the device acts as demultiplexer. That is, an image is read onto the stimulator array. Although the devices discussed here for an IRP will perform demultiplexing operations, they are simply referred to as multiplexers.

Figure 2.4 shows a test device for an IRP positioned against the retina as it would be in a short-term human experiment performed by an ophthalmologist. The experimental procedure uses standard retinal surgical techniques identical to those in an operating room environment. It is necessary that the patient be administered local (rather than general) anesthesia so that he or she is conscious during the procedure.

Figure 2.5 shows a side view of the fully packaged test device. The NCG is hybridized to the multiplexer using indium bump bonds; again, this is similar to hybridization techniques used in IRFPAs. The image is serially input onto the multiplexer through a very narrow, flexible microcable. The ceramic carrier with gold via holes (conducting wires penetrating from the front to the back) provides a mechanically convenient means of routing interconnects from the top side of the device to the back side. By designing the ceramic carrier so that the via holes are in close proximity to the bond pads on the silicon multiplexer, the interconnection can be made with conventional tab bonds (thin gold ribbons fused to interconnects with mechanical pressure). This keeps all the interconnects from protruding above the spherical curved envelope defined by the polished NCG surface and therefore protects the retina from damage and reduces the risk of breaking a tab bond.

As discussed later, a critical issue for any neural prosthesis is biocompatiblilty and safety. Because the durations of any tests with the IRP are very short (less than an

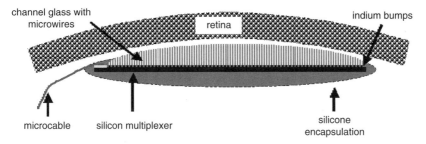

Figure 2.5
Side view of the fully packaged test device for an intraocular retinal prosthesis (IRP). The nanochannel glass (NCG) is hybridized to the multixplexer using indium bump bonds similar to the hybridization techniques used in infrared focal plane arrays (IRFPAs).

hour), biocompatibility issues are primarily reduced to acute effects and need not address the more difficult chronic issues that arise with permanent implants. Note that the surface of the packaging shown in figure 2.5 consists only of glass, platinum electrodes, and silicone encapsulation. However, as with any electronic medical instrumentation, a major safety issue is electrical shock hazard. The objective of the device is to provide minimal electrical stimulation of retinal tissue using very low voltages and the smallest currents possible. During this procedure, the patient must be coupled to the external instrumentation. To protect the patient from any electrical shock, the patient is isolated from high voltages using optocouplers that are powered by low-voltage batteries.

Neurophysiology of an IRP

Many questions and concerns arise when interfacing an electronic device to neural tissue. One fundamental concern is that because the retina is a thin-layered structure, more than one layer may respond to electrical stimulation. Other questions involve electrode configurations, electrical currents, and pulse shapes, as well as the important issues of safety and biocompatibility.

Preferential Stimulation of Retinal Cell Layers
The advantage of stimulating retinal cells other than ganglions was mentioned earlier. Histological analysis of postmortem eyes of RP (Humayun et al., 1999b; Santos et al., 1997; Stone et al., 1992) and AMD patients reveals apparently healthy ganglion and bipolar cells in the macular region. Experimentally, it has been shown that phosphenes could be elicited in patients with advanced outer retinal degeneration via electrical stimulation (Potts and Inoue, 1970; Weiland et al., 1999; Humayun et al., 1996a; Rizzo et al., 2000). These electrically elicited responses require and indicate the presence of functioning retinal cells.

Retinal ganglion cells (RGC) lie close to the surface of the retina facing the vitreous cavity and send mostly unmyelinated axons in a more superficial layer toward the optic disk. As the human RGC axons exit the eye, they become myelinated and form the optic nerve. The cell bodies (somas) of these ganglion cells are mapped over the surface of the retina in a manner that approximates the projection of the visual world onto the surface of the retina. However, at any particular location on the surface of the retina, axons from distant sites overlay the individual ganglion cell bodies. If these superficial passing axons were preferentially stimulated, groups of ganglion cells from large areas of the retina would be excited. One might expect the visual perception of such a stimulus to appear as a wedge. On the other hand, if the ganglion cell bodies or deeper retinal cells were stimulated, one would expect the visual perceptions to be focal spots. RP patients that were stimulated with 50–200-μm-diameter platinum disk electrodes reported seeing spots, not wedges, of light (Humayun et al., 1999; Weiland et al., 1999; Humayun et al., 1996a).

To explore the possibilities of retinal electrical stimulation, a computational model of extracellular field stimulation of the RGC has been constructed (Greenberg et al., 1999). The model predicted that the stimulation threshold of the RGC soma is 58–73% lower than a passing axon, even though the axon was closer to the electrode. Nevertheless, a factor of less than 2 does not explain the source of visual perceptions observed during previous experiments with intraocular patients.

Another possibility was that deeper retinal cells were stimulated. Postmortem morphometric analysis of the retina of RP patients revealed that many more inner nuclear layer cells retain functionality (e.g., bipolar cells and others, with 78.4%) compared with the outer nuclear layer (photoreceptors, 4.9%) and the ganglion cell layer (29.7%) (Santos et al., 1997). Early electrophysiological experiments showed that cathodic stimulation on the vitreous side of the retina depolarizes presynaptic end terminals of the photoreceptors (Knighton, 1975a,b) and bipolar cells (Toyoda and Fujimoto, 1984). Recently, latency experiments in frog retinas showed that higher currents stimulate the RGC directly, while lower currents activate other cells (photoreceptors, bipolar cells) (Greenberg, 1998).

Another finding in those experiments was that shorter stimulating pulses (<0.5 ms) have an effect different than longer stimulating pulses (>0.5 ms). There are well-defined relationships between the threshold current and the duration of the stimulus pulse required for neuronal activation (West and Wolstencroft, 1983). As the duration of the stimulus pulse decreases, the threshold increases exponentially. Also, as the pulse duration increases, the threshold current approaches a minimum value, called the rheobase. A chronaxie is the pulse width for which the threshold current is twice the rheobase current. Greenberg (1998) showed that deeper retinal cells have unusually long chronaxies compared with RGCs. In human experiments, a short stimulation time (<0.5 ms) created elongated phosphene percepts, while longer stimulation (1–8 ms) created rounded percepts (Greenberg, 1998). It can be speculated from these results that there is a preferential stimulation of RGC cells or axons for short pulses and deeper cellular elements for long pulses.

Interfacing IRP Electrodes to Retinal Tissue

A number of basic physiological questions and concerns arise when interfacing an electronic device to neural tissue. Three of these questions are addressed here.

What Is the Minimum Current for Neuron Activation?

In 1939, Cole and Curtis found that during propagation of the action potential in the axon of the giant squid, the conductance of the membrane to ions increases dramatically (Cole and Curtis, 1939). In 1949, Cole designed an apparatus known as the voltage clamp to overcome the problems of experimentally measuring the Na^+ and K^+ currents through the axon's membrane. The amount of current that must be generated by the voltage clamp to keep the membrane potential from changing provides a direct measure of the current flowing across the membrane. Hodgkin and Huxley (1952a,b) used the voltage clamp technique and the squid axon to give the first complete description of the ionic mechanisms underlying the action potential. According to the Hodgkin-Huxley model, an action potential involves the following sequence of events. A depolarization of the membrane causes Na^+ channels to open rapidly, resulting in an inward Na^+ current (because of a higher resting concentration of this ion *outside* the cell membrane). This current causes further depolarization, thereby opening more Na^+ channels, and results in increased inward current; the regenerative process causes the action potential.

Electrical stimulation elicits a neural response by "turning on" the voltage-sensitive ion channels, bypassing the chemically gated channels in the stimulated cell. There are different methods by which neurons can be activated. The first is activation of the cathodic threshold. This is the minimum amplitude and duration of a stimulus required to initiate an action potential. Once the membrane reaches a certain potential, a trigger mechanism is released and an action potential results (an all-or-nothing mechanism). Other methods to stimulate neurons are anodic pulses and biphasic pulses.

There are well-defined relationships between the threshold charge and pulse duration (West and Wolstencroft, 1983). Charge and threshold have different minimum requirements during neuronal stimulation. A minimum charge is required for a shorter pulse duration, in contrast to threshold current, which is minimized at long pulse durations. Experiments were performed at Johns Hopkins University Hospital to define threshold currents for electrical stimulation of the retina. One study assessed the effect of changing the parameters of the stimulating electrode and the stimulus pulse by recording electrically elicited action potential responses from retinal ganglion cells in an isolated rabbit retina (Shyu et al., 2000). It was concluded that the threshold for stimulation from the ganglion side is lower than from the photoreceptor side, especially when using microelectrodes (19.05 μA versus 48.89 μA, with a pulse duration of 0.5 ms). Recently, similar experiments with very small electrodes (10-μm diameter) demonstrated successful stimulations with currents as low as 0.14–0.29 μA (Grumet et al., 1999, 2000).

A second type of experiment compared the electrical stimulation threshold in normal mouse retinas with different aged retinal degenerate (rd) mouse retinas (Suzuki et al., 1999). Retinal ganglion cell recordings were obtained from anesthetized 8- and 16-week-old rd mice, and 8-week-old normal mice in response to a constant current electrical stimulus delivered via a platinum wire electrode on the retinal surface. The excitation thresholds were significantly higher in the 16-week-old rd mouse (0.075 μC for an 0.08-ms square pulse) than in the 8-week-old rd (0.048 μC for an 0.08-ms square pulse) ($p < 0.05$) and the normal mouse (0.055 μC for 0.08-ms square pulse) ($p < 0.05$). In all groups, short-duration pulses were more efficient than longer pulses (lower total charge) ($p < 0.05$). A related experiment involved the electrical stimulation of normal and rd mouse retinas and the visual cortical responses elicited (Chen et al., 1999). A square-wave stimulus (240 ± 58 μA) was more efficient than the sine waveform (533 ± 150 μA) or pulse-train (1000 ± 565 μA) waveform ($p = 0.002$).

In human experiments at Johns Hopkins University Hospital, typical thresholds observed for retinal stimulation of RP patients was 500 μA with a 2-ms half-pulse stimulus duration (1 μC/phase) using electrodes with from 50- to 200-μm-diameter disks that were very near, but not touching the retina (Humayun et al., 1996a). The quantity charge per phase is defined as the integral of the stimulus current over one half-cycle of the stimulus duration. In summary, the measurements that have been made to date serve as useful guides for the threshold levels needed to stimulate retinal neurons; however, a quantitative relationship between minimum currents, electrode size, proximity, and pulse shape is still incomplete.

What Is the Maximum Current That Can Be Used Before Impairing the Physiological Function of Retinal Cells?   Among the early studies that have addressed this issue are the histopathological studies of long-term stimulation by Pudenz et al. (1975a,b,c) as well as the electrochemical studies of the electrode/electrolyte interface by Brummer and Turner (1975). Lilly (1961) demonstrated the relative safety of biphasic, charge-balanced waveforms compared with monophasic waveforms. McCreery et al. (1988) showed that stimulation-induced neural damage derives from processes associated with the passage of stimulus current through tissue, rather than from electrochemical reactions at the electrode/tissue interface.

They also showed that the threshold of tissue damage from electrical stimulation is primarily dependent on charge density and charge per phase (McCreery et al., 1988,

1990). Charge density is defined as charge per phase divided by the electrochemically active electrode surface area. Since total charge density is responsible for the damage of tissue and electrodes, it has been hypothesized that there is a theoretical limit for how small electrodes can be (Brown et al., 1977; Tehovnik, 1996). Using simple waveforms, conservative charge density limits for long-term stimulation with platinum are 100 $\mu C/cm^2$ and 1 μC/phase. For activated iridium oxide electrodes, the limit is 1 mC/cm^2 and 16 nC/phase. Most of the studies that were done to determine these limits were performed with superficial cortical electrodes (McCreery et al., 1988, 1990), or intracortical microstimulation (Bullara et al., 1983). Long-term in vivo retinal stimulation tests still need to be performed to define tissue damage thresholds.

What Are the Optimum Conditions for Stimulating Retinal Neurons and What Is the Desired Response?   One of the conditions for safe electrical stimulation of neural tissue is a reversible faradaic process. These reactions involve electron transfer across the electrode/neuron interface. Some chemicals are either oxidized or reduced during these reactions. These chemicals remain bound to the electrode surface and do not mix with the surrounding solution. It is also necessary to know the chemical reversibility of electrode materials and stimulation protocols. Chemical reversibility requires that all processes occurring at an electrode that are due to an electrical pulse, including H_2 and O_2 evolution, will be chemically reversed by a pulse of opposite polarity.

The two basic waveforms used in electrical neural stimulation to achieve chemical reversibility are sinusoidal and pulsatile. The sinusoidal waveform is completely described by its amplitude and frequency. The pulsatile waveform is completely described by a square-ware pulse amplitude, that is, amplitude, duration, polarity, and repetition frequency (Gorman and Mortimer, 1983).

Over time, any net dc current can lead to charge accumulation and irreversible electrolytic reactions. A biphasic current waveform consisting of two consecutive pulses of equal charge but opposite polarity avoids these problems. A simple monophasic waveform is similarly unacceptable. Studies with isolated rabbit retinas in both normal and rd mice showed that the electrophysiological response has the lowest threshold when a cathodic wave is used first. These studies also showed that the response threshold was lower when a square-wave electrical stimulus was used (Shyu et al., 2000; Suzuki et al., 1999; Chen et al., 1999).

Electrode Biocompatibility

Because any future implantable device would be positioned against neural tissue for very long periods of time, potentially decades, a number of biocompatibility issues need to be addressed. Among them is the following question.

What Kind of Electrode Array and Attachment Methods Should be Used for Minimizing Any Possible Damage to Neural Tissue? The biocompatibility between an implanted medical device and the host tissue is as important as its mechanical durability and functional characteristics. This includes the effects of the implant on the host and vice versa. Effects of the implant on the tissue include inflammation, sensitivity reactions, infections, and carcinogenicity. Effects of the tissue on the implant are corrosion and other types of degradation. Sources of toxic substances are antioxidants, catalysts, and contaminants from fabrication equipment.

Microfabricated electrodes were initially conceived in the early 1970s (Wise et al., 1970). In subsequent years, the dimensions of these electrodes have been decreased, using concurrent advances in the microelectronics industry. Today, micromachined silicon electrodes with conducting lines of 2 μm are standard (Hetke et al., 1994; BeMent et al., 1986; Kovacs et al., 1992; Turner et al., 1999). Methods for depositing thin-film metal electrodes have been established. Long-term implantation and in vitro testing have demonstrated the ability of silicon devices to maintain electrical characteristics for long-periods (Weiland and Anderson, 2000).

Even the "noble" metals (platinum, iridium, rhodium, gold, and palladium) corrode under conditions of electrical stimulation (McHardy et al., 1980; Laing et al., 1967). Platinum and its alloys with iridium are the most widely used. Using simple waveforms, conservative charge density limits for long-term stimulation with platinum are 100 $\mu C/cm^2$. For activated iridium oxide electrodes, the limit is 1 mC/cm^2 (Beebe and Rose, 1988). Platinum-iridium alloys are mechanically stronger then platinum alone.

Iridium oxide electrodes belong to a new category termed "valence change oxides." Iridium oxide layers can be formed by electrochemical activation of iridium metal, by thermal decomposition of an iridium salt on a metal substrate, or by reactive sputtering from an iridium target. Activated iridium is exceptionally resistant to corrosion. It appears to be a promising electrode material. Most neural prostheses use platinum stimulating electrodes, the exception being the BION microstimulator (Advanced Bionics, Sylmar, California), which uses iridium oxide. Iridium oxide has been shown in vitro to have a safe stimulation limit of 3 mC/cm^2 (Beebe and Rose, 1988). Recently, a titanium nitride, thin-film electrode has demonstrated charge injection limits higher than both platinum and iridium oxide, with an in vitro limit of 22 mC/cm^2 (Janders et al., 1996).

Stabilizing the electrode array on the surface of the retina is an especially formidable problem. The biocompatibility and the feasibility of surgically implanting an electrode array onto the retinal surface have been examined at Johns Hopkins University Hospital. In one experiment, a 5×5 electrode array (25 disk-shaped platinum electrodes in a silicone matrix) was implanted on the retinal surface using retinal tacks in each of four mixed-breed sighted dogs for a maximum period of 1 year. No retinal detachment, infection, or uncontrolled intraocular bleeding occurred in any of the animals. Retinal tacks and the retinal array remained firmly affixed to the retina throughout the follow-up period. It was concluded that implantation of an electrode array on the epiretinal side (i.e., the side closest to the ganglion cell layer) is surgically feasible, with little if any significant damage to the underlying retina, and that platinum and silicone arrays as well as the metal tacks are biocompatible in the eye (Majji et al., 1999).

Another method for attaching electrode arrays is by biocompatible adhesives. Nine commercially available compounds were examined for their suitability as intraocular adhesives: commercial fibrin sealant, autologous fibrin, Cell-Tak, three photocurable glues, and three different polyethylene glycol hydrogels. One type of hydrogel (SS-PEG, Shearwater, Inc., Huntsville, AL) proved to be nontoxic to the retina (Margalit et al., 2000). Hydrogels proved superior for intraocular use in terms of consistency, adhesiveness, stability, impermeability, and safety.

IRP Experiments

A number of in vivo and in vitro retinal stimulation studies have been performed in animals and humans at Johns Hopkins University Hospital. The next major step will be long-term implantation of active devices in animal models to examine the efficacy and safety of such devices.

Specific parameters that will be examined during these experiments are the clinical appearance of the retina during the period of the implantation, and electrophysiological responses—electroretinogram (ERG) and visual-evoked potentials (VEP). The VEP can be examined by scalp electrodes, subdural surface electrodes, or intracortical recording of single neurons. These experiments will be conducted in both normal and retinal degenerate animals. After chronic implantation in animal models, the retina and cortex will be examined for any histological damage using optical and electron microscopy. If animal model experiments prove successful, chronic human experiments would follow with blind volunteer patients.

Future devices will contain more electrodes, more advanced electronics, and radiofrequency or other wireless communication links. Proper hermetic sealing and the use of advanced biocompatible materials will improve the host's response and ensure the long-term integrity of the device. After successful demonstration of prototype devices, the issues of biocompatibilty will become the most challenging aspect of this technology.

Research programs to develop retinal and cortical visual prostheses are progressing in parallel tracks, and it is too early to say if either will provide therapeutic benefit. Chronic experiments in animal models and humans will provide some idea of the future of these projects in 5 years. A successful retinal prosthetic device will aid only blind patients affected with outer retinal degenerative diseases such as RP and AMD.

Other blind patients would benefit from a cortical visual prosthesis. It is not clear whether humans who became blind early in life will benefit from either type of prosthesis. The visual cortex is desensitized to visual information if the eyes are deprived of visual stimuli during a critical period during early childhood. This process is called amblyopia. Patients who have been blind from early childhood may have lost their ability ever to process visual stimuli in the visual centers of their cortex and therefore lose their ability to benefit from any type of visual prosthesis.

The cortical visual prosthesis, if and when it proves successful, can provide important information on the mechanisms and development of amblyopia. Patients whose blindness is caused by ischemic events, trauma, tumor, or other destructive processes of the occipital cortex, may also have lost their ability to benefit from the visual prosthesis. These questions will be answered in future experiments.

Conformal Microelectrode Array in Retinal Protheses

Specific requirements for the NCG are that the channels be small enough so that many microwires can be connected to each unit cell. This provides redundancy, but more important, helps simplify the alignment process when the electrode array is hybridized to the silicon multiplexer. If the NCG microwires were to approach the size of the multiplexer unit cells, then a one-to-one alignment would be required. This would be problematic because of irregularities in the channel glass periodicity and the possibility of shorting nearest-neighbor cells. On the other hand, very narrow channels imply very high length-to-width aspect ratios for the channel geometry. This makes it difficult to fabricate large-area NCG samples with the proper thickness. Therefore, a reasonable design goal for the channel width is about a 1-μm diameter.

The NCG channels must be filled with a high-conductivity material to create microwires. The microwires can be fabricated by using electrodeposition or infusion of molten metal under pressure. After the channels have been filled with a conductive material and the continuity of the microwires has been confirmed, one side of the glass must be curved to create a spherical surface. Grinding and polishing techniques similar to those used in lens fabrication can be applied to the NCG pieces. The radius of curvature is nominally half an inch to provide a conformal fit against the inside of the retina. This is critically important because it allows the high-density electrodes to be positioned in direct contact with the retinal tissue. The polishing process will create microwires that are slightly recessed with respect to the curved NCG surface. This is because the metal is softer than the glass. Therefore further processing is necessary to create electrodes that protrude slightly above the curved surface. This can be accomplished by applying a chemical etch to the surface that removes a few micrometers of glass.

In preparation for hybridizing the NCG to the multiplexer, indium bumps can be deposited on the flat side of the NCG. Alternatively, the microwires can be hybridized directly to the indium bumps on the multiplexer if they are formed to protrude slightly from the NCG. Getting the microwires to protrude could again be accomplished by chemical etching like that described for forming protruding electrodes on the curved side of the NCG.

Currently, the electrode arrays that are being fabricated at the U.S. Naval Research Laboratory use a novel approach involving electrodeposition of metals within microchannel glass and nanochannel glass templates. The total number of electrodes in an array that is 2×5 mm can range up to several million. It should be noted that the total number of electrically addressable pixels (or unit cells) on the silicon multiplexer array is in the thousands. Therefore, considerable redundancy is achieved in the number of electrodes associated with each pixel.

Both microchannel and nanochannel glass are fabricated using glass drawing procedures that involve bundled stacks of composite glass fibers. The process is begun by placing an acid-etchable glass rod into an inert glass tube and drawing this pairing of dissimilar glasses at elevated temperature into a fiber of smaller diameter. Several thousand of these fibers are then cut and stacked in a hexagonal close-packed arrangement, yielding a hexagonal bundle. This bundle is subsequently drawn at an elevated temperature, fusing the individual composite fibers together while reducing the overall bundle size. At this stage, the fibers are hexagonal and contain a fine structure of several thousand micrometer-sized (typically 5 to 10 μm in diameter) acid-etchable glass fibers in a hexagonal close-packed pattern. Standard microchannel plate glass is obtained at this point by bundling these fibers together in a twelve-sided bundle and fusing the bundle together at an elevated temperature.

Alternatively, nanochannel glass may be obtained by stacking the hexagonal fibers into a new bundle and then drawing the bundle at an elevated temperature, thereby fusing the individual fibers together and reducing the overall size. In this manner, submicrometer channel diameters and extremely high channel densities can be achieved. After the last draw of the glass, the boules are wafered, polished, and then etched to remove the acid-etchable glass. In this way, a glass with extremely uniform, parallel, hollow channels is obtained (Tonucci et al., 1992). A scanning electron micrograph (SEM) of nanochannel glass having a channel diameter of 0.8 μm is shown in figure 2.6.

The thickness of the polished and etched channel glass wafers is dependent on the diameter of the channels and the etching conditions. Wafers can generally be etched if the thickness is less than 2000 times the channel diameter. For 1-μm diameter channels, this means that a realistic overall thickness is about 2 mm. This is an important parameter since in the fabrication of the electrode array to be used in the IRP, a spherical surface must be ground and polished on one side of the array to

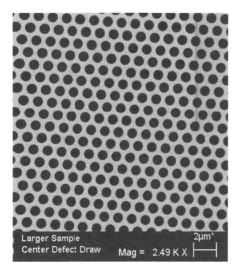

Figure 2.6
Scanning electron microscope (SEM) micrograph of nanochannel glass having 0.8-μm-diameter channels.

conform to the shape of the retina. Since the inner surface of a typical human eyeball has a concave radius of curvature of about 12 mm, it is necessary to grind and polish a convex, 12-mm radius of curvature on the electrode array. To perform such an operation successfully, the array must have a thickness ≥1 mm. If the channel diameter is less than a micrometer, the aspect ratio of the channels is necessarily greater than 1000. Nanochannel glass is the only technology available at present that can provide uniform, hollow channels having such large aspect ratios.

Once a nanochannel glass or microchannel glass template having the desired channel diameter and length is obtained, the next step in the fabrication of an electrode array is the deposition of metal nanowires or microwires in the channels. Electrodeposition of metal nanowire arrays using nanochannel glass templates has been described previously (Nguyen et al., 1998). In this work, arrays of uniform, continuous nickel wires having diameter of 250 nm were fabricated. In addition, nanotubes and nanowires of other metals, including platinum, copper, and cobalt, have been fabricated. Using similar electroplating methods, modified to account for the growth of metal wires with larger cross-sectional areas, arrays of nickel, copper, and platinum microwires have been grown in both microchannel glass and nanochannel glass templates.

Briefly, the etched glass (hollow channels) is prepared for electrodepostion by coating one surface with a thin layer of gold. A film of chromium is first applied to ensure good adhesion of the gold. The gold-coated channel glass is then attached to a gold

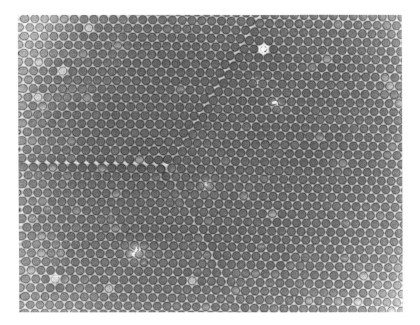

Figure 2.7
Optical photograph of nickel microelectrode array. The channel diameter is 5.6 μm.

electrode that has been similarly coated onto a glass slide. Good electrical contact between the gold films is required. Electrodeposition of metal within the hollow channels of the glass proceeds by immersing the sample in an electroplating solution and applying a voltage using a current-regulated power supply. Growth rates vary between 0.1 and 1 μm per hour, with a noticeable tradeoff between growth rate and deposition quality. High-quality deposition is observed when the growth rate is maintained lower than that commonly used for electrodeposition of bulk metals. The limited growth rate is most likely due to reactant depletion in the channels because diffusion-limited transfer of reactants down the high aspect-ratio channels is unable to maintain an optimum reactant concentration. Following electrodepostition, the piece is removed from the slide and both sides are ground and polished to a smooth finish.

An optical photograph of a microelectrode array of nickel microwires electrodeposited in channel glass is shown in figure 2.7. The microwire diameter is 5.6 μm. The overall sample area is >1 cm^2. A closeup of the nickel microwires is shown in the SEM micrograph of figure 2.8. It is apparent from figure 2.8 that the wires have an extremely uniform shape, are dense, and are well insulated from each other.

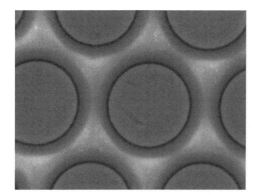

Figure 2.8
SEM micrograph showing a closeup of the 5.6-μm-diameter nickel microwires of figure 2.7.

Microelectronic Multiplexer Design for an Advanced IRP

The silicon multiplexer discussed previously performs several operations in a sequential order. During the first step, an image frame is read onto the multiplexer, pixel-by-pixel, to each unit cell. Row-by-row, each unit cell samples the analog video input and stores the pixel value as a charge on a metal-oxide-semiconductor (MOS) capacitor. A full field is completed every sixtieth of a second in a manner compatible with the RS-170 television format (30 frames per second consisting of two fields per frame); this allows the use of the test prosthesis with standard video equipment.

Figure 2.9 shows the multiplexer jointly developed by the U.S. Naval Research Laboratory and Raytheon RIO Corporation. The digital electronics is of major importance because it generates the switching pulses that route image data into the unit cells. Without the on-chip digital electronics, a dozen or more clocks would have to be input to the device. That would make the cable through the eye wall much larger and more cumbersome. The use of IRFPA multiplexer technology greatly simplifies the cable problems through the eye wall.

After all the unit cells have been loaded with the pixel values for the current frame, the next step is to send a biphasic pulse to each unit cell, which in turn is modulated in proportion to the pixel value stored in each unit cell. The biphasic pulse flows from an external source, through each unit cell, thus stimulating retinal neurons in a simultaneous manner. This is an important feature of the design because it is a synchronistic action analogous to imaged photons stimulating photoreceptors in a normal retina. Finally, the electrodes are all connected to ground to prevent any possible charge buildup at the electrode/neuron interface.

There are several important considerations in designing a device that performs all these operations successfully. First, the multiplexer operation should be designed with

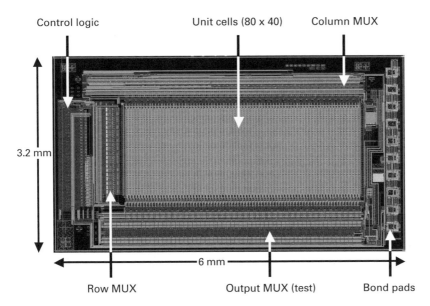

Figure 2.9
The floor plan of the microelectronic test IRP. Mux, multiplexer.

many of the requirements that exist for imaging arrays; for example, good uniformity, low noise, and high dynamic range. Of course, the prosthetic test device moves image data in the direction opposite to that of a conventional imaging multiplexer; that is, the image moves onto the device rather than off it, but otherwise the specifications are analogous. Another consideration is that each unit cell should store an individual pixel value and then use it to modulate the biphasic pulse that is input to the retinal tissue through the NCG.

Figure 2.10 shows a simplified circuit design for such a unit cell. Note that the biphasic pulse and the image data are both generated off-chip. This allows greater flexibility during human testing because any image sequence can be input and combined with any shape of biphasic pulse. The switch at the bottom of figure 2.10 provides the capability to connect the retinal tissue to ground to avoid any possibility of charge buildup.

Ancillary Electronics
The operation of the test device during acute experiments is controlled and powered by external ancillary electronics (figure 2.11). The input signal is an image sequence at data rates fast enough to achieve 60 frames per second. As mentioned earlier, the multiplexer array can be designed to sample the multiplexed input signal in a manner compatible with the RS-170 format. This allows the test prothesis to be interfaced

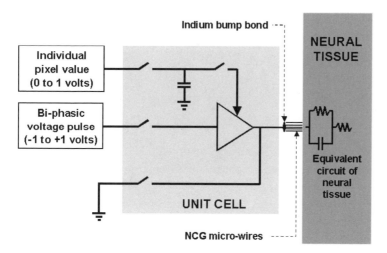

Figure 2.10
Conceptual design of the unit cell for a test device for an IRP showing the external inputs from off-chip. The pixel values are acquired from a camera (or any other video system that generates RS-170 signals) and are routed to each unit cell via a pixel-by-pixel raster scan through the on-chip multiplexer. The biphasic pulse is generated off-chip and delivered to each unit cell via a global connection.

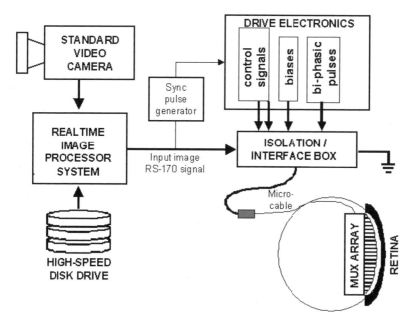

Figure 2.11
Block diagram of ancillary electronics for a test device for an IRP.

directly with any standard video camera. This includes the use of a personal computer that stores digital imagery and can display sequential fields at a 60-Hz rate.

The drive electronics control of the multiplexer array uses precisely timed pulses in a manner similar to that used in typical imaging arrays. The sync pulse generator is used to synchronize the RS-170 signal with the clocking pulses. Briefly, the sync pulse generator detects the beginning of each RS-170 field and then sends a corresponding pulse to the drive electronics box that triggers the clocking signals that control each field of image data input to the multiplexer. The isolation interface box is used to isolate the human subject from any high-voltage power supplies. The box contains optocouplers that isolate the clocks and biphasic pulse signals and low-voltage batteries for supplying bias potentials.

The biphasic pulses used to stimulate the retinal tissue can be programmed so that any pulse shapes can be tested. This has several important implications for the development process. First, because the input impedance to the retinal tissue has both a resistive and capacitive reactance associated with it, a square-wave voltage pulse will not produce the desired square-wave current pulse. Neurobiologists have found that square-wave current pulses are best to achieve effective neural stimulation. With knowledge of the output impedance at the electrode/retina interface, a voltage shape can be computed that will provide a square-wave current pulse, thus providing efficient stimulation. Second, there is evidence that different-shaped pulses will stimulate different layers of the retina—probably because of their differing frequency responses. Specifically, it is expected that either the ganglion or bipolar cells can be selectivity stimulated. Stimulating the bipolar cells instead of the ganglion cells has the advantage of reaching more deeply into the retina, allowing more use of natural signal processing.

Algorithms

As mentioned earlier, direct electrical stimulation of the ganglion cells precludes certain processing functions that normally would have occurred in the earlier layers of the retina. Therefore, it may be necessary to perform certain functions on the incoming imagery before stimulation to compensate for the missing processing. Unfortunately, a detailed model of human retinal functions has never been confirmed. Nevertheless, animal models of retinal processing exist and are suitable for use in defining processing algorithms. In fact, an existing model of the tiger salamander retina (Teeters et al., 1997) has been mapped onto the PC controller shown in figure 2.11.

As a future concept, a permanent IRP that responds to incident photons naturally imaged through the lens of the eye was shown in the bottom half of figure 2.3. It would be surgically implanted, with no external connections passing through the eye wall. The basic design is based extensively on the test IRP described here. Specifically, the permanent implant would use an NCG array hybridized to a silicon chip in a manner identical to that of the test device. However, the unit cell circuitry would need to be redesigned in that the image would no longer be multiplexed onto the chip through an electrical lead from an external camera. Instead, the image would be generated simultaneously within each unit cell through a photon-to-electron conversion using a silicon photodiode. The photons can propagate directly into each unit cell because the silicon chip can be used in a backside illuminated configuration— essentially the photons enter through the back side of the silicon chip. Therefore, the packaging of the device would be different than that shown for the test device. An implanted IRP would need to allow photons to pass through its back side. This is a simple matter of eliminating the ceramic carrier. To improve the quantum efficiency, the silicon chip can be thinned.

Note that because there is no need for any multiplexing functions, that is, input of imagery onto the chip from an external camera, the design of the silicon chip becomes much simpler. There are no ancillary electronics, as was needed in the case of the test device. Although there are no multiplexing requirements, there are two new requirements. Specifically, these are external power and a command link to adjust the operation of the IRP. Power and signals can be transmitted to the IRP with an inductively driven coil or antenna (Liu et al., 1999). The major on-chip electronic controls needed are adjustments of bias supplies and the biphasic pulse generator, plus the standard digital electronics that supply timing for simultaneous operation of the unit cell sequences.

The packaging of the permanent implant is demanding. Along with issues of biocompatiblilty is the question of operational lifetime. Permanent implants might need to operate for several decades. Similar requirements exist for other electronic implants, such as cardiac pacemakers and cochlear prostheses.

Summary

The hope of restoring vision to the blind is now believed to be a real possibility using neural prostheses. However, many technical problems remain and many engineering issues must be resolved before complete clinical success is achieved. Not the least of these problems is solving the issues of biocompatibility and the reliability of a device that will be implanted and expected to function without degradation for decades. Ultimately, the true measure of success will be the acceptance of this approach by the blind community. It is hoped that this success will parallel that of the cochlear implant, which although initially slow, continues to grow exponentially each year and is now a fully commercialized medical product.

Acknowledgments

Work on a test device for an IRP is being sponsored by the Defense Advanced Research Projects Agency Tissue Based Biosensors Program.

References

Agnew, W. F., and McCreery, D. B., eds. (1990) *Neural Prosthesis.* New York: Prentice-Hall.

Beebe, X., and Rose, T. L. (1988) Charge injection limits of activated iridium oxide electrodes with 0.2-ms pulses in bicarbonate-buffered saline. *IEEE Trans. Biomed. Eng.* 135: 494–495.

BeMent, S. L., Wise, K. D., Anderson, D. J., Najafi, K., and Drake, K. L. (1986) Solid-state electrodes for multichannel multiplexed intracortical neuronal recording. *IEEE Trans. Biomed. Eng.* 33: 230–241.

Brown, W. J., Babb, T. L., Soper, H. V., Lieb, J. P., Ottino, C. A., and Crandall, P. H. (1977) Tissue reactions to long-term electrical stimulation of the cerebellum in monkeys. *J. Neurosurg.* 47: 366–379.

Brummer, S. B., and Turner, M. J. (1975) Electrical stimulation of the nervous system: The principle of safe charge injection with noble metal electrodes. *Bioelectrochem. Bioenerg.* 2: 13–25.

Bullara, L. A., McCreery, D. B., Yuen, T. G., and Agnew, W. F. (1983) A microelectrode for delivery of defined charge densities. *J. Neurosci. Meth.* 9: 15–21.

Chen, S. J., Humayun, M. S., Weiland, J. D., Margalit, E., Shyu, J. S., Suzuki, S., and de Juan, E. (2000) Electrical stimulation of the mouse retina: A study of electrically elicited visual cortical responses. *Invest. Ophthalmol. Vis. Sci.* 41 (suppl): 4724B671.

Chow, A. Y., and Chow, V. Y. (1997) Subretinal electrical stimulation of the rabbit retina. *Neurosci. Lett.* 225: 13–16.

Chow, A. Y., and Peachey, N. S. (1998) The subretinal microphotodiode array retinal prosthesis [letter; comment]. *Ophthalmic Res.* 30: 195–198.

Cole, J., and Curtis, H. (1939) Electric impedance of the squid giant axon during activity. *J. Gen. Physiol.* 22: 649–670.

de Juan, E., Humayun, M. S., Hatchell, D., and Wilson, D. (1989) Histopathology of experimental retinal neovascularization. *Invest. Ophthamol.* 30: 1495.

Djourno, A., and Eyries, C. (1957) Prothese auditive par excitation electrique a distance du nerf sensorial a l'aide d'un bobinage inclus a demeure. *Presse Med.* 35: 14–17.

Eckmiller, R. (1997) Learning retina implants with epiretinal contacts. *Ophthalmic Res.* 29: 281–289.

Fritsch, G., and Hitzig, J. (1870) Ueber die elecktrische erregbarkeit des grosshirns. *Arch. Anat. Physiol.* 37: 300–332.

Galvani, L. (1791) De viribus electricitatis in motu musculary, commentarius. *De Bononiensi Scientiarum et Artium Instituto atque Academia* 7: 363–418.

Glenn, W., Mauro, E., Longo, P., Lavietes, P. H., and MacKay, F. J. (1959) Remote stimulation of the heart by radio frequency transmission. *N. Engl. J. Med.* 261: 948.

Gorman, P. H., and Mortimer, J. T. (1983) The effect of stimulus parameters on the recruitment characteristics of direct nerve stimulation. *IEEE Trans. Biomed. Eng.* 30: 407–414.

Greenberg, R. J. (1998) Analysis of electrical stimulation of the vertebrate retina-work towards a retinal prosthesis. Ph.D. dissertation, Johns Hopkins University, Baltimore, Md.

Grumet, A. E., Rizzo, J. F., and Wyatt, J. L. (1999) Ten-micron diameter electrodes directly stimulate rabbit retinal ganglion cell axons. ARVO abstracts, Ft. Lauderdale, Fla., p. 3883.

Grumet, A. E., Rizzo, J. F., and Wyatt, J. (2000) In-vitro electrical stimulation of human retinal ganglion cell axons. ARVO abstracts, Ft. Lauderdale, Fla., p. 50.

Guenther, E., Troger, B., Schlosshauer, B., and Zrenner, E. (1999) Long-term survival of retinal cell cultures on retinal implant materials. *Vision Res.* 39: 3988–3994.

Heetderks, W. J. (1988) RF powering of millimeter and submillimeter sized neural prosthetic implants. *IEEE Trans. Biomed. Eng.* 35: 323–326.

Heiduschka, P., and Thanos, S. (1998) Implantable bioelectronic interfaces for lost nerve functions. *Prog. Neurobiol.* 55: 433.

Hetke, J. F., Lund, J. L., Najafi, K., Wise, K. D., and Anderson, D. J. (1994) Silicon ribbon cables for chronically implantable microelectrode arrays. *IEEE Trans. Biomed. Eng.* 41: 314–321.

Hodgkin, A., and Huxley, A. (1952a) Currents carried by sodium and potassium ions through the membrane of the giant axon of *Loligo*. *J. Physiol.* 116: 449–472.

Hodgkin, A., and Huxley, A. (1952b) A quantitative description of membrane current and its application to conduction and excitation in nerve. *J. Physiol.* 116: 500–544.

Humayun, M., Propst, R., de Juan, E. J., McCormick, K., and Kickingbotham, D. (1994) Bipolar surface electrical stimulation of the vertebrate retina. *Arch. Ophthalmol.* 112: 110–116.

Humayun, M. S., de Juan, E. J., Dagnelie, G., Greenberg, R., Propst, R. H., and Phillips, D. H. (1996a) Visual perception elicited by electrical stimulation of retina in blind humans. *Arch. Ophthalmol.* 114: 40–46.

Humayun, M., de Juan, E., Jr., Dagnelie, G., Greenberg, R., Propst, R., and Phillips, H. (1996b) Visual perception elicited by electrical stimulation of retina in blind humans. *Arch. Ophthalmol.* 114: 40–46.

Humayun, M. S., de Juan, E. J., Weiland, J. D., Dagnelie, G., Katona, S., Greenberg, R., and Suzuki, S. (1999a) Pattern electrical stimulation of the human retina. *Vision Res.* 39: 2569–2576.

Humayun, M. S., Prince, M., de Juan, E. J., Barron, Y., Moskowity, M., Klock, I. B., and Milam, A. H. (1999b) Morphometric analysis of the extramacular retina from postmortem eyes with retinitis pigmentosa. *Invest. Ophthalmol. Vis. Sci.* 40: 143–148.

Janders, M., Egert, U., Stelze, M., and Nisch, W. (1996) Novel thin-film titanium nitride micro-electrodes with excellent charge transfer capability for cell stimulation and sensing applications. In *Proceedings of the 19th International Conference IEEE/EMBS*. New York: Institute of Electrical and Electronics Engineers, pp. 1191–1193.

Knighton, R. W. (1975a) An electrically evoked slow potential of the frog's retina. I. Properties of response. *J. Neurophysiol.* 38: 185–197.

Knighton, R. W. (1975b) An electrically evoked slow potential of the frog's retina. II. Identification with PII component of electroretinogram. *J. Neurophysiol.* 38: 198–209.

Kolb, H., Fernandez, E., and R. Nelson, *Web Vision* an internet resource, located at http://webvision. med.utah.edu.

Kovacs, G. T., Storment, C. W., and Rosen, J. M. (1992) Regeneration microelectrode array for peripheral nerve recording and stimulation. *IEEE Trans. Biomed. Eng.* 39: 893–902.

Laing, P. G., Ferguson, A. B., Jr., and Hodge, E. S. (1967) Tissue reaction in rabbit muscle exposed to metallic implants. *J. Biomed. Mater. Res.* 1: 135–149.

Lilly, J. C. (1961) Injury and excitation by electric currents: The balanced pulse-pair waveform. In: D. E. Sheer, ed., *Electrical Stimulation of the Brain*. Hogg Foundation for Mental Health, University of Texas Press, Austin, Texas.

Liu, W., McGucken, E., Clements, M., DeMarco, S. C., Vichienchom, K., Hughes, C., Humayun, M., de Juan, E., Weiland, J., and Greenberg, R. (1999) An implantable neuro-stimulator device for a retinal prosthesis. In *Proceedings of the IEEE International Solid-State Circuits Conference*. New York: Institute of Electrical and Electronics Engineers.

Majji, A. B., Humayun, M. S., Weiland, J. D., Suzuki, S., D'anna, S. A., and de Juan, E. (1999) Long-term histological and electrophysiological results of an inactive epiretinal electrode array implantation in dog. *Invest. Ophthalmol. Vis. Sci.* 40: 2073–2081.

Margalit, E., Fujii, G., Lai, J., Gupta, P., Chen, S. J., Shyu, J. S., Piyathaisere, D. V., Weiland, J. D., de Juan, E., and Humayun, M. S. (2000) Bioadhesives for intraocular use. *Retina* 20: 469–477.

McCreery, D. B., Agnew, W. F., Yuen, T. G., and Bullara, L. A. (1988) Comparison of neural damage induced by electrical stimulation with faradaic and capacitor electrodes. *Ann. Biomed. Eng.* 16: 463–481.

McCreery, D. B., Agnew, W. F., Yuen, T. G. H., and Bullara, L. (1990) Charge density and charge per phase as cofactors in neural injury induced by electrical stimulation. *IEEE Trans. Biomed. Eng.* 37: 996–1001.

McHardy, J., Robblee, L. S., Marston, J. M., and Brummer, S. B. (1980) Electrical stimulation with Pt electrodes. IV. Factors influencing Pt dissolution in inorganic saline. *Biomaterials* 1: 129–134.

Nguyen, P. P., Pearson, D. H., and Tonucci, R. J. (1998) Fabrication and characterization of uniform metallic nanostructures using nanochannel glass. *J. Electrochem. Soc.* 145: 247–251.

Normann, R. A. (1999) MERPWD. A neural interface for a cortical vision prothesis. *Vision Res.* 39: 2577–2587.

Ogden, T. E. (1989) *Retina: Basic Science and Inherited Retinal Disease*, vol 1. St. Louis: C.V. Mosby.

Peyman, G., Chow, A. Y., Liang, C., Perlman, J. I., and Peachey, N. S. (1998) Subretinal semiconductor microphotodiode array. *Ophthalmic Surg. Lasers* 29: 234–241.

Polyak, S. L. (1941) *The Retina.* Chicago: University of Chicago Press.

Potts, A. M., and Inoue, J. (1970) The electrically evoked response of the visual system (EER) III. Further consideration to the origin of the EER. *Invest. Ophth.* 9: 814–819.

Pudenz, R. H., Bullara, L. A., Dru, D., and Talalla, A. (1975a) Electrical stimulation of the brain. II. Effects on the blood-brain barrier. *Surg. Neurol.* 4: 265–270.

Pudenz, R. H., Bullara, L. A., Jacques, S., and Hambrecht, F. T. (1975b) Electrical stimulation of the brain. III. The neural damage model. *Surg. Neurol.* 4: 389–400.

Pudenz, R. H., Bullara, L. A., and Talalla, A. (1975c) Electrical stimulation of the brain. I. Electrodes and electrode arrays. *Surg. Neurol.* 4: 37–42.

Rizzo, J., and Wyatt, J. (1997) Prospects for a visual prosthesis. *Neuroscientist* 3: 251–262.

Rizzo, J., Wyatt, J., Loewenstein, J., and Kelly, S. (2000) Acute intraocular retinal stimulation in normal and blind humans. ARVO abstracts, Ft. Lauderdale, Fla., p. 532.

Santos, A., Humayun, M. S., de Juan, E. J., Greenberg, R. J., Marsh, M. J., Klock, I. B., and Milam, A. H. (1997) Preservation of the inner retina in retinitis pigmentosa. A morphometric analysis. *Arch. Ophthalmol.* 115: 511–515.

Scribner, D. A., Kruer, M. R., and Killiany, J. M. (1991) Infrared focal plane array technology. *Proc. IEEE* 79: 65–85.

Shyu, J., Maia, M., Weiland, J., Humayun, M., Chen, S., Margalit, E., Suzuki, S., de Juan, E., and Piyathaisere, D. (2000) Electrical stimulation of isolated rabbit retina. Paper presented at the Biomedical Engineering Society Annual Meeting.

Stone, J. L., Barlow, W. E., Humayun, M. S., de Juan, E., and Milam, A. H. (1992) Morphometric analysis of macular photoreceptors and ganglion cells in retinas with retinitis pigmentosa. *Arch. Ophthalmol.* 110: 1634–1639.

Suzuki, S., Humayun, M., de Juan, E., Weiland, J. D., and Barron, Y. (1999) A comparison of electrical stimulation threshold in normal mouse retina vs. different aged retinal degenerate (rd) mouse retina. ARVO abstracts, Ft. Lauderdale, Fla., p. 3886.

Teeters, J., Jacobs, A., and Werblin, F. (1997) How neural interactions form neural responses in the salamander retina. *J. Comp. Neurosci.* 4: 5.

Tehovnik, E. (1996) Electrical stimulation of neural tissue to evoke behavioral responses. *J. Neurosci. Meth.* 65: 1–17.

Tonucci, R. J., and Justus, B. L. (1993a) Nanochannel Glass Matrix Used in Making Mesoscopic Structures. U.S. Patent 5,264,722, issued November 1993.

Tonucci, R. J., and Justus, B. L. (1993b) Nanochannel Filter. U.S. Patent 5,234,594, issued August 1993.

Tonucci, R. J., Justus, B. L., Campillo, A. J., and Ford, C. E. (1992) Nanochannel array glass. *Science* 258: 783–785.

Toyoda, J., and Fujimoto, M. (1984) Application of transretinal current stimulation for the study of bipolar-amacrine transmission. *J. Gen. Physiol.* 84: 915–925.

Troyk, P., and Schwan, M. (1992) Closed-loop class E transcutaneous power and data link for microimplants. *IEEE Trans. Biomed. Eng.* 39: 589–599.

Turner, J. N., Shain, W., Szarowski, D. H., Andersen, M., Martins, S., Isaacson, M., and Craighead, H. (1999) Cerebral astrocyte response to micromachined silicon implants. *Exp. Neurol.* 156: 33–49.

Veraart, C., Raftopoulos, C., Mortimer, J. T., Delbeke, J., Pins, D., Michaux, G., Vanlierde, A., Parrini, S., and Wanet-Defalque, M. C. (1998) Visual sensations produced by optic nerve stimulation using an implanted self-sizing spiral cuff electrode. *Brain Res.* 813: 181–186.

Weiland, J. D., and Anderson, D. J. (2000) Chronic neural stimulation with thin-film, iridium oxide stimulating electrodes. *IEEE Trans. Biomed. Eng.* 47: 911–918.

Weiland, J. D., Humayun, M. S., Dagnelie, G., de Juan, E., Greenberg, R. J., and Iliff, N. T. (1999) Understanding the origin of visual percepts elicited by electrical stimulation of the human retina. *Graefes Arch. Clin. Exp. Ophthalmol.* 237: 1007–1013.

West, D. C., and Wolstencroft, J. H. (1983) Strength-duration characteristics of myelinated and nonmyelinated bulbospinal axons in the cat spinal cord. *J. Physiol.* (*London*) 337: 37–50.

Wise, K. D., Angell, J., and Starr, A. (1970) An integrated-circuit approach to extracellular microelectrodes. *IEEE Trans. Biomed. Eng.* BME-17: 238–247.

Wyatt, J., and Rizzo, J. F. (1996) Ocular implants for the blind. *IEEE Spectrum* 112: 47–53.

Yagi, T., and Hayashida, Y. (1999) Implantation of the artificial retina. *Nippon Rinsho* 57: 1208–1215.

Yagi, T., Ito, N., Watanabe, M. A., and Uchikawa, Y. (1998) A computational study on an electrode array in a hybrid retinal implant. In *Proceedings of the 1998 IEEE International Joint Conference on Neural Networks*. New York: Institute of Electrical and Electronics Engineers, pp. 780–783.

Zrenner, E., Stett, A., Weiss, S., et al. (1999) Can subretinal microphotodiodes successfully replace degenerated photoreceptors? *Vision Res.* 39: 2555–2567.

The checkerboard pattern consisted of a number of 1.1×1.1-degree squares. Using a pseudorandom number generator, each square was set to one of three intensities: white with 15% probability, off with 15% probability, or background with 70% probability. The logical origin of the screen was selected randomly. This allowed the entire checkerboard to be shifted both vertically and horizontally by 0.14-degree steps. A new checkerboard with a new logical screen offset was displayed at a rate of 25 Hz. For all stimuli, the difference between the most intense white and darkest black was selected to give a 50% contrast, with the background intensity set halfway through the intensity range. In addition, all stimuli completely filled the entire screen.

Data Analysis

The optimal orientation was calculated from the drifting sine wave gratings by the method described by Orban (1991). For each orientation tested, a peristimulus time histogram (PSTH) was calculated for the activity recorded on each electrode. The optimal orientation for each multiunit was selected as the orientation giving the largest firing rate for that unit.

The recently introduced method of electrophysiological imaging (Diogo et al., 2003) was utilized to estimate the optimal orientation at locations between electrodes. In this method, one interpolates activity-level maps for each of the conditions tested; here it was the orientation of a drifting sine wave grating. The condition maps are then combined using the same methods used by the optical imaging community to give a single response map. Their finding that the map of activity for a single condition is relatively smooth supports the validity of interpolating the condition maps. The same method was also used to estimate the ocular dominance.

A reverse correlation method was used to estimate the receptive field size and position from the random checkerboard stimulus (Jones and Palmer, 1987; Eckhorn et al., 1993). In brief, this method performs a cross-correlation between the occurrence of a spike and the state of each of the pixels of the computer monitor. Since there is a delay between changing the visual stimulus and the resulting spike, the cross-correlation is typically only examined over a period of 100–20 ms before the spike. After normalization, the result is a three-dimensional array of t-scores, with two of the dimensions representing the vertical and horizontal extent of the computer monitor and the third the latency from the state of the display to a spike. Since the result is presented as a t-score, typically out of a distribution with a very large number of degrees of freedom, the magnitude of the cross-correlation has units of standard deviations. A more complete description of the statistical interpretation of the cross-correlation as well as the spatial and temporal criteria that we apply before accepting a region as being a receptive field are detailed elsewhere (Warren et al., 2001).

In this chapter, we defined the receptive field to be the contiguous region having a magnitude greater than 4.3 standard deviations (SD). The size of the receptive field was calculated as the area bounded by this region. The location of the receptive field was defined as the center of mass of the region. Both the size and position were calculated at the latency having the peak magnitude.

Fitting Receptive Fields

To analyze the visuotopic organization of the primary visual cortex, we compared the position of the receptive field with fields estimated by an affine coordinate transformation of the locations of the electrode array onto its visual space representation. The particular affine transformation provides 5 degrees of freedom: magnification (SF_x and SF_y), the rotation (θ), and translation (OFF_a and OFF_e). A nonlinear, least-mean-squares minimization method (FMINS function in MATLAB) was used to minimize the difference between the coordinate transform and the measured receptive fields. The electrode position (E_x and E_y) was related to the visual space position by the equation

$$\begin{bmatrix} V_h \\ V_v \end{bmatrix} = \begin{bmatrix} SF_x \cos\theta & SF_y \sin\theta \\ -SF_x \sin\theta & SF_y \cos\theta \end{bmatrix} \begin{bmatrix} E_x \\ E_y \end{bmatrix} + \begin{bmatrix} OFF_a \\ OFF_e \end{bmatrix},$$

where V_h and V_v are the horizontal and vertical positions of the receptive field in degrees, respectively. We interpreted our results in terms of both linear and conformal mapping. A conformal map is one that preserves angles. For example, a transformation on a grid printed on a rubber diaphragm that has been stretched is a conformal operation.

Results

The use of the UEA requires a new approach to electrophysiological measurements, and it offers distinct advantages and disadvantages over the conventional single-electrode technique. The problem of inserting 100 electrodes simultaneously into the cortex precludes the possibility of positioning each electrode individually so that it is recording optimally from a well-isolated single unit. Rather, the entire array must be rapidly inserted (Rousche and Normann, 1992) to a precisely determined cortical depth. The recordings are then made from the electrodes that have either multiunit or single-unit activity on them. Thus, the number of electrodes having single- or multiunit recording capability varies considerably from experiment to experiment, and the quality of the recordings varies from electrode to electrode in each implantation.

Because the position of the electrode cannot be adjusted to optimize recordings, the length of its exposed tip has been increased to improve the likelihood of record-

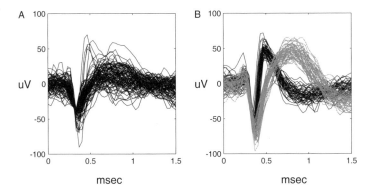

Figure 3.2
Specimen records of (*A*) typical mixture of multiunit wave forms recorded with the UEA, and (*B*) two single units that were isolated and classified (offline) from the multiunit records of Figure 2A. The gray unit was an "on-center" cell and the black unit was an "off-center" cell.

ing useful neural activity from as many electrodes as possible, yet still preserving an adequate signal-to-noise ratio for the units that are recorded. Thus the impedances of the UEA electrodes are lower than those of conventional single microelectrodes and range from 200 to 400 kΩ. An example of recordings we made with the UEA is shown in figure 3.2A, where we have superimposed responses from an electrode that recorded a mixture of well-isolated multiple and single units. Note that for reasons of clarity, only 100 of the 24,000 spikes recorded on this electrode during a half hour trial are shown. Figure 3.2B shows 50 superimposed responses after offline identification and classification of two distinct single units that were readily isolated from the multiunit records of figure 3.2A. Unit classification was done by a mixture of Gaussian methods (Sahani et al., 1997; Lewicki, 1998; Jain et al., 2000).

The size of the single units recorded with the UEA varies substantially from electrode to electrode. In this experiment, one electrode recorded single units that had an amplitude of 700 μV. The mean, isolated single-unit amplitude was 110 $\pm$ 50 μV, and the median single-unit amplitude was 95 μV.

Single- versus Multiunit Response Characteristics
The recordings described in this chapter were obtained in our best experiment to date. Of the 100 electrodes in the array, only two had unrecordable neural activity, owing to two nonfunctioning channels in our multichannel amplifier. Of the 98 recording electrodes, 29 had clearly visible single units and 57 had isolatable single units using a mixture of Gaussian approaches. The remainder recorded only nonisolatable multiunit activity. In order to produce the most complete electrophysiologically determined maps, we used the multiunit recordings to determine orientation,

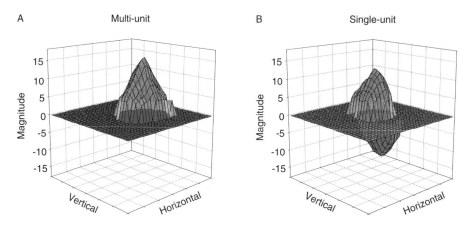

Figure 3.3
Receptive field plots generated with the reverse correlation technique from data recorded from one of the 100 electrodes in the UEA (the multi- and single-unit data shown in figure 3.2). (*A*) Plot generated from multiunit data. (*B*) Plot generated from the two single units shown in figure 3.2B. The upward-plotted unit is the "on" unit and the downward-plotted unit is the "off" unit of figure 3.2B. The horizontal and vertical grids on each plot are built from 1-degree squares. The magnitude is represented in terms of "*t*-scores."

ocular dominance, and visuotopic organization. We justify this simplification because the receptive field properties measured with both multiple and single units recorded with the same electrode had very similar spatial properties. This comparison of multi- and single-unit receptive field properties is illustrated in figure 3.3, where we plotted the receptive fields measured with spike-triggered averaging (the reverse correlation technique) from multiple and single units recorded with one of the 100 electrodes in the UEA (the units illustrated in figure 3.2).

The two receptive field plots were made using the same absolute visual space coordinates. As expected, the size of the multiunit receptive field is larger (5.2 degrees^2) than that measured from the single-unit data (3.4 and 2.6 degrees^2), and the centers of mass of the two receptive fields in figure 3.3B differ from the center of mass of the multiunit receptive field by 21 and 32 seconds of arc. The lack of an "off" component in the multiunit receptive field in figure 3.3A is due to the much larger number of spikes used to generate the receptive field plot in that figure compared with the number of identified spikes used to generate the receptive field map of figure 3.3B. The estimated ocular dominance and the measured orientation sensitivity of the two measures were very similar. We have performed similar comparisons in five other well-isolated single units, and reached similar conclusions: the spatial properties of the multi- and single-unit data are sufficiently similar to justify the use of multiunit data in the genesis of the functional maps described here.

Summary of Receptive Field Properties

We used spike-triggered averaging to determine the receptive field properties of the multiple and single units recorded with each electrode. We measured the "on" and/or "off" nature of the receptive fields, the ocular dominance, the orientation sensitivity, and the receptive field areas of the multiunits recorded on all 98 electrodes. One significant advantage of using microelectrode arrays in such experiments is that one can measure receptive field data from all 100 electrodes in the time it takes to measure the same data from a single electrode. We have summarized these receptive field data in the histograms of figure 3.4.

About half of the cells were of the "on" type; 6% responded mainly to the "off" of the stimuli; and 21% responded to both "on" and "off" components of the stimuli. Eighteen percent of the cells did not have a receptive field that could be revealed using spike-triggered averaging, but these cells responded well to moving bars. The ocular dominance histogram showed that most multiunits were binocularly stimulated. Eighty-two of the 98 multiunits showed significant orientation sensitivity, with half of the cells being most sensitive to vertical lines. However, all orientations were represented in the 98 multiunits studied. Finally, the mean receptive field size of all 98 multiunits was 5.6 ± 3.4-degree^2 (SD).

Ocular Dominance Maps

A fundamental organizational feature of the primary visual cortex is the representation of visual input from each eye. This feature was originally studied electrophysiologically (Hubel and Wiesel, 1962), and subsequently histologically (LeVay et al., 1975). Both techniques reveal a segregation of inputs from each eye in layer IV, where the ipsilateral and contralateral inputs alternate in a striped pattern. While input from each eye is delivered to the visual cortex as an independent message, the layers of visual cortex manifest binocular responses to varying degrees. Ocular dominance was readily mapped using the UEA by recording the responses from all electrodes in the array to sinusoidal grating stimulation delivered sequentially to each eye. The ocular dominance for each electrode was quantified by the following relation:

$$\text{ocular dominance factor} = [(N_c - N_o) - (N_i - N_o)]/[(N_c - N_o) + (N_i - N_o)],$$

where N_c is the average firing rate for contralateral stimulation, N_i is the average firing rate for ipsilateral stimulation, and N_o is the average firing rate in the absence of stimulation. If the differences between contra- or ipsilateral firing rates during stimulation and the firing rates in the absence of stimulation were negative, this difference was set to zero. Thus, if the multiunit activity is exclusively driven by the contralateral eye, the ocular dominance will be approximately $+1$, and if it is driven exclusively by the ipsilateral eye, the ocular dominance will be approximately -1.

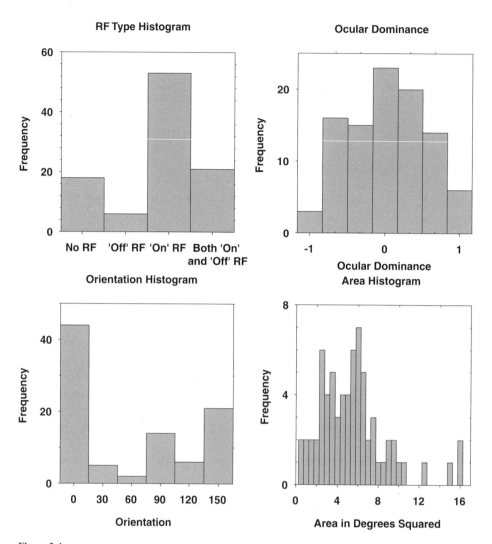

Figure 3.4
Receptive field properties of the multiunits recorded with the UEA. Measurements were made simultaneously in all 98 electrodes.

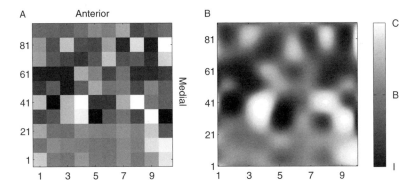

Figure 3.5
Ocular dominance map of the cat area 17. (*A*) Raw map. (*B*) Electrophysiological imaging map generated from the same data. The numbers surrounding the map represent electrode coordinates and are separated by 400 μm.

Multiunits driven equally by both eyes will have an ocular dominance factor of approximately 0.

An ocular dominance factor was calculated for the multiunits recorded on each electrode, and the resulting ocular dominance map is reproduced in gray scale in figure 3.5. In this and all subsequent maps, the activity maps represent neural activity on each electrode as viewed looking down on the top of the array. The anterior and medial directions of the brain are indicated on the map of figure 3.5A, and this convention has been followed in all subsequent maps.

The raw ocular dominance map of figure 3.5A has been created from discrete recordings from electrodes separated by 400 μm. This map preserves the discrete 400-μm sampling of the UEA, but the sharp boundaries between adjacent map regions make patterns present in the overall ocular dominance image difficult to appreciate. In order to compare this map with maps made using other spatially averaged imaging techniques (histological or optical techniques), we used electrophysiological imaging methods to develop an estimate of the ocular dominance in the region sampled by the array, as shown in figure 3.5B. The estimated ocular dominance image retains the raw data of figure 3.5A, but more closely resembles the patterns found with histochemical or optical imaging techniques.

Orientation Sensitivity Maps
Another general organizational feature of the primary visual cortex is that many of the cells in this area manifest orientation sensitivity (as shown in figure 3.4). These cells are particularly sensitive to bars of a particular width and contrast, oriented in a particular direction, and moving through the cell's receptive field with a particular velocity. Furthermore, the preferred orientation of these cells seems to vary in a

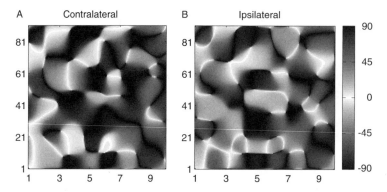

Figure 3.6
The orientation sensitivity organization of cat area 17 as measured with the UEA. (*A*) Map produced by contralateral stimulation, and (*B*) map produced by ipsilateral stimulation. The numbers surrounding the map represent electrode coordinates and are separated by 400 μm. The scale indicating the principal angle orientation of multiunits in maps is given on the right.

rational fashion as one records from a linear sequence of cells (Hubel and Wiesel, 1962).

We used the multiunit recordings obtained with the UEA in combination with electrophysiological analysis methods to create orientation sensitivity maps of the cat visual cortex. Sine wave patterns of various orientations were drifted across the stimulation monitor and the responses of all multiunits recorded. This procedure was repeated in 30-degree increments. Since we were demonstrating orientation sensitivity, not directional selectivity, we combined the data for 30 and 210 degrees, 60 and 240 degrees, etc. Thus, the orientation angle was converted to the principal angle through a modulo 180 function. The maximum multiunit response from each electrode for the principal angle orientation was determined from the combined data. Figure 3.6A shows the maximum orientation sensitivities for all electrodes for contralateral stimulation. In figure 3.6B we show the same procedure, but for stimulation delivered via the ipsilateral eye.

The ipsilateral and contralateral maps of figure 3.6 manifest similar periodicity, but they differ in their detailed structure. This difference does not seem to be due to eye rotation caused by the paralytic agent because the two maps cannot be made identical by a simple redefinition of the stimulus bar angle by any given amount for one eye. Thus it appears that while a given unit generally is activated by bars of a particular orientation for monocular stimulation, the optimal orientation for stimulation via the other eye is often not the same orientation. This difference in the contra- and ipsilateral orientation sensitivity of the visual cortex has been noted by others (Hubener et al., 1997) and raises questions about how the higher visual centers decompose binocularly viewed images (Hubel, 1988).

Visuotopic Organization

The visuotopic organization of the visual cortex has been studied by many investigators (Hubel and Wiesel, 1962; Tusa et al., 1978; Dow et al., 1985), but these studies have been complicated by problems of eye fixation and imprecision in the location of recording electrodes. However, the UEA is particularly well suited to the task of studying the visuotopic organization of the cat primary visual cortex. Because receptive fields are measured simultaneously with this approach, any eye drift that occurs during the course of the measurement is a common-mode interferent, and the consequences of such eye drift are significantly reduced by differential measurements of the receptive field properties (Warren et al., 2001).

We have measured the visuotopic organization of area 17 by simultaneously recording the responses of all multiunits to our ternary checkerboard stimulus. We then used the spike-triggered averaging technique to determine the receptive field properties of the multiunits recorded with each electrode. To analyze the visuotopic organization of receptive fields, we collapsed the three-dimensional representation of each receptive field (the two spatial dimensions and the strength of the excitation) into a two-dimensional point in visual space by calculating the center of mass of the region contained within its boundary. We then applied a least-mean-squared-error fit to a linear transformation of the electrode loci to their respective representation in visual space.

Figure 3.7A illustrates the results of this visuotopic mapping procedure. The rectangle of small, filled circles represents the outline of the UEA as mapped in visual space, with each symbol indicating the location of an electrode along the periphery of the UEA. The filled diamond and squares represent the electrode sites at the most rostral-lateral and rostral-medial corners of the UEA, respectively. The visual space representations of electrode sites having reliable receptive fields are represented by crosses. Each of these crosses is connected to an open square that represents the location in visual space of the center of the mass of the receptive field mapped at the electrode site. The vectors connecting these sets of points are the result of performing a least-mean-squared-error fit that minimizes the root-sum-squared length of these vectors.

The global visuotopic organization of this region of area 17 is in general agreement with the findings of Tusa (Tusa et al., 1978) and Albus (1975). We have determined the global magnification of this region of the cortex by measuring the area in visual space that is represented by the multiunits recorded by our electrode array. This value, 16 degree^2/13 mm^2 or 1.2 square degree per square millimeter on the cortex is also in approximate agreement with these previous studies for the particular region of visual space addressed by the array.

It is clear from figure 3.7A that the visuotopic map of the cat primary visual cortex is not conformal. Electrodes that are adjacent to each other can record from

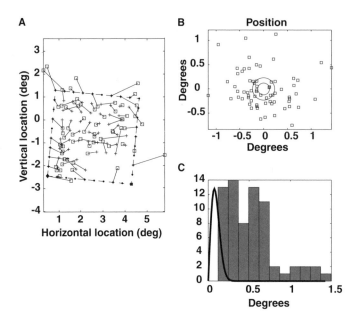

Figure 3.7
(*A*) The visuotopic map of area 17, measured from simultaneous recordings of multiunit activity on 98 of the 100 electrodes of the UEA (note that only 67 electrodes had sufficiently well-defined receptive field properties to be included in this plot). Activity was evoked by checkerboard stimulation and spike-triggered averaging. (*B*) Plot of residuals (vectors of *A*) with the electrode sites superimposed on the origin. (*C*) Distribution of residuals (histogram), and predicted distribution of residuals based on estimates of the error in our measurement technique (solid curve, scaled to fit the histogram).

multiunits with receptive fields that can be separated by as much as 2 degrees, while electrodes that are separated by as much as 1.4 mm can have virtually overlapping receptive fields. We have attempted to quantify the degree of this visuotopic non-conformality in figure 3.7B, which shows the residual errors from the least-mean-squared-error fit of the electrode positions to their respective receptive fields. This was done by translating all electrode sites to the origin of this plot, and plotting all receptive field sites with respect to this point. The resulting map of residual errors shows no apparent bias along any preferred direction. Figure 3.7C is a histogram of the residual length. The continuous curve is a plot of the estimated distribution of residuals that would result from errors in the measurement of the receptive field position. It is clear that the 0.53 ± 0.31-degree (SD) mean error in the residuals reflects an inherent nonconformality in the visuotopic map.

Response to Moving Bars
One unique capability of monitoring cortical activity with microelectrode arrays is visualizing ensemble responses to simple patterned stimuli. We used the UEA to vi-

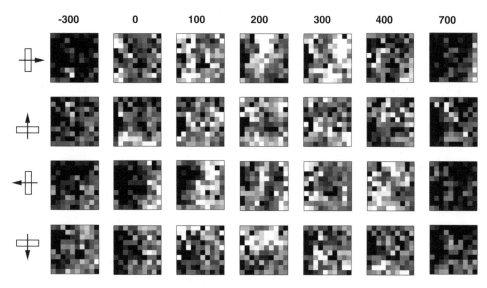

Figure 3.8
The multiunit activity, recorded at 98 sites in area 17, evoked by a single passage of a bar at four different orientations, moving through the receptive fields of the recording sites. Each frame is a 100-ms sum of the multiunit activity on each electrode. The numbers above each column indicate the time of the frame when time zero was selected to maximize the activity in the 100-, 200-, and 300-ms frames. Each movie (row) shows a total of 1s of cortical activity.

sualize the neural pattern associated with bars of light moving through the global receptive field of the ensemble at each of four orthogonal orientations. The results of these experiments are illustrated in the activity "movies" of figure 3.8. The speed and width of the bar used in this experiment, 8 degrees/s and 2 degrees, respectively, and the 4-degree spatial window sampled by the UEA (figure 3.7), suggests that the activity pattern should be present for about 0.75 s. To allow the visual system to recover from each sweeping bar, we initiated a new sweeping bar every 4 s.

In this figure, each frame shows the summated firing at all 98 electrode sites for a 100-ms period. Above each column is the time, in milliseconds, of the frame where time zero was selected to maximize the activity in the 100-, 200-, and 300-ms frames. The bar to the left of each movie shows the orientation of the moving bar, and the arrow indicates its direction of motion through the visual field. Close inspection of the movies reveals the following patterns: For the 0-degree orientation (top movie), there is a wave of activity that appears at the left for the 100-ms frame and progresses to the right. In the 90-degree orientation (second movie from the top), there is a subtler wave of activity that starts at the bottom of the frames and moves upward. In the 180-degree orientation (third movie from the top), there is a wave of activity that enters from the right and moves to the left. Finally, in the 270-degree orientation (bottom movie), there is a wave of activity that enters from the top and progresses downward. This wave of activity, like that for the 90-degree orientation, is subtler. Each of these frames was made using the spatiotemporal activity pattern for only a single passage of the bar.

The activity patterns shown in figure 3.8 were made by normalizing the activity for each orientation. That is, the firing rate at each electrode was normalized to the maximum firing rate over the 4-s period of the passage of the bar. Thus the maps indicate that the multiunits recorded on each electrode generally modulate their firing activity as the bar sweeps through the receptive fields of the recorded units, regardless of the orientation of the bar and the principal angle orientations of the units.

Discussion

The goals of this chapter are twofold: to demonstrate the use of microelectrode arrays to achieve high-resolution, spatiotemporal imaging of the activity patterns of neural ensembles in the sensory cortex, and to use an electrode array to record the activity patterns that are produced by single presentations of simple, moving visual stimuli. We are using these maps and activity patterns to model how patterned visual stimuli could be encoded by the firing properties of cortical neurons (Normann et al., 2001), but this analytical focus goes beyond the scope of this chapter.

The Functional Architecture of the Cat Visual Cortex

Before one can model encoding strategies that could be used by the vertebrate visual system to represent spatiotemporal patterns of retinal illumination, one needs to characterize the receptive field properties of the units upon which the models are built. The three organizational maps described in this chapter provide such a functional characterization. The maps also extend the one-dimensional descriptions of the functional organization made with single-electrode "tracks" to two-dimensional maps. Because the 98 parallel measurements from which the maps have been made were performed simultaneously, any distortions in the maps that are due to eye drift or uncertainties in electrode position are significantly reduced. Furthermore, because the maps were made directly from multi- and single-unit activity, they did not require the inferences of causality that are necessary with some optical techniques.

However, one significant limitation of this multielectrode technique is the spatial sampling imposed by the 400-μm spacing of the electrodes in the UEA. This is contrasted with the optical visualization techniques that provide a virtually continuous image of the cortex, with spatial optical sampling on the order of 10 μm (Shtoyerman et al., 2000). The recently introduced method of electrophysiological imaging (Diogo et al., 2003) allows the electrophysiologist to begin to study the regions left unsampled. The low-pass filtering associated with the interpolation of a single condition map is justifiable only in the context of the low spatial frequency periodicity of the columnar organization of the cortex.

As was shown in the early work of Hubel and Wiesel (1962), single-electrode tracks of the orientation sensitivity of complex cells in monkey area 17 show an orderly progression of preferred orientation with distance across the cortex. Cells separated by approximately 20 μm will have their orientation sensitivity changed by 5 to 10 degrees. Thus, a trajectory approximately 1 mm long will encounter a set of units that encompasses a full 360 degrees of orientation sensitivity. When this architecture has been studied with optical visualization (Blasdel, 1992; Arieli et al., 1995), or with various histological techniques using visual stimulation with only horizontal or vertical lines (LeVay et al., 1975), one observes a set of stained orientation bands in a field of unstained cortex (much like stripes on a zebra's coat). The periodicity of these stripes is on the order of 1 mm. Based upon the Nyquist sampling theorem, the minimum spacing required to sample this spatial information is half of this spatial period, or 0.5 mm. Thus, the 0.4-mm spacing of the UEA would seem to be just barely adequate to sample the orientation and functional architecture of ocular dominance. Clearly, more closely spaced electrodes would provide an even better sampling of these architectures, and work is underway in our laboratory to develop electrode arrays with closer spacing.

Multiunit Activity Patterns Produced by Moving Bars

The second goal of this chapter is to demonstrate the neural activity pattern produced by simple visual stimuli. While optical techniques with extrinsic dye-enhanced signal-to-noise ratios can begin to reveal single-trial-evoked activity patterns, the recording of single- and multiunit activity with an electrode array directly enables the visualization of such single-trial-evoked activity. This capability is particularly important in light of the variability that has been described in cortical responses (Abeles, 1991; Rieke et al., 1997). In figure 3.8 we illustrated the activity patterns produced by the movement of a single bar of light in front of the animal. The bar was oriented in one of four orthogonal directions. We stress that these data were obtained from single passes of the bar and that the 98 single-unit responses have not been temporally averaged over multiple passes of the bar to enhance the signal-to-noise ratio of the measurement. While a subsequent report will focus on our ability to use these firing patterns to estimate the nature of the visual stimulus that evoked the patterns, we show these response patterns to make a few simple points regarding spatial information processing by the visual cortex.

First, the nonconformal visuotopic organization of area 17 shown in figure 3.7A, and the complex distribution of orientation sensitivities of the units that make up the map (figure 3.6), result in a complex firing pattern in area 17 to even a simple patterned stimulus such as a moving bar. While the activity pattern does not directly resemble a moving bar of evoked activity, careful observation of the four movies indicates that each bar produces a diffuse wave of activity that generally moves across the cortex in a pattern consistent with the gross visuotopy of the cortex (Tusa et al., 1978).

Second, the movies of figure 3.8 indicate that the response patterns to vertical bars moving either to the left or to the right are more robust than the response patterns evoked by horizontally oriented bars moving either up or down. This is most likely a manifestation of the larger number of multiunits with a preferred vertical orientation sensitivity seen in the histogram of figure 3.4 and reported by others (Leventhal, 1983).

Finally, it is noted that while most recorded units manifested a preferred orientation (see figure 3.4), most units also responded to each of the four moving bars. The movie for each moving bar was not composed exclusively of activity evoked in units with a preference for that particular orientation. This observation, and the data of figure 3.6 showing that the principal angle orientation generally differed for ipsi- and contralateral stimuli, suggest that the visual cortex may not primarily decompose images incident on the retina into a set of oriented line-basis vectors (Hubel, 1988).

Implications for a Visual Prosthesis

The data presented in this chapter have relevance for the emerging field of sensory and motor neuroprosthetics. While most work in this area is still focused on animal experimentation, researchers are beginning to use electrode arrays to selectively excite and record from neural ensembles in human volunteers as a means to restore lost sensory or motor function (Veraart et al., 1998; Humayun et al., 1999; Grumet et al., 2000; Kennedy et al., 2000). One example of a sensory application that would use an array of penetrating electrodes such as the UEA is a visual neuroprosthesis. The electrodes in the UEA could provide the means to selectively excite large numbers of neurons in the visual cortex of individuals with profound blindness. A complete cortically based visual neuroprosthesis would consist of a video camera in a pair of eyeglasses and signal-processing electronics to convert the output of the video camera into a signal that could be delivered transdermally to an implanted very large scale integrated stimulator that would be directly interfaced to an electrode array implanted in the visual cortex.

While each of the elements in such a visual neuroprosthesis offers significant design challenges to the electrical, mechanical, and bioengineer, we believe that there are two main issues that must be resolved before this approach to restoring sight can be entertained seriously. First, the safety of the implanted electrode array and the implantation procedure must be rigorously demonstrated in animal studies, and second, the efficacy of this implant system must be demonstrated in human volunteers. Specifically, it must be shown that patterned electrical stimulation of the visual cortex via an array of implanted, penetrating electrodes does evoke discriminable patterned percepts.

Much of the animal experimental work we have conducted to date has focused on the former issue. Colleagues have implanted the UEA in the motor cortex of primates that have been trained to play a simple video game. For periods up to 3 years, we have been able to record the single- and multiunit responses of the neurons in the hand representation of the motor cortex as the animal "plays" the video game (Maynard et al., 1999). This 3-year recording capability provides a proof-of-concept that the UEA can be implanted safely in the primate cerebral cortex and that it can perform stably over extended periods. We have yet to conduct long-term electrical stimulation experiments to document that neither the electrode materials nor the cortical tissues are significantly affected by chronic current injections, but work in other laboratories indicates that current injections into neural tissues can be performed safely. McCreery has shown that currents that are expected to evoke sensory percepts when injected into the sensory cortex through penetrating electrodes can be delivered with little consequence on neural tissues (McCreery et al., 1995).

We have conducted short-term chronic experiments with intermittent current injections via UEAs implanted into the auditory cortex (Rousche and Normann, 1999). These experiments, and additional acute experiments conducted in sciatic nerves of cats (Branner et al., 2001), have allowed us to measure the current thresholds required to evoke a behavioral or motor response. We find that as little as 5 to 10 μA of current injection (delivered in a 200-μs, biphasic pulse) can evoke behavioral responses or muscle twitches. These current levels are regarded as modest, and provide further evidence of the potential safety and efficacy of the UEA as a chronic neural interface. When detailed animal experiments have been performed, we will be in a position to use the UEA in basic human experimentation.

Thus, the major barrier to the development of a cortically based visual neuroprosthesis is the demonstration that patterned electrical stimulation of the visual cortex evokes patterned, discriminable percepts. Evidence suggesting that this might be expected to be the case dates back to the early work on cortical electrical stimulation by Brindley (Brindley and Lewin, 1968), and Dobelle (Dobelle and Mladejovsky, 1974). Schmidt and his co-workers (Schmidt et al., 1996) have more recently conducted a series of experiments in which they stimulated the visual cortex of a blind human volunteer with currents passed through an assortment of small penetrating electrodes. They demonstrated that stimulation of a sequence of five electrodes in a line evoked the percept of a line. Clearly, this is a rather primitive pattern, but it supports the hypothesis.

On the other hand, the organization of the primary visual cortex into numerous superimposed maps makes it difficult to fully embrace this hypothesis without more detailed experimentation. Because the visual cortex contains both "on" and "off" center cells, if injected currents excite an ensemble of cells containing an equal number of "on" and "off" center cells, one might expect that this current might not evoke an apparent percept. Another possibility is that patterned current injections might evoke general "blobs" of light, and not be useful in generating patterned percepts. Much basic experimentation will have to be conducted with human volunteers before these basic issues can be resolved.

If patterned current injections do evoke discriminable patterned percepts in human volunteers, then significant engineering problems must still be resolved. The problem of converting a video signal into patterns of electrical stimulation that evoke appropriate percepts must be addressed. The results described in this chapter (and previously demonstrated by others), allow us to anticipate two potential problems. First, the visuotopic organization of the primary visual cortex illustrated in figure 3.8 is quite nonconformal. This suggests that the phosphene space evoked by an implanted electrode array is also not likely to be conformal. If this were the case, then in order to evoke the percept of a line, a complex pattern of electrode excitation would have to be effected. This in turn would require that the signals produced by the video camera be remapped to produce a phosphene perceptual space that was conformally related to the visual world encoded by the video camera (Eckmiller, 1997). Of course, if the perceptual nonconformality were not large, then the plasticity of the visual pathways might be sufficient to recreate a conformal perceptual space with time and training of the implanted subject.

Finally, in order to produce useful visual percepts, one might be required to decompose a recorded video image into an image composed of sets of oriented lines located at specific points in the visual space. This possibility is suggested by figures 3.4 and 3.6, which show that the visual cortex is composed of cells that manifest orientation sensitivity. Once the input images are decomposed, a visual percept could be recreated by stimulating the neurons with the correct visuotopic location and the appropriately oriented receptive field.

This notion has been suggested by a number of basic visual neuroscientists and researchers working in the area of visual neuroprosthetics. However, there is little evidence to suggest that such a complex signal-processing scheme would be needed to evoke patterned percepts. First, in all the studies done to date on intracortical microstimulation, it has generally been observed that microstimulation evokes point percepts, not percepts of lines (Brindley and Lewin, 1968; Dobelle and Mladejovsky, 1974; Bak et al., 1990; Schmidt et al., 1996). Second, the suggestion is based upon the character of receptive fields, where the receptive field of a neuron reflects its presynaptic organization. While it is indisputable that the optimum stimulus to excite a cortical complex cell will be a line of a particular orientation, such a line will also excite a complex pattern of activity in the visual cortex. It is this pattern of activity that will be interpreted by higher visual centers, not simply the firing pattern of the single recorded neuron. We believe that this question, as well as the feasibility of this approach to restoring lost visual function, can be fully answered only with human experimentation. We believe that the development of new arrays of penetrating electrodes, like the UEA, can provide the tools that will make this new class of psychophysical experiments possible.

References

Abeles, M. (1991). *Corticonics: Neural Circuits of the Cerebral Cortex*. Cambridge: Cambridge University Press.

Albus, K. (1975). A quantitative study of the projection area of the central and the paracentral visual field in area 17 of the cat. I. The precision of the topography. *Exp. Brain. Res.* 24(2): 159–179.

Arieli, A., Shoham, D., Hildesheim, R., and Grinvald, A. (1995). Coherent spatiotemporal patterns of ongoing activity revealed by real-time optical imaging coupled with single-unit recording in the cat visual cortex. *J. Neurophysiol.* 73(5): 2072–2093.

Bak, M., Girvin, J. P., Hambrecht, F. T., Kufta, C. V., et al. (1990). Visual sensations produced by intracortical microstimulation of the human occipital cortex. *Med. Biol. Eng. Comput.* 28(3): 257–259.

Bishop, P., Kozak, W., and Vakkur, G. J. (1962). Some quantitative aspects of the cat's eye: Axis and plane of reference, visual field co-ordinates and optics. *J. Physiol.* 163: 466–502.

Blasdel, G. G. (1992). Differential imaging of ocular dominance and orientation selectivity in monkey striate cortex. *J. Neurosci.* 12(8): 3115–3138.

Blasdel, G. G., and Salama, G. (1986). Voltage-sensitive dyes reveal a modular organization in monkey striate cortex. *Nature* 321(6070): 579–585.

Branner, A., Stein, R. B., and Normann, R. A. (2001). Selective stimulation of cat sciatic nerve using an array of varying-length microelectrodes. *J. Neurophysiol.* 85(4): 1585–1594.

Brindley, G. S., and Lewin, W. S. (1968). The visual sensations produced by electrical stimulation of the medial occipital cortex. *J. Physiol. (London)* 194(2): 54–5P.

Diogo, A. C., Soares, J. G., Koulakov, A., Albright, T. D., and Gattass, R. (2003). Electrophysiological imaging of functional architecture in the cortical middle temporal visual area of *Cebus apella* monkey. *J. Neurosci.* 23(9): 3881–3898.

Dobelle, W. H., and Mladejovsky, M. G. (1974). Phosphenes produced by electrical stimulation of human occipital cortex, and their application to the development of a prosthesis for the blind. *J. Physiol. (London)* 243(2): 553–576.

Dow, B. M., Vautin, R. G., and Bauer, R. (1985). The mapping of visual space onto foveal striate cortex in the macaque monkey. *J. Neurosci.* 5(4): 890–902.

Eckhorn, R., Krause, F., and Nelson, J. I. (1993). The RF-cinematogram. A cross-correlation technique for mapping several visual receptive fields at once. *Biol. Cybern.* 69(1): 37–55.

Eckmiller, R. (1997). Learning retina implants with epiretinal contacts. *Ophthalmic Res.* 29(5): 281–289.

Gray, C. M., Maldonado, P. E., Wilson, M., and McNaughton, B. (1995). Tetrodes markedly improve the reliability and yield of multiple single-unit isolation from multi-unit recordings in cat striate cortex. *J. Neurosci. Meth.* 63(1–2): 43–54.

Grinvald, A., Lieke, E., Frostig, R. D., Gilbert, C. D., and Wiesel, T. N. (1986). Functional architecture of cortex revealed by optical imaging of intrinsic signals. *Nature* 324(6095): 361–364.

Grinvald, A. D., Shoham, A., Schmuel, A., Glaser, D., et al. (1999). *In vivo* optical imaging of cortical architecture and dynamics. In U. Windhorst and H. Johansson, eds., *Modern Techniques in Neuroscience Research*. Berlin: Springer-Verlag, pp. 893–969.

Grumet, A. E., Wyatt, J. L., Jr., and Rizzo, J. F. (2000). Multi-electrode stimulation and recording in the isolated retina. *J. Neurosci. Meth.* 101(1): 31–42.

Guillory, K. S., and Normann, R. A. (1999). A 100-channel system for real-time detection and storage of extracellular spike waveforms. *J. Neurosci. Meth.* 91(1–2): 21–29.

Hubel, D. H. (1988). *Eye, Brain, and Vision*. New York: Scientific American Library.

Hubel, D. H., and Wiesel, T. N. (1962). Receptive fields, binocular interaction and functional architecture in the cat's visual cortex. *J. Physiol. (London)* 160: 106–154.

Hubener, M., Shoham, D., Grinvald, A., and Bonhoeffer, T. (1997). Spatial relationships among three columnar systems in cat area 17. *J. Neurosci.* 17(23): 9270–9284.

Humayun, M. S., de Juan, E., Jr., Wieland, J. D., Dagnelie, G., et al. (1999). Pattern electrical stimulation of the human retina. *Vision Res.* 39(15): 2569–2576.

Jain, A. K., Duin, R. P. W., and Mao, J. C. (2000). Statistical pattern recognition: A review. *IEEE Trans. Pattern Anal. Machine Intelli.* 22(1): 4–37.

Jones, J. P., and Palmer, L. A. (1987). The two-dimensional spatial structure of simple receptive fields in cat striate cortex. *J. Neurophysiol.* 58(6): 1187–1211.

Jones, K. E., Campbell, P. K., and Normann, R. A. (1992). A glass/silicon composite intracortical electrode array. *Ann. Biomed. Eng.* 20(4): 423–437.

Kennedy, P. R., Bakay, R. A., Moore, M. M., Adamo, K., and Goldthwaite, J. (2000). Direct control of a computer from the human central nervous system. *IEEE Trans. Rehabil. Eng.* 8(2): 198–202.

Kruger, J., and Aiple, F. (1988). Multimicroelectrode investigation of monkey striate cortex: Spike train correlations in the infragranular layers. *J. Neurophysiol.* 60(2): 798–828.

LeVay, S., Hubel, D. H., and Wiesel, T. N. (1975). The pattern of ocular dominance columns in macaque visual cortex revealed by a reduced silver stain. *J. Comp. Neurol.* 159(4): 559–576.

Leventhal, A. G. (1983). Relationship between preferred orientation and receptive field position of neurons in cat striate cortex. *J. Comp. Neurol.* 220(4): 476–483.

Lewicki, M. S. (1998). A review of methods for spike sorting: The detection and classification of neural action potentials. *Network* 9(4): R53–78.

Masland, R. H. (1996). Processing and encoding of visual information in the retina. *Curr. Opin. Neurobiol.* 6(4): 467–474.

Maynard, E. M., Hatsopoulos, N. G., Ojakangas, C. L., Acuna, B. D., et al. (1999). Neuronal interactions improve cortical population coding of movement direction. *J. Neurosci.* 19(18): 8083–8093.

McCreery, D. B., Agnew, W. F., Yuen, T. G. H., and Bullara, L. A. (1995). Relationship between stimulus amplitude, stimulus frequency and neural damage during electrical stimulation of sciatic nerve of cat. *Med. Biol. Eng. Comput.* 33(3 special issue): 426–429.

Meister, M., Pine, J., and Baylor, D. A. (1994). Multi-neuronal signals from the retina: Acquisition and analysis. *J. Neurosci. Meth.* 51(1): 95–106.

Nicolelis, M. A., Lin, R. C., Woodward, D. J., and Chapin, J. K. (1993). Dynamic and distributed properties of many-neuron ensembles in the ventral posterior medial thalamus of awake rats. *Proc. Natl. Acad. Sci. U.S.A.* 90(6): 2212–2216.

Nikara, T., Bishop, P. O., and Pettigrew, J. D. (1968). Analysis of retinal correspondence by studying receptive fields of binocular single units in cat striate cortex. *Exp. Brain Res.* 6(4): 353–372.

Nordhausen, C. T., Maynard, E. M., and Normann, R. A. (1996). Single unit recording capabilities of a 100 microelectrode array. *Brain Res.* 726(1–2): 129–140.

Normann, R. A., Warren, D. J., Ammermuller, J., Fernandez, E., and Guillory, S. (2001). High-resolution spatiotemporal mapping of visual pathways using multi-electrode arrays. *Vision Res.* 41(10–11): 1261–1275.

Orban, G. A. (1991). Quantitative electrophysiology of visual cortex neurons. In A. G. Leventhal, ed., *The Neural Basis of Visual Function*. Boca Raton, Fla.: CRC Press.

Rieke, F., Warland, D., de Ruyter van Steveninck, R., and Bialek, W. (1997). *Spikes*. Cambridge, Mass.: MIT Press.

Rousche, P. J., and Normann, R. A. (1992). A method for pneumatically inserting an array of penetrating electrodes into cortical tissue. *Ann. Biomed. Eng.* 20(4): 413–422.

Rousche, P. J., and Normann, R. A. (1999). Chronic intracortical microstimulation (ICMS) of cat sensory cortex using the Utah Intracortical Electrode Array. *IEEE Trans. Rehabil. Eng.* 7(1): 56–68.

Sahani, M., Pezaris, J. S., et al. (1997). On the separation of signals from neighboring cells in tetrode recordings. In *Advances in Neural Information Processing Systems*, vol. 11. Denver, Colo. Cambridge, MA: MIT Press.

Schmidt, E. M., Bak, M. J., Hambrecht, F. T., Kufta, C. V., et al. (1996). Feasibility of a visual prosthesis for the blind based on intracortical microstimulation of the visual cortex. *Brain* 119(pt. 2): 507–522.

Shtoyerman, E., Arieli, A., Slovin, H., Vanzetta, I., and Grinvald, A. (2000). Long-term optical imaging and spectroscopy reveal mechanisms underlying the intrinsic signal and stability of cortical maps in V1 of behaving monkeys. *J. Neurosci.* 20(21): 8111–8121.

Singer, W. (1993). Synchronization of cortical activity and its putative role in information processing and learning. *Ann. Rev. Physiol.* 55: 349–374.

Stanley, G. B., Li, F. F., and Dan, Y. (1999). Reconstruction of natural scenes from ensemble responses in the lateral geniculate nucleus. *J. Neurosci.* 19(18): 8036–8042.

Tusa, R. J., Palmer, L. A., and Rosenquist, A. C. (1978). The retinotopic organization of area 17 (striate cortex) in the cat. *J. Comp. Neurol.* 177(2): 213–235.

Veraart, C., Raftopoulos, C., Mortimer, J. T., Delbeke, J., et al. (1998). Visual sensations produced by optic nerve stimulation using an implanted self-sizing spiral cuff electrode. *Brain Res.* 813(1): 181–186.

Warland, D. K., Reinagel, P., and Meister, M. (1997). Decoding visual information from a population of retinal ganglion cells. *J. Neurophysiol.* 78(5): 2336–2350.

Warren, D. J., Fernandez, E., and Normann, R. A. (2001). High-resolution two-dimensional spatial mapping of cat striate cortex using a 100-microelectrode array. *Neuroscience* 105(1): 19–31.

Wise, K. D., and Najafi, K. (1991). Microfabrication techniques for integrated sensors and microsystems. *Science* 254(5036): 1335–1342.

II NEURAL REPRESENTATIONS

4 Brain Parts on Multiple Scales: Examples from the Auditory System

Ellen Covey

What Is a Brain "Part"?

Before considering the possibility of replacing defective parts of the brain with analog or digital hardware, transplanted neural tissue, or hybrid devices that include both hardware and biological tissue, we first need to have a clear and specific idea of what "part" is being replaced, what function that part serves, and whether that part is a stand-alone item or a component of a larger integrated system. To date, the most successful case in which a nervous system-related structure has been replaced by hardware is the cochlear implant. It is likely that this technology is successful partly because the cochlear hair cell array is a discrete and relatively independent structure, and we have a good idea of what the cochlear hair cells are designed to do. Perhaps the biggest factor contributing to the success of the cochlear implant, however, is the fact that all of the neural structures in the auditory system remain intact, starting with the peripherally located ganglion cells, and the brain continues to do its job as usual.

Once we enter the domain of the brain, it is no longer apparent exactly what constitutes a brain "part," or what function any part by itself might serve. In reality, the brain operates as a single dynamic integrated system that could be subdivided into "parts" using a variety of different temporal, anatomical, and functional criteria, with each criterion yielding a different set of putative "parts." In order to successfully replace a part of the brain, it would presumably be necessary to integrate the prosthetic part with other parts, starting with the appropriate neural inputs and outputs. The replacement part would probably also need to be adaptable, changing its properties in response to the overall state of the organism, the sensory or behavioral context, or other factors.

The subcortical portion of the central auditory system (figure 4.1) contains a highly complex network of cell groups and fiber pathways. The success of the cochlear implant can probably be attributed to the exquisitely adaptable operation of this system, which can take the highly artificial, impoverished, and distorted input

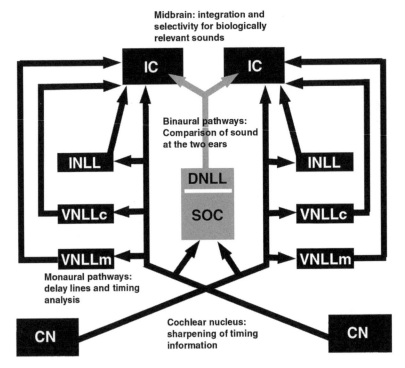

Figure 4.1
Schematic diagram showing the main brainstem pathways of the central auditory system. Crossed monaural pathways are shown in black; binaural pathways are indicated in gray. CN, cochlear nucleus; DNLL, dorsal nucleus of the lateral lemniscus; IC, inferior colliculus; SOC, superior olivary complex; INLL, intermediate nucleus of the lateral lemniscus; VNLLc, ventral nucleus of the lateral lemniscus, columnar division; VNLLm, ventral nucleus of the lateral lemniscus, multipolar cell division (from Covey, 2001).

provided by patterned electrical stimulation of ganglion cells using one or a few electrodes and interpret it in a way that is useful for the organism. This chapter uses the central auditory pathways to illustrate some of the many ways in which we can subdivide the brain into "parts," and considers the utility of each viewpoint for conceptualizing and designing technology that might someday replace brain structures or other functional units within the central nervous system.

Molecules as Brain "Parts"

If we choose to take a bottom-up approach and start with the smallest brain "parts" that are practical to consider, a logical place to begin would be with the molecules that make up the brain and the genes that code for these molecules. A great deal is known about the function of brain molecules, especially those involved in neurotransmission and neuromodulation. These classes of molecules include neurotransmitters, receptors, second messengers, ion channel subunits, etc. Although perhaps not directly relevant to the theme of this book, replacement of brain molecules through pharmacology, transplantation of cells, or gene therapy is clearly an area in which the strategy of replacement has met with considerable success and is likely to be a major area of research and development for therapeutic treatments in the future.

Although the molecular level might appear to be the smallest common denominator when it comes to brain "parts," it could also be considered one of the largest, since a given neurotransmitter, ion channel, or other molecule is likely to be found throughout large regions of the brain, or even throughout the brain as a whole. Thus, replacement of a molecule is likely to affect global aspects of brain function as well as specific ones. Here we will consider just two examples of molecules that are distributed rather ubiquitously within the central nervous system but that are essential for proper auditory system function on a cellular, circuit, and global level.

Inhibitory Neurotransmitters, γ-Aminobutyric Acid and Glycine

Throughout the central auditory system, a large number of neurons synthesize and release γ-aminobutyric acid (GABA). Below the level of the midbrain, there are not only many GABAergic neurons, but also many neurons that synthesize and release glycine (e.g., Mugnaini and Oertel, 1985; Peyret et al., 1987; Fubara et al., 1996). Thus, cells in structures up through the auditory midbrain center, the inferior colliculus (IC), may receive two different types of inhibitory input, each of which presumably serves a different function. Moreover, the same neurotransmitter may serve both a specific and a global function at any given neuron. The function of GABA in the IC provides a good example of this principle.

The mammalian IC contains a higher density of GABAergic terminals and receptors than any other part of the brain except the cerebellum (e.g., Fubara et al., 1996). The nature of GABA's action on cells depends on the type of receptors present on the postsynaptic membrane. The IC contains both $GABA_A$ receptors, which provide rapid, short-acting inhibition, and $GABA_B$ receptors, which provide delayed, long-acting inhibition. Activation of these two receptor types by GABA release may be one of the factors that provide a restricted temporal window during which ongoing excitatory input can depolarize a cell to threshold, with $GABA_A$ activation limiting the early part of the response and $GABA_B$ activation limiting the late part of the response. The characteristics of the window during which excitation may occur would be expected to vary as a function of the relative proportions of the two receptor types on the cell membrane.

There is evidence that individual IC neurons not only possess $GABA_A$ and $GABA_B$ receptors in different ratios, but that they also receive varying amounts of glycinergic inhibition. Moreover, electrophysiological studies show that the different

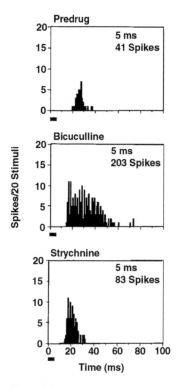

Figure 4.2
Responses of a neuron in the IC of the bat before and during local application of bicuculline, a blocker of GABAergic inhibition, and strychnine, a blocker of glycinergic inhibition. (*Top*) In response to a 5-ms tone, the neuron discharged a short burst of spikes at a latency of approximately 20 ms. (*Middle*) During application of bicuculline, the latency shortened to about 15 ms; firing rate increased; and the period during which action potentials were fired increased to more than 40 ms, far outlasting the duration of the stimulus. (*Bottom*) During application of strychnine, latency shortened to less than 15 ms and spike rate increased, but there was no lengthening of the response period (adapted from Casseday et al., 2000).

sources of inhibition act together to create specialized response properties of IC cells, including the ability to select for behaviorally relevant features of sound. Studies of IC neurons in which $GABA_A$ receptors are blocked by bicuculline show that the magnitude and duration of sound-evoked responses greatly increase, suggesting that long-lasting GABAergic input normally suppresses a long-lasting excitatory input to the cell. In the same neuron, blocking glycinergic input with strychnine typically causes first-spike latency to decrease and total spike count to increase, but the duration of the response remains short (Casseday et al., 2000; figure 4.2). These findings suggest that glycine acts mainly to suppress responses to the early part of a prolonged sound-evoked excitatory input, whereas GABA suppresses responses to a large portion of the sound-evoked excitation, especially the later part. These findings are consistent with the idea that there is a narrow temporal window within which the cell can respond to a sustained excitatory input.

Because different inputs to the IC neuron have different thresholds, rate-intensity functions, frequency tuning, spatial tuning, and other properties, the temporal relationship among the multiple excitatory and inhibitory inputs to an IC neuron changes parametrically as a function of physical parameters of the sound, such as its intensity or duration. This variable relationship is important for creating selectivity to behaviorally relevant sound features such as its duration (e.g., Casseday et al., 1994, 2000; Covey et al., 1996; Ehrlich et al., 1997) or the location from which the sound originates (e.g., Vater et al., 1992; Park and Pollak, 1994).

There is a large body of evidence indicating that inhibitory neurotransmitters are involved in the specific processing mechanisms that allow auditory midbrain neurons to select specific types of information for transmission to the thalamocortical system and/or motor systems (e.g., Casseday and Covey, 1996). However, it is likely that the massive amount of inhibition in the IC also serves some more global functions. One of these has to do with slowing the cadence of processing from that of the inputs from lower centers that are time locked to the fine structure of the stimulus to a slower rate that is matched to the rate at which motor actions are performed (Casseday and Covey, 1996).

A second global function has to do with keeping the amount of excitation that reaches the IC in check. In the lower brainstem, the auditory nerve diverges to create a number of different parallel pathways, all of which then converge at the IC (figure 4.1). If the outputs of all of these pathways were excitatory, the activity arriving via the auditory nerve would be amplified many times over. It seems reasonable to suppose that inhibition helps maintain the amount of neural activity at a relatively constant level while allowing the IC to integrate many streams of information processed in parallel.

Evidence to support this idea comes from studies of audiogenic seizures, which can occur when there is an abnormally high amount of activity in the IC that is due to a pharmacologically or genetically induced deficit in GABAergic inhibition (e.g., Frye et al., 1983, 1986; Millan et al., 1986, 1988; Faingold and Naritoku, 1992). Clearly, this is a case in which a brain "part" at the molecular level, that is, GABAergic inhibition at the IC, has a global effect that it might be possible to mimic by a uniform increase in GABA across space and time. However, GABA also plays a specific role at each neuron that depends on the precise ratio and timing of GABAergic input relative to other inputs, as well as the adjustment of this ratio and timing according to the physical parameters of the stimulus. This specific function would be difficult to duplicate in a "replacement" system without knowing in detail the mechanisms and outcomes of stimulus-specific processing. To some extent this information can be obtained by considering individual neurons as brain "parts."

Single Neurons as "Parts"

With few exceptions, the groups of cells and fibers that we typically think of as anatomically distinct brain structures such as the hippocampus, neocortex, inferior colliculus, or cochlear nucleus, are all made up of multiple neuron types, each of which performs a different class of function. It is quite clear from electrophysiological studies that single neurons throughout the brain function as complex computational, decision-making devices and could therefore be thought of as brain "parts."

In the auditory system, the response to sound by a neuron at any level is determined by a number of interactive factors. The factors that determine a neuron's sound-evoked response start with the neuron's intrinsic properties, as determined by the subset of receptor sites for neurotransmitters and neuromodulators expressed on its cell membrane, and the subset of ion channels and second messenger systems expressed by the neuron. Responses to sensory stimuli are also determined by the number, morphology, location, chemical makeup, and temporal properties of synaptic inputs from different sources, and the spatiotemporal pattern of activity of those synaptic inputs. A few good examples of the ways in which auditory neurons transform and integrate synaptic inputs include sharpening of the temporal precision of phase-locked responses in some classes of neurons in the anteroventral cochlear nucleus, comparison of input from the two ears to provide an estimate of the location of a sound source along the horizontal plane in neurons in the superior olive, and tuning to a specific duration of sound in one population of neurons in the IC.

Intrinsic Properties and Temporal Precision

As the auditory nerve enters the brain, each of its component fibers branches to innervate three major subdivisions of the cochlear nucleus, creating three separate representations of the frequency organization produced by the cochlea. Within each of these central representations of the cochlea are multiple cell types, each with a characteristic morphology and biochemical makeup (for review, see Oertel, 1991; Trussell, 1999).

The input transmitted by the branches of a given auditory nerve fiber to the different types of neuron is essentially identical, consisting of an initial high frequency burst of action potentials followed by steady-state sustained firing at a rate that, at least over the fiber's dynamic range, is proportional to the intensity of the sound. In response to a low-frequency tone or amplitude-modulated sound, auditory nerve fiber responses are phase-locked (i.e., correlated in time) with a specific point in each cycle of a low frequency pure tone or each peak in an amplitude modulation pattern. It has been shown that "bushy" neurons in the cochlear nucleus take this information and sharpen its temporal precision so that phase locking is greatly enhanced (e.g., Frisina et al., 1990; Joris et al., 1994a, b). An example of this enhancement is shown in figure 4.3.

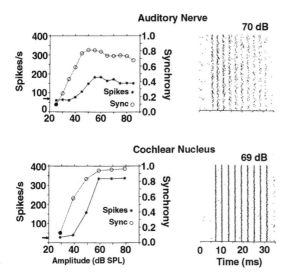

Figure 4.3
Dot rasters (*right*) and plots of spike count and synchronization coefficient as a function of sound level (*left*) to illustrate enhancement of the auditory nerve's temporal precision by a neuron in the cochlear nucleus of the cat. The top panels illustrate the phase-locked response of an auditory nerve fiber to a low frequency tone. The bottom panels illustrate the responses of a fiber in the trapezoid body, originating in the cochlear nucleus, to the same low frequency tone (adapted from Joris et al., 1994a).

   Intracellular recordings from neurons in the cochlear nucleus have shown that the intrinsic properties of those types of neurons that preserve fine timing information or provide temporal enhancement differ in some respects from the intrinsic properties of other cell types in the cochlear nucleus (e.g., Smith and Rhode, 1987; Manis and Marx, 1991; Trussell, 1997). When depolarizing current steps are applied to bushy cells, they typically discharge only one or two action potentials in response to the onset of the current step, after which a voltage-gated outward current is activated that brings the cell's membrane potential to an equilibrium value just below the threshold for spike generation, as shown in figure 4.4. This means that the cell does not fire again as long as the depolarization step is maintained. Hyperpolarization typically results in a rebound and spike at the offset of the current step (e.g., Oertel, 1983; Manis and Marx, 1991).

   These same cells also exhibit a low-threshold outward current that greatly reduces the excitatory postsynaptic potential (EPSP) time constant, limiting to less than a millisecond the time window over which successive EPSPs can sum (e.g., Oertel, 1983, 1985; Manis and Marx, 1991). Given these properties, the bushy cells are able to follow high frequency input with great temporal precision. Because these cells receive synaptic endings from multiple auditory nerve fibers (Oertel, 1999), they receive multiple estimates of the onset time of a sound or other auditory event. Because of

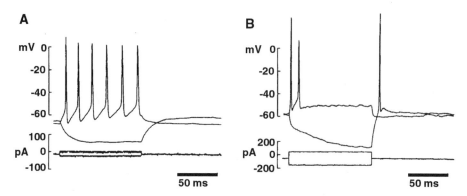

Figure 4.4
Responses of two types of cochlear nucleus neurons to depolarizing and hyperpolarizing current steps. Intracellular recordings were obtained in guinea pig brain slices. (*A*) This neuron fires a regular train of action potentials throughout the duration of the depolarizing step. (*B*) This neuron, characteristic of "bushy" cells, fires one or two action potentials at the beginning of the depolarizing step and maintains a membrane potential just below threshold for the remainder of the step. Following a hyperpolarizing step, there is a rebound accompanied by an action potential. After hyperpolarization, there is no overshoot (adapted from Manis and Marx, 1991).

the bushy cell's limited integration window, it will fire at the temporal peak of the input distribution, thus providing a high degree of temporal enhancement. The output of the bushy cells is subsequently used for tasks that require fine timing analysis, including the measurement of phase differences between low-frequency sounds at the two ears.

The bushy cell provides an example of a neuron in which much of the processing is accomplished through an excitatory input interacting with the cell's intrinsic properties. However, there are many other neurons whose processing depends on the interaction of excitatory and inhibitory synaptic inputs. One of the simplest examples is provided by neurons in the pathway for comparison of sound at the two ears.

Interaction of Synaptic Excitation and Inhibition Leading to Simple Computation
Inputs from the two cochlear nuclei first come together at the superior olivary complex, located in the lower brainstem (figure 4.1). The lateral superior olive (LSO) is one component of the pathway that computes the location of a sound source based on a comparison of the physical properties of the sound that reaches the two ears. Each neuron in the LSO receives excitatory input directly from the ipsilateral cochlear nucleus. It also receives inhibitory input indirectly from the contralateral cochlear nucleus via a synapse in the medial nucleus of the trapezoid body (MNTB), a group of glycinergic neurons with properties similar to those of bushy cells in the cochlear nucleus (Brew and Forsythe, 1994). Figure 4.5A shows the details of the LSO circuitry.

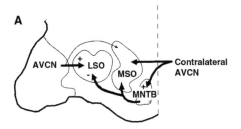

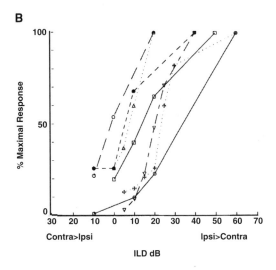

Figure 4.5
(*A*) Inputs to the lateral superior olive (LSO) in the mustached bat as seen in a schematic frontal section through the lower left side of the brainstem. The left anteroventral cochlear nucleus (AVCN) contributes ipsilaterally evoked excitatory input to the left LSO. The right cochlear nucleus provides contralateral excitatory input to the left medial nucleus of the trapezoid body (MNTB), which in turn provides inhibitory input to the left LSO. The vertical dashed line indicates the midline. (*B*) Examples of seven different LSO neurons' responses as a function of interaural level difference (ILD). To facilitate comparison among neurons, the response magnitude is normalized to the maximal response. The response of all of the neurons is maximal when the ipsilateral sound is louder than the contralateral one. As the ILD approaches zero (equal sound amplitude at the two ears), the response of all the neurons declines, starting at different ILDs, but with similar slopes. When the amplitude of the contralateral sound exceeds that of the ipsilateral sound by about 30 dB, all of the neurons' responses have declined to a spontaneous rate. (*A* and *B* adapted from Covey et al., 1991.)

For sounds with wavelengths shorter than the distance between the ears, the head creates a sound shadow that is more or less pronounced, depending on the azimuthal location of the sound source. As a result, there is an interaural level difference (ILD) that varies from zero (both sides equal) when the sound source is straight ahead, to maximal (ipsi louder than contra) when the sound source is located 90 degrees to the right or left. Consequently, a sound source 90 degrees to the right provides strong excitation and weak inhibition to a neuron in the right LSO, so the neuron will respond. When the sound source is straight ahead, the sound level at the two ears is equal, so excitation will equal inhibition and the neuron will respond weakly or not respond. When the sound source is anywhere on the left, then inhibition to the right LSO will exceed excitation, and the neuron will not respond.

In reality, different LSO neurons appear to have slightly different weights of excitation and inhibition. This can be seen by plotting the responses of LSO neurons as a function of ILD (figure 4.5B). Each neuron's response is maximal when the ipsilateral sound is much louder than the contralateral, but at some point it begins to decline as the ILD approaches zero. LSO neurons typically have dynamic ranges that correspond to a range of ILDs produced by sound sources within the 45-degree space just ipsilateral to the midline. As figure 4.5 shows, different LSO neurons' dynamic ranges differ somewhat, suggesting that the relative weights of excitation and inhibition differ. Each LSO neuron functions as a computational device that provides an output proportional to the location of a sound source relative to the midline, but the response of each neuron declines over a slightly different range of ILDs.

The fundamental mechanism by which an LSO neuron performs its computation is quite straightforward since it essentially involves only the algebraic summation of simultaneous excitatory and inhibitory inputs. Neurons that act as analyzers of the temporal structure of sound, duration, for example, need an added temporal dimension in their processing. The convergence of inputs from multiple sources at the midbrain provides an ideal substrate for a temporal analysis of sound.

Complex, Multicomponent Computation and Duration Tuning
Neurons in the midbrain auditory center, the inferior colliculus, receive direct projections from the cochlear nucleus as well as from subsequent stages of processing, including the cell groups of the superior olivary complex and the nuclei of the lateral lemniscus (figure 4.1). Because each stage of processing introduces a time delay of a millisecond or more, even a brief stimulus such as a click that lasts a fraction of a millisecond can cause a cell in the IC to receive a complex series of excitatory and inhibitory inputs that extend over many tens of milliseconds (e.g., Covey et al., 1996; Covey and Casseday, 1999). Since each input neuron has its own sensitivity profile and repertoire of response properties, the magnitude and time course of synaptic input from each source will vary systematically, but in a different pattern, in response

to parametric changes in the auditory stimulus. Thus, the IC neuron functions as a sort of "readout" of activity across the population from which it receives input (Covey, 2000, 2001). This integrative function is especially obvious in intracellular recordings in which it is possible to follow the changes in synaptic inputs that occur as a stimulus parameter is varied (e.g., Nelson and Erulkar, 1963; Covey et al., 1996; Kuwada et al., 1997).

Many neurons in the IC exhibit bandpass tuning to sound duration (figure 4.6) in that they fail to respond if the sound is too short or too long and respond best to a specific duration (Pinheiro and Jen, 1991; Casseday et al., 1994; Ehrlich et al., 1997; Chen, 1998; Fuzessery and Hall, 1999; Brand et al., 2000). Duration tuning is largely independent of sound intensity (Fremouw et al., 2000; Zhou and Jen, 2001). The finding that blocking synaptic inhibition eliminates duration tuning (Casseday et al., 2000) indicates that this form of response selectivity is created through the interaction of excitatory input with inhibitory input. Intracellular recordings (figure 4.7) show that duration-tuned neurons always receive some inhibition regardless of stimulus duration, that the inhibition is sustained for the duration of the stimulus,

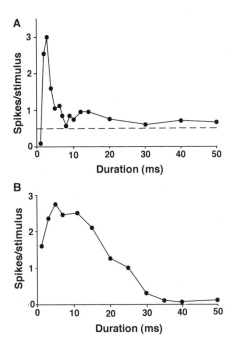

Figure 4.6
Two examples of duration-tuned cells in the IC of the big brown bat. The response magnitude is plotted as a function of stimulus duration, showing that there is a specific duration at which the response is maximal and that the neuron's response declines to a spontaneous rate at longer durations. (Adapted from Ehrlich et al., 1997.)

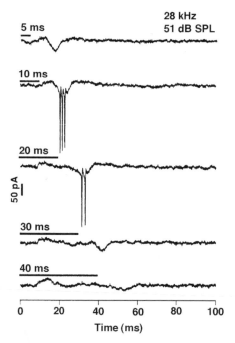

Figure 4.7
Sound-evoked postsynaptic currents recorded intracellularly from a duration-tuned neuron in the IC of the big brown bat. The neuron's best duration was about 10 ms. The recordings were obtained in voltage-clamp mode using whole-cell patch-clamp recording in an awake, intact animal. In this and figure 4.11, the outward current, indicative of an inhibitory postsynaptic current (IPSC), is an upward deflection of the trace and the inward current, indicative of an excitatory postsynaptic current (EPSC), is a downward deflection. At each duration there is a long-lasting IPSC locked in time to stimulus onset and a short EPSC or rebound associated with the offset of the stimulus. (From Covey et al., 1996.)

and that it arrives with a relatively short latency. These recordings further suggest that a transient, onset-related excitatory input is partially cancelled and rendered subthreshold by the sustained inhibition, and that the cell only responds when the duration of the sound is such that the transient onset excitation coincides in time with a rebound from inhibition correlated with stimulus offset. Figure 4.8 shows how a model neuron with these characteristics would respond to different sound durations.

Duration-tuned neurons thus appear to depend on an intrinsic property—rebound from inhibition—for part of their processing capability and on temporally distributed patterns of excitatory and inhibitory synaptic inputs for another part of their processing capability. Although the basic function of a duration-tuned neuron is clear, the mechanism underlying this function depends on a highly structured spatio-temporal pattern of inputs. If the characteristics of even one of these inputs is altered

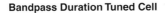

Bandpass Duration Tuned Cell

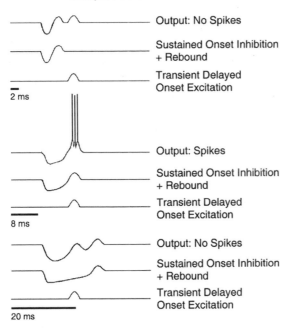

Figure 4.8
A hypothetical model for bandpass duration tuning, based on data from duration-tuned neurons in the IC of the bat. The cell's output in response to three different durations of sound is shown in the top trace of each group. The cell receives a sustained, onset-evoked inhibitory postsynaptic potential with a depolarizing rebound at sound offset (middle trace of each group). It also receives a short excitatory postsynaptic potential evoked by the onset of the sound, but rendered subthreshold by the simultaneously occurring IPSP (lower trace of each group). The cell reaches threshold only if the onset EPSP coincides with the offset rebound. In response to a 2-ms sound (upper group of three traces), the rebound occurs before the EPSP, so the stimulus is too short to elicit a response. In response to an 8-ms sound (middle group of three traces), the rebound and EPSP coincide, causing the cell to fire a burst of action potentials. In response to a 20-ms sound (bottom group of three traces) the EPSP occurs before the rebound, so the duration is too long to elicit a response. (From Casseday et al., 2001.)

(e.g., by blocking GABAergic transmission), the neuron ceases to perform its function. On a more subtle level, if the spatiotemporal pattern of inputs is faulty, the output of the neuron will also be faulty even though its internal mechanism is functioning perfectly. Thus, for any brain part, including a single neuron, it is essential to have the right information going in, in the right format, if an appropriate output is to result.

Clearly, neurons do not act in isolation since they require patterned input from multiple sources and in turn typically provide divergent input to multiple other neurons. However, before considering multilevel neural systems as brain "parts," it is useful to consider the function of populations of neurons at a single level.

Morphologically Distinct Cell Groups as "Parts"

Probably the most common definition of a brain "part" is an anatomically distinguishable group of cell bodies and associated fibers within the brain. In their simplest form, brain structures are homogeneous groups of cells such as the glycinergic
"bushy"-type neurons that comprise the MNTB or the columnar subdivision of
the ventral nucleus of the lateral lemniscus in echolocating animals (e.g., Covey and
Casseday, 1986, 1991). In their most complex form, brain structures consist of many
different cell types and connectional relationships, and perform multiple functions.
Examples include the hippocampus, cerebral cortex, and inferior colliculus. We will
begin by considering a small homogeneous group of neurons in the lower brainstem
of echolocating bats, the function of which is relatively straightforward.

**The Columnar Subdivision of the Ventral Nucleus of the Lateral Lemniscus as a Set
of Time-Marking Frequency Filters**

In the auditory brainstem of all mammals, "bushy"-type neurons are not confined to
the cochlear nucleus; they are also present in the MNTB and the ventral nucleus of
the lateral lemniscus (VNLL). In the MNTB and VNLL, these neurons stain for glycine, indicating that their output is inhibitory. In the VNLL of most mammals, the
"bushy"-type neurons are intermingled with other cell types, but in echolocating bats
they are segregated and neatly arranged in columns (figure 4.9). This part of the
VNLL is referred to as the columnar subdivision, or VNLLc (Covey and Casseday,
1986). Connectional and electrophysiological studies have shown that the VNLLc
contains a complete tonotopic map of the cochlea projected onto the height of
the columns, each of which contains about 20–30 cells (Covey and Casseday, 1986,
1991). When presented with pure tones, neurons in the VNLLc respond over a broad
range of frequencies. Each neuron responds with one spike that is tightly locked in
time to the onset of the stimulus. The latency of response remains constant across
sound frequency and amplitude (Covey and Casseday, 1991). Each isofrequency
sheet within the columnar organization of the VNLLc projects heavily throughout a
broad frequency range within the IC (Covey and Casseday, 1986). VNLLc neurons
respond best to downward frequency sweeps that are similar to the echolocation calls
that the bat emits, firing one spike that is tightly locked in time to the point at which
the frequency enters the upper border of the neuron's response area and remaining
silent for the remainder of the sweep (Huffman et al., 1998).

Given these characteristics, it seems likely that the population of VNLLc neurons
together function as a set of broadband frequency filters that apportion the echolocation call into approximately 25–30 discrete frequency segments. Each time the
emitted vocalization or the echo reflected from an object reaches the bat's ear, neurons in the isofrequency sheets of the VNLLc are successively activated, starting with

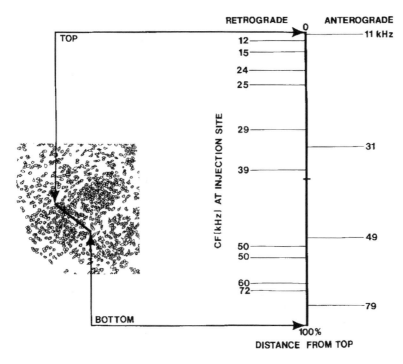

Figure 4.9
Drawing of cells in the VNLLc of the big brown bat illustrating columnar organization and tonotopic representation within a column as seen by anterograde transport of tracer from tonotopically characterized sites in the cochlear nucleus and retrograde transport from tonotopically organized regions of the IC. Each column contains a highly organized sequence from low to high frequencies that spans the extent of the bat's audible range. (From Covey and Casseday, 1986.)

the highest frequencies and progressing to the lowest ones, transmitting a precise time marker for the onset of each frequency segment. Because VNLLc cells appear to be glycinergic, it may be that the function of the time marker is to "initialize" the IC cells that encode information within a frequency segment, preparing them to receive information within that band. It is known that in at least some auditory neurons, the discharge patterns and latencies of responses to a given stimulus can vary greatly, depending on what the membrane potential of the cell is when it receives the stimulus (e.g., Kanold and Manis, 1999). Therefore, for precise time-coding tasks such as the measurement of the time between the vocalization and the echo, it might be advantageous to have uniform starting conditions that are replicated from one measurement to the next.

A second function for the VNLLc output might be to provide a rebound from inhibition evoked by one stimulus (e.g., the vocalization) that would coincide with excitation evoked by a second stimulus (e.g., the echo), allowing the IC neuron to respond when the two stimuli are separated by a specific time interval. Neurons tuned to the delay between two stimuli are found in the IC, and their delay tuning is eliminated when inhibition is blocked (Portfors and Wenstrup, 2001), suggesting that VNLLc neurons may indeed play a role in the circuitry that computes the distance of an object relative to the bat.

In the auditory system, tonotopic organization is a ubiquitous feature of brain structures. Not only does it provide a way of segmenting a complex auditory stimulus into discrete frequency bands, each of which is analyzed in a separate channel, it also provides a substrate upon which other parameters can be represented and compared across frequency channels. The LSO provides a simple example of how such a system might work.

The LSO as a System of ILD Maps

Complex sounds typically consist of multiple frequency components mixed together. Often different sets of frequency components originate from different locations in space. The LSO of all mammals is tonotopically organized with regard to its inputs, outputs, and electrophysiological response properties. As described earlier, the population of LSO neurons is relatively homogeneous; nevertheless, individual LSO neurons have dynamic ranges that span somewhat different ranges of ILDs, corresponding to different regions of azimuthal space. Although it has not been demonstrated conclusively, it is likely that each isofrequency sheet within the LSO contains neurons with different ILD functions, so that the population activity within an isofrequency sheet would provide an accurate estimate of the azimuthal location of the source of that frequency component, which could then be compared with population activity in other isofrequency sheets to ultimately provide a profile of which frequencies belong together.

The VNLLc and LSO are both relatively easy to characterize in terms of tasks that their constituent neurons might perform together as a population. For a nonhomogeneous structure such as the IC, where there is a large amount of convergent input from other structures as well as large numbers of interneurons, the tasks that they perform are not as easy to characterize.

The IC as an Integrative Center

The IC receives ascending input from virtually every one of the lower brainstem auditory nuclei as well as descending input from the auditory cortex, crossed input from the opposite IC, and internal connections from other neurons within the IC. It also receives input from motor-related structures such as the substantia nigra and globus pallidus. The dendrites of some of its neurons are confined to an isofrequency sheet, whereas the dendrites of other neurons span many frequency sheets. The main outputs of the IC are to the thalamocortical system and motor-related systems, including the superior colliculus and cerebellum, via the pontine gray (for a detailed review of IC connections, see Covey and Casseday, 1996; Casseday et al., 2000). Because of the structural and connectional complexity of the IC, it is difficult to assign it a single function on either a specific or a global level. In fact, the IC, like any system with highly divergent output, may perform multiple functions, depending on which output path we consider, with the same output taking on very different and even unrelated "meanings" that are determined by the other information with which it is combined (Covey, 2001).

Because the IC receives input from so many sources, ranging from monosynaptic input from the cochlear nucleus to polysynaptic pathways from the neocortex, the input in response to a single "instantaneous" stimulus onset could be spread over a hundred milliseconds or even more. Because the time scale of the fine structure of auditory stimuli is on the order of a millisecond or so, this means that IC neurons integrate information about fine structure over a time window that is roughly comparable to the rate at which motor activity occurs. For speech sounds, for example, the integration performed by IC neurons could accomplish the transition from analysis of fine structure to analysis on the time scale of phonemes, syllables, or even words.

There is considerable evidence that certain populations of IC neurons are selective for sound features that are behaviorally relevant to the species. For example, the range of durations to which IC neurons in bats are tuned corresponds closely to the range of durations of their echolocation signals (Ehrlich et al., 1997). Analysis of sound patterns on a scale of tens or even hundreds of milliseconds obviously requires integration of information over time. As a consequence, the neurons performing the analysis do not respond until the integration period is over and the proper conditions have been met. This lengthening of the analysis period is reflected in IC neurons' wide range of response latencies and inability to respond to stimuli presented at a rapid repetition rate (Casseday and Covey, 1996).

The IC contains multiple populations of neurons that are tuned to different aspects of sound and apparently perform different types of analysis. Parameters to which IC neurons are sensitive include duration, amplitude (Casseday and Covey, 1992), direction, depth and slope of frequency modulation, repetition rate of periodic amplitude or frequency modulation (Langner and Schreiner, 1988; Casseday et al., 1997), and the interval between two sounds (Mittmann and Wenstrup, 1995). These forms of sensitivity are not mutually exclusive and are usually accompanied by other forms of sensitivity, such as frequency tuning and sensitivity to the location of a sound source in space. Because of the heterogeneity and complexity of the IC, we still have a long way to go before we fully understand its function either in terms of the operation of its individual neurons in sound analysis or its role as a population of neurons in providing outputs to sensory and motor systems.

Although a population of neurons that forms a visual grouping for the neuroana-
tomist is the most obvious brain "part," it is also possible to think of "parts" in
strictly functional terms that transcend the anatomical boundaries of nuclei or other
cell groupings based on proximity.

Functional Modules or Channels as "Parts"

Because the auditory system is tonotopically organized at all levels, there must be a
close functional relationship between a given isofrequency contour in one cell group
and the same isofrequency contour in the cell groups to which it sends information
(figure 4.10). Thus, the representation of a specific frequency range across brain
levels, starting at the cochlea and progressing through the auditory cortex, could be
thought of as a cohesive brain "part." In this sense, a person with a hearing loss
restricted to a specific frequency range could be thought of as missing a "part" of
the auditory system that could be replaced by supplying the missing frequency-
specific input.

Multicomponent Loops as "Parts"

No part of the brain functions in isolation. Cell groups are connected with other cell
groups, not just in a feedforward pattern of hierarchical processing, but also in feedback loops. The inferior colliculus is a good example of a structure that not only
receives a massive amount of ascending input which it processes through the intrinsic
properties of its cells, through convergence of ascending inputs with one another, and
through internal circuitry, but also through the action of descending inputs from
some of the same structures to which it sends output. For example, the range of
latencies in the auditory cortex of the bat is about 4–50 ms. The range of latencies
in the IC is about the same, 3–50 ms (Simmons et al., 1995). This means that feedback from short latency neurons in the auditory cortex could reach the longer latency
neurons in the inferior colliculus and influence their responses to the same sound that
evoked the cortical feedback. If the longer latency IC neurons also project to the feedback neurons, this would create a reverberation that could persist for some time and
influence the responses of neurons in both the IC and cortex to subsequent sounds.

Intracellular recording shows that sound can evoke long-lasting oscillatory activity
in IC neurons (figure 4.11), but the origin of the oscillations is not known. Recent
evidence suggests that cortical stimulation or inactivation can influence the responses
of IC neurons on a stimulus-by-stimulus basis, but it is not known to what extent
cortical input contributes to shaping the responses of IC neurons.

What is clear is that the IC does not function alone. It is a the hub of a highly
distributed and interactive system. It requires multiple inputs, including ongoing

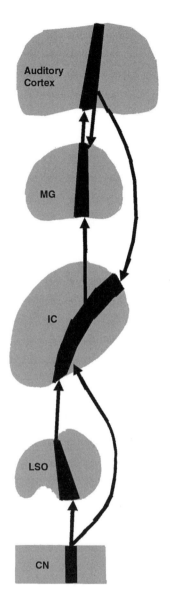

Figure 4.10
Diagram showing a multilevel isofrequency module that includes direct input from the cochlear nucleus (CN) to the inferior colliculus (IC); input from the CN to the lateral superior olive (LSO) and thence to the IC; ascending input from the IC to the medial geniculate nucleus of the thalamus (MG) and thence to the cortex; descending input from the cortex to the MG and IC. All of these connections and others that are not shown remain within their frequency channel or module.

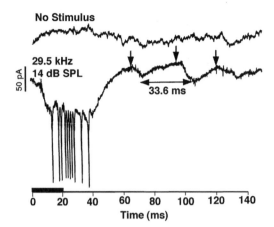

Figure 4.11
Sound-evoked postsynaptic currents recorded intracellularly from a neuron in the IC of the big brown bat showing a series of oscillating currents (arrows) that last for more than 100 ms after the offset of the stimulus. The top trace shows that there are no oscillations in the absence of sound. (From Covey et al., 1996.)

feedback from the auditory cortex, as well as multiple outputs to sensory and motor structures. The highly interdependent and interactive nature of the IC, its inputs, and its outputs, suggests that perhaps the entire central auditory system could be thought of as a brain "part," and that any attempt to reduce it to smaller components is unrealistic.

Acknowledgments

Many thanks to Kimberly Miller for expert technical assistance. This research is supported by the National Institute on Deafness and Other Communication Disorders, grants DC-00607 and DC-00287.

References

Brand, A., Urban, R., and Grothe, B. (2000) Duration tuning in the mouse auditory midbrain. *J. Neurophysiol.* 84: 1790–1799.

Brew, H. M., and Forsythe, I. D. (1999) Auditory neurons of the rat MNTB posess potassium conductances that aid high-fidelity, high-frequency synaptic transmission. *J. Physiol. Lond.* 480P: P109.

Casseday, J. H., and Covey, E. (1992) Frequency tuning properties of neurons in the inferior colliculus of an FM bat. *J. Comp. Neurol.* 319: 34–50.

Casseday, J. H., and Covey, E. (1996) A neuroethological theory of the operation of the inferior colliculus. *Brain Behav. Evol.* 47: 311–336.

Casseday, J. H., Ehrlich, D., and Covey, E. (1994) Neural tuning for sound duration: Role of inhibitory mechanisms in the inferior colliculus. *Science* 264: 847–850.

Casseday, J. H., Covey, E., and Grothe, B. (1997) Neurons specialized for periodic frequency modulations in the inferior colliculus of the big brown bat, *Eptesicus fuscus. J. Neurophysiol.* 77: 1595–1605.

Casseday, J. H., Ehrlich, D., and Covey, E. (2000) Neural measurement of sound duration: Control by excitatory-inhibitory interactions in the inferior colliculus. *J. Neurophysiol.* 84: 1475–1487.

Chen, G. D. (1998) Effects of stimulus duration on responses of neurons in the chinchilla inferior colliculus. *Hearing Res.* 122: 142–150.

Covey, E. (2000) Neural population coding in auditory temporal pattern analysis. *Physiol. Behav.* 69: 211–220.

Covey, E. (2001) Neural population coding in the auditory system. In M. A. L. Nicolelis, ed., *Progress in Brain Research: Advances in Neural Population Coding*, vol. 130. Amsterdam: Elsevier, pp. 205–220.

Covey, E., and Casseday, J. H. (1986) Connectional basis for frequency representation in the nuclei of the lateral lemniscus of the bat, *Eptesicus fuscus. J. Neurosci.* 6: 2926–2940.

Covey, E., and Casseday, J. H. (1991) The ventral lateral lemniscus in an echolocating bat: Parallel pathways for analyzing temporal features of sound. *J. Neurosci.* 11: 3456–3470.

Covey, E., and Casseday, J. H. (1999) Timing in the auditory system of the bat. *Annu. Rev. Physiol.* 61: 457–476.

Covey, E., Vater, M., and Casseday, J. H. (1991) Binaural properties of single units in the superior olivary complex of the mustached bat. *J. Neurophysiol.* 66: 1080–1094.

Covey, E., Kauer, J. A., and Casseday, J. H. (1996) Whole-cell patch clamp recording reveals subthreshold sound-evoked postsynaptic currents in the inferior colliculus of awake bats. *J. Neurosci.* 16: 3009–3018.

Ehrlich, D., Casseday, J. H., and Covey, E. (1997) Neural tuning to sound duration in the inferior colliculus of the big brown bat, *Eptesicus fuscus. J. Neurophysiol.* 77: 2360–2372.

Faingold, C. L., and Naritoku, D. K. (1992) The genetically epilepsy-prone rat: Neuronal networks and actions of amino acid neurotransmitters. In C. L. Faingold and G. H. Fromm, eds., *Drugs for Control of Epilepsy: Actions on Neuronal Networks Involved in Seizure Disorders.* Boca Raton, Fla.: CRC Press, pp. 227–308.

Fremouw, T., Covey, E., and Casseday, J. H. (2000) Duration-tuned units in the inferior colliculus are tolerant to changes in sound level. *Soc. Neurosci. Abstr.* 26: 161.14.

Frisina, R. D., Smith, R. L., and Chamberlain, S. C. (1990) Encoding of amplitude modulation in the gerbil cochlear nucleus. I. A hierarchy of enhancement. *Hear. Res.* 44: 99–122.

Frye, G. D., McCown, T. J., and Breese, G. R. (1983) Characterization of susceptibility to audiogenic seizures in ethanol-dependent rats after microinjection of γ-aminobutyric acid (GABA) agonists into the inferior colliculus, substantia nigra or medial septum. *J. Pharmacol. Exp. Therap.* 227: 663–670.

Frye, G. D., McCown, T. J., Breese, G. R., and Peterson, S. L. (1986) GABAergic modulation of inferior colliculus excitability: Role in ethanol withdrawal audiogenic seizures. *J. Pharmacol. Exp. Therap.* 237: 478–542.

Fubara, B. M., Casseday, J. H., Covey, E., and Schwartz-Bloom, R. D. (1996) Distribution of $GABA_A$, $GABA_B$ and glycine receptors in the central auditory system of the big brown bat, *Eptesicus fuscus. J. Comp. Neurol.* 369: 83–92.

Fuzessery, Z. M., and Hall, J. C. (1999) Sound duration selectivity in the pallid bat inferior colliculus. *Hear. Res.* 137: 137–154.

Huffman, R. F., Argeles, P. C., and Covey, E. (1998) Processing of sinusoidally frequency modulated signals in the nuclei of the lateral lemniscus of the big brown bat, *Eptesicus fuscus. Hear. Res.* 126: 161–180.

Joris, P. X., Carney, L. H., Smith, P. H., and Yin, T. C. T. (1994a) Enhancement of neural synchronization in the anteroventral cochlear nucleus. I. Responses to tones at the characteristic frequency. *J. Neurophysiol.* 71: 1022–1036.

Joris, P. X., Smith, P. H., and Yin, T. C. T. (1994b) Enhancement of neural synchronization in the anteroventral cochlear nucleus. II. Responses in the tuning curve tail. *J. Neurophysiol.* 71: 1037–1051.

Kanold, P. O., and Manis, P. B. (1999) Transient potassium currents regulate the discharge patterns of dorsal cochlear nucleus pyramidal cells. *J. Neurosci.* 19: 2195–2208.

Kuwada, S., Batra, R., Yin, T. C. T., Oliver, D. L., Haberly, L. B., and Stanford, T. R. (1997) Intracellular recordings in response to monaural and binaural stimulation of neurons in the inferior colliculus of the cat. *J. Neurosci.* 17: 7565–7581.

Langner, G., and Schreiner, C. E. (1988) Periodicity coding in the inferior colliculus of the cat I. Neuronal mechanisms. *J. Neurophysiol.* 60: 1799–1822.

Manis, P. B., and Marx, S. O. (1991) Outward currents in isolated ventral cochlear nucleus neurons. *J. Neurosci.* 11: 2865–2880.

Millan, M. H., Meldrum, B. S., and Faingold, C. L. (1986) Induction of audiogenic seizure susceptibility by focal infusion of excitant amino acid or bicuculline into the inferior colliculus of normal rats. *Exp. Neurol.* 91: 634–639.

Millan, M. H., Meldrum, B. S., Boersma, C. A., and Faingold, C. L. (1988) Excitant amino acids and audiogenic seizures in the genetically epilepsy-prone rat. II. Efferent seizure propagating pathway. *Exp. Neurol.* 99: 687–698.

Mittmann, D. H., and Wenstrup, J. J. (1995) Combination-sensitive neurons in the inferior colliculus. *Hear. Res.* 90: 185–191.

Mugnaini, E., and Oertel, W. H. (1985) An atlas of the distribution of GABAergic neurons in the rat CNS as revealed by GAD immunohistochemistry. In A. Björklund and T. Hökfelt, eds., *Handbook of Chemical Neuroanatomy*, vol. 4. *GABA and Neuropeptides in the CNS*, Part I. Amsterdam: Elsevier Neuroscience, pp. 436–553.

Nelson, P. G., and Erulkar, S. D. (1963) Synaptic mechanisms of excitation and inhibition in the central auditory pathway. *J. Neurophysiol.* 26: 908–923.

Oertel, D. (1983) Synaptic responses and electrical properties of cells in brain slices of the mouse anteroventral cochlear nucleus. *J. Neurosci.* 3: 2043–2053.

Oertel, D. (1985) Use of brain slices in the study of the auditory system: Spatial and temporal summation of synaptic inputs in the anteroventral cochlear nucleus of the mouse. *J. Acoust. Soc. Am.* 78: 328–333.

Oertel, D. (1991) The role of intrinsic neuronal properties in the encoding of auditory information in the cochlear nuclei. *Curr. Opin. Neurobiol.* 1: 221–228.

Oertel, D. (1999) The role of timing in the brainstem auditory nuclei of vertebrates. *Annu. Rev. Physiol.* 66: 497–519.

Park, T. J., and Pollak, G. D. (1994) Azimuthal receptive fields are shaped by GABAergic inhibition in the inferior colliculus of the mustache bat. *J. Neurophysiol.* 72: 1080–1102.

Peyret, D., Campistron, G., Geffard, M., and Aran, J.-M. (1987) Glycine immunoreactivity in the brainstem auditory and vestibular nuclei of the guinea pig. *Acta Otolaryngol. (Stockholm)* 104: 71–76.

Pinheiro, A. D., Wu, M., and Jen, P. H. (1991) Encoding repetition rate and duration in the inferior colliculus of the big brown bat, *Eptesicus fuscus. J. Comp. Physiol. A* 169: 69–85.

Portfors, C. V., and Wenstrup, J. J. (2001) Topographical distribution of delay-tuned responses in the mustached bat inferior colliculus. *Hear. Res.* 151: 95–105.

Simmons, J. A., Saillant, P. A., Ferragamo, M. J., Haresign, T., Dear, S. P., Fritz, J., and McMulllen, T. (1995) Auditory computations for biosonar target imaging in bats. In *Auditory Computation*, H. L. Hawkins, T. A. McMullen, A. N. Popper and R. R. Fay, eds. New York: Springer-Verlag, pp. 401–468.

Smith, P. H., and Rhode, W. S. (1987) Characterization of HRP-labeled globular bushy cells in the cat anteroventral cochlear nucleus. *J. Comp. Neurol.* 266: 360–375.

Trussell, L. O. (1997) Cellular mechanisms for preservation of timing in central auditory pathways. *Curr. Opin. Neurobiol.* 7: 487–492.

Trussell, L. O. (1999) Synaptic mechanisms for coding timing in auditory neurons. *Ann. Rev. Physiol.* 61: 477–496.

Vater, M., Habbicht, H., Kössl, M., and Grothe, B. (1992) The functional role of GABA and glycine in monaural and binaural processing in the inferior colliculus of horseshoe bats. *J. Comp. Physiol. A* 171: 541–553.

Zhou, X., and Jen, P. H. (2001) The effect of sound intensity on duration-tuning characteristics of bat inferior collicular neurons. *J. Comp. Physiol. A* 187: 63–73.

5 A Protocol for Reading the Mind

Howard Eichenbaum

A major overall goal of neuroscience is the development of prostheses that can interpret neural signals in a way that helps individuals with disorders accommodate their limitations of perception or action. This chapter considers the long-range goal of "reading the mind," or more specifically, the development of devices that may allow us to interpret the brain activity associated with conscious recollections and the formulation of explicit intentions. Imagine a situation where a patient has severe limitations in the capacity to express behavior overtly, while retaining perception, memory, and cognition—the condition of cerebral palsy is a particularly striking case. Wouldn't it be wonderful if we could develop a means for interpreting the patients' recollections and plans so that artificial speech and other robotic devices could express his memories and intentions? Such a development is not practical at present, but it is not too soon to begin thinking about the design requirements for a device that could perform this function.

In my view, we now have sufficient data on the anatomy and physiology of the brain to encourage optimism that such a device could be developed. Furthermore, the findings allow us to set the goals and identify the challenges that have to be met as we look forward to this sort of development. These data fall into three main domains, each of which addresses a major question about the relevant brain circuitry and operation. First, what is the brain system that mediates conscious recollection and explicit expression of intentions? Specifically, what brain structures are involved in these functions, how are they connected, and what are the individual roles of each structure involved? Second, what are the coding elements in these brain structures? Specifically, what kind of information is reflected in the firing patterns of individual neurons in each component of this functional system? Third, what do we know about the functional organization of the neural networks in these brain areas? That is, how do the neural elements act in concert beyond merely the sum of their independent information-coding properties? We now have preliminary answers to each of these questions. How these findings can be extended toward the development of a future "mind-reading" prosthetic device will be my final consideration in this chapter.

The System: A Brain Circuit for Conscious Recollection and Explicit Memory Expression

There are now considerable convergent data indicating that the brain system that mediates conscious recollection as well as the explicit expression of intentions is composed of widespread cortical areas acting in concert with the hippocampus and neighboring cortex of the medial temporal lobe. In particular, the hippocampal region has been identified as central to conscious recollection, and the prefrontal cortex as central to the higher-order cognitive functions associated with the development of intentions and plans. This section considers the brain system that encompasses the hippocampal region and prefrontal cortex, as well as other cortical areas, specifically with regard to their interactions in memory functions.

The Hippocampus and Conscious Recollection

Scoville and Milner's (1957) initial report of memory loss in humans following removal of the hippocampal region demonstrated that this area is dedicated to memory independently of other cognitive functions. Early observations suggested that the involvement of the hippocampal region was "global," that is, critical to the mediation of all kinds of memory. However, it has become clear that there are multiple memory systems in the brain, of which the hippocampal system is only one (Eichenbaum and Cohen, 2001).

As Cohen and Squire (1980) first recognized, the hippocampal region plays a selective role in declarative memory. Although the terminology used to characterize this kind of memory has varied, there is consensus on the phenomenology of declarative memory as being composed of our capacity for episodic and semantic memory and our ability for conscious recollection and "flexible" memory expression (Schacter and Tulving, 1994). By contrast, the hippocampal region is not required for the acquisition of a variety of skills and biases that can be expressed unconsciously through alterations in performance on a broad variety of tasks. These kinds of memory are instead mediated by pathways through the neostriatum, cerebellum, amygdala, and other brain areas.

Through the use of animal models, we are beginning to characterize the neural circuitry and information-processing mechanisms that mediate the capacity for conscious recollection. Recent studies have shown that the general pattern of memory deficits and spared capacities following damage to the hippocampal region in monkeys and rats parallels the phenomenology of amnesia in humans (for a full review, see Squire, 1992; Eichenbaum, 2000). Sensory, motor, motivational, and cognitive processes are intact following hippocampal damage, confirming that this region serves a selective role in memory in animals as it does in humans.

In addition, as in humans, the scope of memory that depends on the hippocampal region in animals is broad but selective to a particular type of memory processing. It is impossible to assess in animals some aspects of declarative memory, such as conscious recollection. Nevertheless, several studies have been successful in demonstrating a selective role for the hippocampal region in mediating other central features of declarative memory, including the linking of memories within a network of semantic knowledge and flexible, inferential expression of memories, as outlined later. By contrast, there is abundant evidence that other brain systems in animals mediate other types of learning (for reviews, see McDonald and White, 1993; Eichenbaum and Cohen, 2001). These findings validate the use of animal models to study memory and set the stage for a detailed neurobiological analysis aimed at identifying the relevant pathways and functional mechanisms of the declarative memory system that mediates conscious memory.

A Brain System for Conscious Recollection

The full system of brain structures that mediate conscious recollection is composed of three major components: cerebral cortical areas, the parahippocampal region, and the hippocampus itself (figure 5.1; Burwell et al., 1995; Suzuki, 1996), and the major pathways of the system are very similar in rats and monkeys. The cerebral cortical areas consist of diverse and widespread "association" regions that are both the

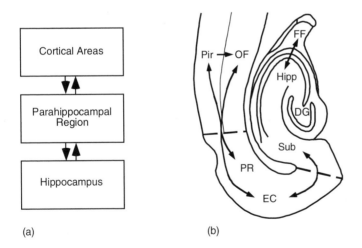

(a) (b)

Figure 5.1
The cortical-hippocampal system. (*A*) Flowchart of two-directional connections between the cortex and hippocampus. (*B*) Outline of a horizontal rat brain section illustrating the locations and flow of information between components of the hippocampus, parahippocampal region, and adjacent cortical areas. DG, dentate gyrus; EC, entorhinal cortex; FF, fimbria-fornix; Hipp, hippocampus proper; OF, orbitofrontal cortex; Pir, piriform cortex; PR, perirhinal cortex; Sub, subiculum.

source of information to the hippocampal region and the targets of hippocampal output. They project in different ways to the parahippocampal region, a set of interconnected cortical areas immediately surrounding the hippocampus that in turn project into the hippocampus itself. The main outputs of the hippocampus return to the parahippocampal region, which sends back projections broadly to the same cortical association areas that provided the inputs to the parahippocampal region. This pattern of anatomical organization complements the findings from studies of amnesia, leading to the working hypothesis that the parahippocampal region and hippocampus make their contributions to memory by altering the nature, persistence, and organization of memory representations within the cerebral cortex.

There is emerging evidence that neocortical association areas, the parahippocampal region, and the hippocampus play distinct and complementary roles in this memory system. The roles of these areas may be best contrasted in the results of studies on a simple recognition memory task, called delayed nonmatch-to-sample (DNMS), where subjects must remember a single stimulus across a variable memory delay.

The prefrontal cortex plays an especially important role in the acquisition and implementation of task rules. For example, in rats performing an odor-guided version of the DNMS task, damage to the orbitofrontal cortex resulted in a deficit in the acquisition of the task when the memory delay was minimal, suggesting an important role in perceptual processing or in learning the nonmatching rule (Otto and Eichenbaum, 1992; Ramus and Eichenbaum, 2000). Consistent with this conclusion, many other studies on humans, monkeys, and rats have led to a broad consensus that the prefrontal cortex performs a critical role in "working memory," the capacity to hold items and manipulate them in consciousness. The prefrontal cortex is parcellated into several distinct areas that have different inputs and whose functions can be dissociated according to different modalities of stimulus processing. However, they share common higher-order functions in working memory and strategic processing, which is reflected in perseveration and other common strategic disorders following damage to any of the subdivisions (Eichenbaum and Cohen, 2001; Miller, 2000; Fuster, 1995; Goldman-Rakic, 1996).

The parahippocampal region plays a different role. In contrast to the effects of prefrontal damage, rats with damage to the parahippocampal region acquired the DNMS task at the normal rate and performed well at brief memory delays. However, their memories declined abnormally rapidly when the memory delay was extended beyond a few seconds, indicating a selective role in maintaining a persistent memory of the sample stimulus (see also Young et al., 1997). Little if any deficit in nonspatial DNMS is observed following damage to the hippocampus or its connections via the fornix, indicating that the parahippocampal region itself mediates the persistence of memories for single items needed to perform the DNMS task.

Parallel results have been obtained in monkeys performing visually guided versions of the DNMS task. Similar to rats, monkeys with damage to the parahippocampal region perform well when the memory delay is brief. However, when the memory demand is increased by extending the delay period, severe deficits in DNMS are observed (Meunier et al., 1993; Zola-Morgan et al., 1989), and these impairments are much more severe than those following damage to the hippocampus (Murray and Mishkin, 1998) or its connections via the fornix (Gaffan, 1994a). The parahippocampal region may also play a role in the intersection of perception and memory, in situations where perceptual processes depend on learned associations among complex stimulus elements (Eichenbaum and Bunsey, 1995; Murray and Bussey, 1999).

The Role of the Hippocampus Itself
It is notable that memory mediated by the hippocampus itself contributes very little to performance in standard DNMS tasks, in that the deficits observed are modest at most compared with the effects of damage to the cortex or parahippocampal region. However, the hippocampus may play an essential role in other types of simple recognition memory tests (Zola et al., 2000; Rampon et al., 2000; see later discussion) and in recognition memory for configurations of items within scenes or places (Gaffan, 1994b; Wan et al., 1999; Cassaday and Rawlins, 1995).

Instead, the findings from studies using animal models point to a critical role for the hippocampus itself in central aspects of declarative memory. To understand this role, it is important to consider the fundamental properties of declarative memory, as introduced by Cohen and Squire (1980) and subsequently elaborated by many investigators. We acquire our declarative memories through everyday personal experiences, and in humans the ability to retain and recall these "episodic" memories is highly dependent on the hippocampus (Vargha-Khadem et al., 1997). But the full scope of hippocampal involvement also extends to semantic memory, the body of general knowledge about the world that is accrued by linking multiple experiences that share some of the same information (Squire and Zola, 1998). For example, we learned about our relatives via personal episodes of meeting and talking about family members, and then weaving this information into a body of knowledge constituting our family tree. Similarly, we learned about the geographies of our neighborhood and home town by taking trips through various areas and eventually interconnecting the information in cognitive maps.

In addition, declarative memory for both episodic and semantic information is special in that the contents of these memories are accessible through various routes. Most commonly in humans, declarative memory is expressed through conscious, effortful recollection. This means that one can access and express declarative memories to solve novel problems by making inferences from memory. Thus, even without ever explicitly studying your family tree and its history, you can infer indirect

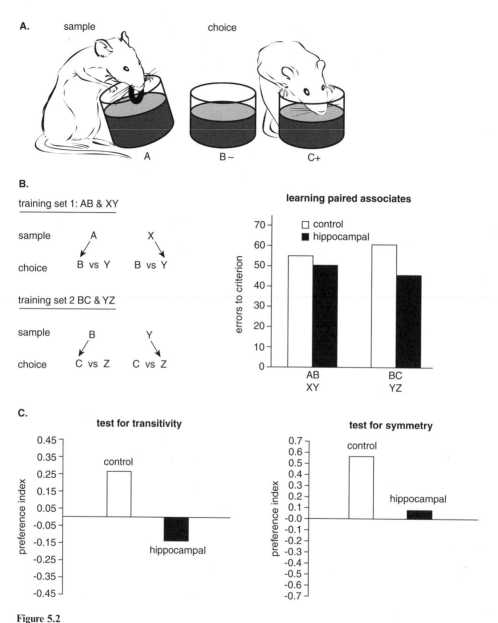

Figure 5.2
Paired associate learning and inferential expression of odor-odor associations. (*A*) Training on odor-odor paired associates. Each training trial consisted of two phases. In the sample phase, the subject was presented with a cup containing a scented mixture of sand and ground rat chow with a buried reward. In the subsequent choice phase, two scented choices were presented. Both choice items involved odors that were different from the sample odor, and which item was baited depended on the identity of the sample. (*B*) Paired associate training and performance in learning paired associates. *Left*: Rats are first trained on two overlapping sets of paired associates. Letters represent odor stimulus items; arrows indicate the correct

relationships, or the sequence of central events in the family history, from the set of episodic memories about your family. Similarly, without ever studying the map of your neighborhood, you can make navigational inferences from the synthesis of many episodic memories of previous routes taken. Family trees and city layouts are but two examples of the kind of "memory space" proposed for mediation by the hippocampal system (Eichenbaum et al., 1999). Within this view, a broad range of such networks can be created, with their central organizing principle the linkage of episodic memories by their common events and places, and a consequent capacity to move among related memories within the network.

These properties of declarative memory depend on the functions of the hippocampus itself. Several experiments have shown that the hippocampus is required in situations where multiple and distinct, but overlapping experiences must be combined into a larger representation that mediates expression of flexible, inferential memory. For example, in one experiment, rats initially learned a series of distinct but overlapping associations between odor stimuli (Bunsey and Eichenbaum, 1996; figure 5.2). On each trial one of two odors was initially presented, followed by a choice between two odors, one of which was baited as the assigned "associate" for a particular initial odor (A goes with B, not Y; X goes with Y, not B). Following training on two sets of overlapping odor-odor associations (A-B and X-Y, then B-C and Y-Z), subsequent probe tests were used to characterize the extent to which learned representations could be linked to support expression of inferential memory. The control rats learned paired associates rapidly and hippocampal damage did not affect the acquisition rate on either of the two training sets. The intact rats also showed that they could link the information from overlapping experiences and employ this information to make inferential judgments in two ways. First, normal rats showed strong transitivity across odor pairings that contained a shared item. For example, having learned that odor A goes with odor B, and B goes with C, they could infer that A goes with C. Second, control rats could infer symmetry in paired associate learning. For example, having learned that B goes with C, they could infer that C goes with B. By contrast, rats with selective hippocampal lesions were severely impaired, showing no evidence of transitivity or symmetry.

A similar characterization accounts for the common observation of deficits in spatial learning and memory following hippocampal damage. For example, in the

choice following each sample. *Right*: Performance on learning the two lists of paired associates. (*C*) Tests for inferential memory expression. For both tests a preference score was calculated as $(\alpha - \beta)/(\alpha + \beta)$, where α and β were the digging times in the appropriate and alternate choices, respectively. *Left*: In the test for transitivity, rats are presented with one of two sample cues from the first training set (A or X) and then required to select the appropriately matched choice cue from the second set (C or Z, respectively), based on the shared associates of these items. *Right*: In the test for symmetry or "reversibility" of the associations, rats are presented with one of two choice cues from the second set (C or Z) and required to select the appropriate sample cue from that set (B or Y, respectively).

Morris water maze test, rats or mice learn to escape submersion in a pool by swimming toward a platform located just underneath the surface. It is important to note that training in the conventional version of the task involves an intermixing of four different kinds of trial episodes that differ in the starting point of the swim. Under this condition, animals with hippocampal damage typically fail to acquire the task (Morris et al., 1982). However, if the demand for synthesizing a solution from four different types of episodes is eliminated by allowing the animal to repeatedly start from the same position, animals with hippocampal damage acquire the task almost as readily as normal rats and use the same distant spatial clues in identifying the escape site (Eichenbaum et al., 1990). Nevertheless, even when rats with hippocampal damage are successful in learning to locate the escape platform from a single start position, they are unable to use this information for expression of flexible, inferential memory. Thus, once trained to find the platform from a single start position, normal rats readily locate the platform from any of a set of novel start positions. However, under these same conditions, rats with hippocampal damage fail to readily locate the platform, often swimming endlessly and unsuccessfully in a highly familiar environment.

The view that has emerged from these and many other studies is that the hippocampus plays a central role in the creation of a broad range of memory networks, with their central organizing principle the linkage of episodic memories by their common events and places, and a consequent capacity to move among related memories within the network. The scope of such a network reaches to various domains relevant to the lives of animals, from knowledge about spatial relations among stimuli in an environment, to categorizations of foods, to learned organizations of odor or visual stimuli or social relationships.

The Elements: Memory-Coding Properties of Cortical and Hippocampal Neurons

Parallel electrophysiological studies that involve recording from single cells throughout this brain system have provided a preliminary understanding of the neural coding mechanisms that underlie different aspects of memory performance that contribute to conscious recollection and explicit expression of memory. In particular, many studies have focused on simple recognition tasks, such as delayed nonmatch-to-sample, which allow analysis of the neural firing patterns associated with perception, maintenance of memory representations, and cognitive judgments and actions based on memory. These studies have examined the firing patterns of neurons in several cortical areas, including the prefrontal cortex, inferotemporal cortex, and parahippocampal region, as well as the hippocampus.

In a variety of cortical areas, and in both monkeys and rats, three general responses have been observed (figure 5.2; Brown and Xiang, 1998; Desimone et al.,

1995; Fuster, 1995; Suzuki and Eichenbaum, 2000). First, many cells exhibited selective tuning to sample stimuli during the initial perception of the stimulus, indicating that these areas encode specific stimulus representations. Second, some cells continued firing in a stimulus-specific fashion during a memory period when the cue was no longer present, indicating the persistence of a representation of the sample. Third, many cells showed enhanced or suppressed responses to the familiar stimuli when they reappeared in the memory test phase of the task, indicating involvement in the match-nonmatch judgment.

All three types of representations have been found in prefrontal areas and in the parahippocampal region, suggesting that information about all aspects of the task is shared among these areas. However, it is likely that each area makes a distinct contribution to the performance of the task. For example, in rats we found that more cells in the orbitofrontal area exhibited stimulus-selective match enhancement or suppression, whereas more cells in the parahippocampal region exhibited sustained stimulus-specific activity during the delay (figure 5.3; Ramus and Eichenbaum, 2000; Young et al., 1997). In monkeys, a greater proportion of cells in the lateral prefrontal region showed sustained responses during the delay and conveyed more information about the match-nonmatch status of the test stimuli than the perirhinal cortex in a task where the memory delay was filled with interpolated material (Miller et al., 1996). By contrast, more neurons in the perirhinal cortex and inferotemporal cortex showed greater stimulus selectivity. Furthermore, in a recognition task where the memory delay was not filled with interpolated material, a large fraction of temporal neurons showed sustained stimulus-specific delay activity (Miyashita and

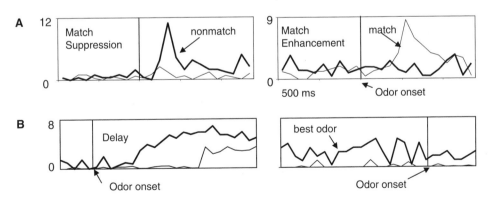

Figure 5.3
Examples of firing patterns of cells from animals performing the delayed nonmatch-to-sample (DNMS) task. (*A, left*) An orbitofrontal cell that fires robustly to an odor when it is a nonmatch and barely fires when it is a match. *Right*: An orbitofrontal cell that fires robustly when an odor is a match and barely fires when it is a nonmatch. (*B*) An entorhinal cell that fires selectively for one odor late in the odor-sampling period (left panel) and throughout the delay period (right panel).

Chang, 1988). In addition, neurons in perirhinal and inferotemporal cortex areas showed long-lasting decrements in responsiveness to highly familiar stimuli, which could provide signals about familiarity for extended periods (Brown et al., 1987; Miller et al., 1991).

It is difficult at this time to directly compare the data across species from studies that use different experimental strategies, focus on different components of the prefrontal and temporal cortices, and use different variants of recognition memory tests. However, the evidence is generally consistent with the notion that several neocortical and parahippocampal areas serve distinct functions in recognition memory. Neocortical areas play specific roles in the perceptual or cognitive processing required to perform the task, and are sufficient to mediate some aspects of working or short-term memory; these functions are localized in the processing by the prefrontal cortex. The parahippocampal region makes a different contribution. This region appears to be critical in extending the persistence of memory for single stimuli over brief periods in the absence of interference, and in maintaining information about stimulus familiarity for prolonged periods, even with interference.

Memory Coding in the Hippocampus

Neurons in the hippocampus also fire in response to a broad range of stimuli and events. Indeed, research on hippocampal neuronal firing patterns has generated considerable controversy with regard to the correct characterization of the functional coding properties of these neurons. However, recent observations from extracellular recordings in behaving animals suggest a reconciliation of various views, implying that hippocampal neuronal networks may represent sequences of events and places that compose episodic memories (Eichenbaum, 1993; Eichenbaum et al., 1999). The content of information encoded by the firing patterns of these neurons includes both specific conjunctions of events and places unique to particular experiences, and features that are common to overlapping experiences. Indeed, there is now evidence that the hippocampus creates separate and linked episodic-like representations even when the overt behaviors and places where they occur are the same, but the events are parts of distinct experiences.

Hippocampal principal cells exhibit firing patterns that are readily related to a broad range of events that occur during sequences of behavior in all tasks examined. For example, as rats perform spatial tasks where they are required to shuttle between a common starting location and one or more reward locations, hippocampal "place" cells fire during each moment as the animal traverses its path, with each neuron activated when the animal is in a particular place and moving toward the goal (figure 5.4A). A largely different set of cells fires similarly in sequence as the rat returns to the starting point, such that each cell can be characterized as an element of a network representing an outbound or inbound part of the episode (Gothard et al., 1996;

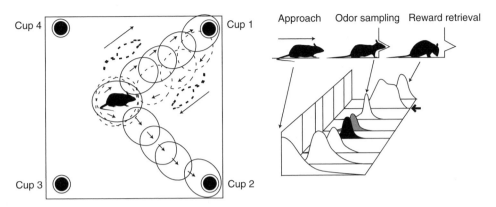

A. Spatial Working Memory

Cup 4

Cup 3

Cup 1

Cup 2

B. Odor Guided Memory

Approach   Odor sampling   Reward retrieval

Figure 5.4
Idealized neuronal firing patterns of an ensemble of hippocampal neurons. (*A*) Firing patterns of place cells from a rat performing a spatial working memory task in an open arena (from Wiener et al., 1989). The arrows indicate the directionality of each place cell. (*B*) Nonspatial firing patterns of cells from a rat performing an olfactory discrimination task (from Eichenbaum et al., 1987). Each panel illustrates the increased firing of a cell at a particular time during the trial. The filled and open curves indicate cells that fire only during the presentation of a particular odor configuration. The thick arrow at the right of one curve indicates a cell that encodes the sequence of odor sampling and the behavioral response.

McNaughton et al., 1983; Muller et al., 1994; Wiener et al., 1989). One can imagine the network activity as similar to a videoclip of each trial episode, with each cell capturing the information about where the rat is and what it is doing in each sequential "frame" of the clip.

Similarly, in both simple and complex learning tasks, hippocampal cells fire at virtually every moment associated with specific relevant events (e.g. Berger et al., 1976; Hampson et al., 1993). For example, in an experiment where rats performed an odor discrimination task, hippocampal cells fired during each sequential event, with different neurons firing during the approach to the odor stimuli, sampling of odors, execution of a behavioral response, and reward consumption (Wiener et al., 1989; figure 5.4B). Again, it is as if each hippocampal cell encodes one of the sequential trial events, with its activity reflecting both aspects of the ongoing behavior and the place where that behavior occurred. In all of these situations, some cells fire during common events or places that occur on every trial, whereas the firing of other cells is associated with events that occurred only during a particular type of episode, such as sampling a particular configuration of two odors presented on that trial.

In an extension of these studies, we were recently able to distinguish hippocampal neurons that encoded both specific combinations of events and places that were unique to particular experiences as well as particular features that were common

A. delayed non-match-to-sample task

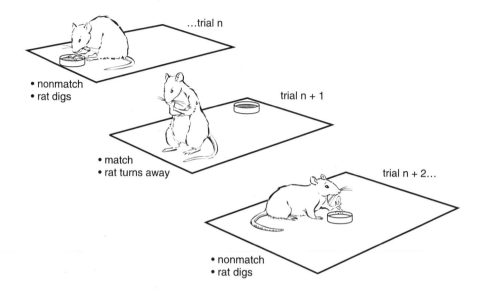

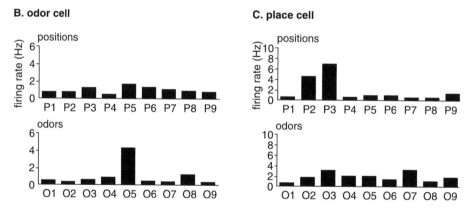

Figure 5.5
Firing patterns of hippocampal neurons associated with performance in the delayed nonmatch-to-sample task. (*A*) Illustration of trials in the continuous delayed nonmatch-to-sample task. On trial *n* the odor was different from that on the previous trial (a nonmatch), so the rat dug in the cup and found a reward. On trial *n* + 1, the odor was the same as on the previous trial (a match), so no reward was available and the rat appropriately turned away. On trial *n* + 2, the odor was a nonmatch, and the rat dug for and found the reward. (*B*) Analyses of the firing patterns of two hippocampal neurons in rats performing an odor-guided recognition memory task. The stimuli were nine different odors (O1–O9) and they appeared randomly at nine different positions (P1–P9). In addition, each odor could appear as a match or nonmatch with the odor on the previous trial.

across many related experiences (Wood et al., 1999). In this experiment, rats performed a variant of the DNMS task at several locations in an open field (figure 5.5). Again, different cells fired during each sequential trial event. Some cells were activated only by an almost unique event, for example, when the rat sniffed a particular odor at a particular place and it was a nonmatch with the odor presented on the previous trial. Other cells fired in response to features of the task that were common across many trials. Some cells fired as the rat approached the odor stimulus, or as it sniffed a particular odor, regardless of where the trial was performed, and other cells fired as the rat performed the trial at a particular location regardless of what odor was presented.

Finally, there is emerging evidence of coding for information specific to particular types of episodes, even in situations where the overt behavioral events and the locations in which they occur are identical for multiple types of experience. For example, as rats performed a spatial DNMS task, some hippocampal cells were activated when the rat pressed one of two levers only during the sample phase or only during the test phase of the task (Hampson et al., 1999). These cells can be characterized as elements encoding one temporally, spatially, and behaviorally defined event in the network representation of a particular trial type. The firing of other cells was associated with common events—a particular lever position regardless of trial phase, or during the sample or test phase regardless of location; these cells could be used to link the separate representations of different trial phases or episodes, and these codings were topographically segregated within the hippocampus.

More direct evidence of episodic-like coding was found in a recent preliminary study in which rats performed a spatial alternation task on a T-maze. Each trial began when the rat traversed the stem of the T and then selected either the left- or the right-choice arm (Wood et al., 2000). To alternate successfully, the rats were required to distinguish between their left-turn and right-turn experiences and to use their memory for the most recent previous experience to guide the current choice. Different hippocampal cells fired as the rats passed through the sequence of locations within the maze during each trial. Most important, the firing patterns of most cells depended on whether the rat was in the midst of a left- or right-turn episode, even when the rat was on the stem of the T and running similarly on both types of trials. Minor variations in the animal's speed, direction of movement, or position within areas on the stem did not account for the different firing patterns on left-turn and right-turn trials (figure 5.6). Also, most of these cells fired at least to some extent when the rat was at the same point in the stem on either trial type, proving that a degree of coding for the set of locations is shared between the two types of episodes. Thus, the hippocampus encoded both the left-turn and right-turn experiences using distinct representations, and included elements that could link them by their common features. In each of these experiments, the representations of event sequences, linked

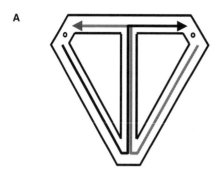

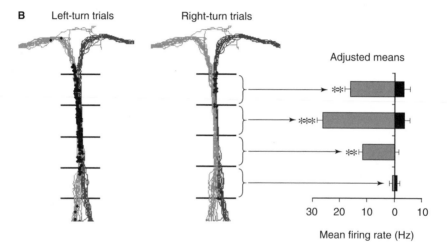

Figure 5.6
Firing patterns of hippocampal neurons associated with performance in the T-maze alternation task. (*A*)
The maze was composed of a T-shaped stem and choice arms, plus return arms that allowed the rat to return to the beginning of the stem on each trial. (*B*) Examples of a hippocampal cell that fired almost exclusively as the rat performed left-turn trials as it traversed the last sectors of the stem of the T-maze. The left
and middle panels show the paths taken by the animal for both types of trials. The location of the rat when
individual spikes occurred is indicated separately for left-turn trials (on the left panel), and right-turn trials
(middle panel). The far right panel shows the mean firing rate of the cell for each of four indicated sectors
of the stem, adjusted for variations in firing associated with the animal's speed, direction, and horizontal
location. **$p < 0.01$, ***$p < 0.001$.

by codings of their common events and places, could constitute the substrate of a network of episodic memories that could mediate performance on this kind of memory task.

The Network: Functional Organization of Cortical and Hippocampal Neural Networks

The foregoing review summarizes the brain structures and pathways that mediate conscious recollection and cognition of intentions, the distinct roles of different components of this system, and the coding properties of its neural elements. Additional information that will be critical to the development of a device that interprets neural activity in this system includes a consideration of the functional organization of the network properties. Efforts to understand network properties in brain structures are still in their infancy. Nevertheless, considerable information has been acquired about ensemble activity in cortical and hippocampal brain areas, much of which is covered in other chapters in this book. Here I will summarize a few aspects of network coding, particularly focusing on the issue of the organization of the neural networks in the cortex and hippocampus that mediate memory.

Considerable preliminary progress has been made in outlining the organization of coding by populations of cells in cortical areas, and there has been recent progress in the hippocampus as well. Cell populations in sensory and motor cortical areas involve a succession of sequential (as well as parallel) areas constituting a hierarchy of processing stages in which early encoded detail is combined (or filtered) in successive stages to achieve the identification of complex objects at the highest stages. In the earliest stage of cortical processing, the main principles for the population code are the specificity of single-cell responses characterized as feature detection or filtering, and topographical organization of these representations along multiple orthogonal dimensions. This scheme breaks down at higher stages of cortical processing where elemental features are not identifiable and topographic organization is lost. Instead, single-cell firing patterns reflect a coarse encoding of complex but meaningful objects or combinations of features, and the organization involves a "clustering" of cells with similar response properties (Tanaka, 1993; Perret et al., 1982).

Ultimately, the outputs of all the cortical modalities converge on the hippocampal region, where the response properties of the cell population are strikingly different. In the hippocampus, cellular activity can reflect quite complex conjunctions of multiple cues and actions, and specific or abstract relationships among them relevant to ongoing behavior. At the same time, hippocampal cellular responses change dramatically whenever the animal seems to perceive any change in the environment or task demands, and during different experiences associated with the same behaviors and places (see earlier discussion). Whether or not the functional characteristics of hippo-campal cells have a systematic organization is currently being investigated.

Early evidence suggested that hippocampal cells with similar response characteristics tend to "cluster" as they do in the afferent cortical areas (Eichenbaum et al., 1989). A recent study has extended this finding and has indicated a clear topographical organization that accommodates both distinct task demands and spatial features of the environment (Hampson et al., 1999). The activity of multiple neurons in a broad area of the hippocampus was monitored in rats performing a version of the delayed nonmatch-to-sample test using spatial cues. On each trial, the animal initially pressed a sample lever presented in one of two positions in a test chamber, then maintained the memory for several seconds, and then finally demonstrated the memory by choosing the alternative lever when both were presented in the nonmatch phase of the trial. The activity of some hippocampal neurons was associated with the position of the lever being pressed, regardless of whether this occurred during the sample or nonmatch trial phase. Conversely, other cells fired during the trial phase, independent of the lever position. Yet other cells fired when there were conjunctions of lever position and trial phase (e.g., left-match), or multiple events that composed a specific type of trial (e.g., right-sample then left-nonmatch). So, hippocampal neuronal activity represented both the relevant aspects of space and the relevant nonspatial features of the task, which is consistent with the mixture of spatial and nonspatial coding observed in other situations described earlier.

Moreover, by collapsing the data across several animals, Hampson et al. (1999) found a set of regular anatomical patterns. Lever position codings were segregated so that alternating longitudinal segments of the hippocampus contained clusters of "left" or "right" codings. Also, trial phase codings were segregated in alternating longitudinal clusters of "sample" and "nonmatch" responses. The two topographies were interleaved so that each lever position cluster contained clusters for both trial phases. Furthermore, the clusterings of lever position and trial phase specificity followed the known anatomical organization in which neurons are more closely interconnected within cross-sectional segments.

An additional finding provided by Hampson et al. (1999) offers a further clue that may relate the organization of these networks to their operation. Hippocampal neurons that encoded combinations of the lever position and trial phase were localized at the borders of appropriate codings for position and trial phase. Considering the "linking" role for the hippocampus outlined earlier, it is possible that these conjunctive cells represent events unique to particular types of trial episodes, whereas the lever position and trial phase cells encode events that are common to the representations of different episodes and therefore might serve to link them. A memory network based on these linked episodic codings could mediate the rat's ability to remember recent past trials based on present events. Of course, this is the critical memory demand in the task. The same kind of functional organization could mediate the linking of episodic memories, and access to them via present cues, across many domains of memory in humans as well as in animals.

The Future: How to Proceed in Developing a Device for Mind Reading

A major guiding theory for information-processing and memory in neural networks was proposed by Hebb in 1949. In his treatise on brain function and behavior, Hebb proposed the existence of "cell assemblies," groups of cells linked to subserve the representation of specific stimuli and behavioral events. He conceived of single cells as having unique coding properties, not as feature detectors, but more as distinct in their differential encoding of a variety of features of information. His proposals about higher-order behavior focused on two closely related properties. One property, widely known as the Hebb learning rule, is that coactivity strengthens existing synaptic connections between neurons.

The other property, following from the first, is that such coactivities and enhanced functional connectivities lead to networks, or assemblies, of cells that fire cooperatively in similar contexts. Thus, complex real-world stimuli come to activate a large assembly of cells whose coactivity constitutes the representation of that stimulus event. Within this framework, each cell can represent only small bits of the total information and fire maximally for a highly specific configuration of information. This property of sparse coding is complemented by the participation of large numbers of cells in any particular assembly. Each cell may represent many dimensions of information while it is coarsely tuned; that is, it contributes only a little accuracy to any one of them. At the same time, many such cells can participate in a variety of assemblies that involve the domain of information that particular cells encode.

In addition, Hebb suggested, once constructed, these assemblies have the ability to show persistent "reverberatory" activity even after the stimulus has turned off, and can reactivate the entire assembly when only part of the input is re-presented. These properties address all of the limitations of the single cell as a feature detector and satisfy the demands for representation of nearly infinite amounts of information. Hebb even speculated further on the possibility that overlapping cell assemblies could be the basis of insightful behavior, supporting logical inferences from only indirectly related experiences.

This review indicates that we can indeed describe superficial aspects of important biological neural networks, and these descriptions are generally consistent with Hebb's account of cell assemblies. In addition, the earlier characterization of a brain circuit that mediates conscious recollection also indicates that the details of the information contained in this system are distributed among systematically organized networks in widespread brain regions, each of which makes a distinct functional contribution. Therefore, future analyses of conscious recollection must include the simultaneous monitoring of activity in multiple brain areas.

This chapter provides some valid reasons for optimism when we can record a good sampling of brain cells in the functionally distinct components of this system. First, we are beginning to understand the contributions of the different parts of the system. Second, single neurons in each area contain specific information that the brain area contributes, and there is considerable sharing and coordination of information among all these areas. Third, there are guiding principles for the sampling of cells in these areas—they all use a kind of topography to segregate the relevant dimensions of information processing. Combining all of these observations, it seems reasonable to expect that simultaneous sampling of the topographic representation from each area can provide a basis for "mind reading" in this brain system.

References

Berger, T. W., Alger, B. E., and Thompson, R. F. (1976) Neuronal substrates of classical conditioning in the hippocampus. *Science* 192: 483–485.

Brown, M. W., and Xiang, J. Z. (1998) Recognition memory: Neuronal substrates of the judgement of prior occurrence. *Prog. Neurobiol.* 55: 1–67.

Brown, M. W., Wilson, F. A. W., and Riches, I. P. (1987) Neuronal evidence that inferomedial temporal cortex is more important than hippocampus in certain processes underlying recognition memory. *Brain Res.* 409: 158–162.

Bunsey, M., and Eichenbaum, H. (1996) Conservation of hippocampal memory function in rats and humans. *Nature* 379: 255–257.

Burwell, R. D., Witter, M. P., and Amaral, D. G. (1995) Perirhinal and postrhinal cortices in the rat: A review of the neuroanatomical literature and comparison with findings from the monkey brain. *Hippocampus* 5: 390–408.

Cassaday, H. J., and Rawlins, J. N. P. (1995) Fornix-fimbria section and working memory deficits in rats: Stimulus complexity and stimulus size. *Behav. Neurosci.* 109: 594–606.

Cohen, N. J., and Squire, L. R. (1980) Preserved learning and retention of a pattern-analyzing skill in amnesia: Dissociation of knowing how and knowing that. *Science* 210: 207–210.

Desimone, R., Miller, E. K., Chelazzi, L., and Lueschow, A. (1995) Multiple memory systems in the visual cortex. In M. S. Gazzaniga, ed., *The Cognitive Neurosciences.* Cambridge, Mass.: MIT Press, pp. 475–486.

Eichenbaum, H. (1993) Thinking about brain cell assemblies. *Science* 261: 993–994.

Eichenbaum, H. (2000) A cortical-hippocampal system for declarative memory. *Nat. Rev. Neurosci.* 1: 41–50.

Eichenbaum, H., and Bunsey, M. (1995) On the binding of associations in memory: Clues from studies on the role of the hippocampal region in paired-associate learning. *Curr. Dir. Psychol. Sci.* 4: 19–23.

Eichenbaum, H., and Cohen, N. J. (2001) *From Conditioning to Conscious Recollection: Memory Systems of the Brain.* New York: Oxford University Press.

Eichenbaum, H., Kuperstein, M., Fagan, A., and Nagode, J. (1987) Cue-sampling and goal-approach correlates of hippocampal unit-activity in rats performing an odor-discrimination task. *J. Neurosci.* 7: 716–732.

Eichenbaum, H., Wiener, S. I., Shapiro, M. L., and Cohen, N. J. (1989) The organization of spatial coding in the hippocampus—a study of neural ensemble activity. *J. Neurosci.* 9: 2764–2775.

Eichenbaum, H., Stewart, C., and Morris, R. G. M. (1990) Hippocampal representation in spatial learning. *J. Neurosci.* 10: 331–339.

Eichenbaum, H., Dudchenko, P., Wood, E., Shapiro, M., and Tanila, H. (1999) The hippocampus, memory, and place cells: Is it spatial memory or memory space? *Neuron* 23: 1–20.

Fuster, J. M. (1995) *Memory in the Cerebral Cortex: An Empirical Approach to Neural Networks in the Human and Nonhuman Primate.* Cambridge, Mass.: MIT Press.

Gaffan, D. (1994a) Dissociated effects of perirhinal cortex ablation, fornix transection and amygdalectomy: Evidence for multiple memory systems in the primate temporal lobe. *Exp. Brain Res.* 99: 411–422.

Gaffan, D. (1994b) Scene-specific memory for objects: A model of episodic memory impairment in monkeys with fornix transection. *J. Cognitive Neurosci.* 6: 305–320.

Goldman-Rakic, P. S. (1996) The prefrontal landscape: Implications of functional architecture for understanding human mentation and the central executive. *Phil. Trans. R. Soc. Lond. Ser. B* 351: 1445–1453.

Gothard, K. M., Skaggs, W. E., Moore, K. M., and McNaughton, B. L. (1996) Binding of hippocampal CA1 neural activity to multiple reference frames in a landmark-based navigation task. *J. Neurosci.* 16: 823–835.

Hampson, R. E., Heyser, C. J., and Deadwyler, S. A. (1993) Hippocampal cell firing correlates of delayed-match-to-sample performance in the rat. *Behav. Neurosci.* 107: 715–739.

Hampson, R. E., Byrd, D. R., Konstantopoulos, J. K., Bunn, T., and Deadwyler, S. A. (1996) Hippocampal place fields: Relationship between degree of field overlap and cross-correlations within ensembles of hippocampal neuroses. *Hippocampus* 6: 281–293.

Hampson, R. E., Simeral, J. D., and Deadwyler, S. A. (1999) Distribution of spatial and nonspatial information in dorsal hippocampus. *Nature* 402: 610–614.

Hebb, D. O. (1949) *The Organization of Behavior.* New York: Wiley.

McDonald, R. J., and White, N. M. (1993) A triple dissociation of memory systems: Hippocampus, amygdala, and dorsal striatum. *Behav. Neurosci.* 107: 3–22.

McNaughton, B. L., Barnes, C. A., and O'Keefe, J. (1983) The contributions of position, direction, and velocity to single unit activity in the hippocampus of freely-moving rats. *Exp. Brain Res.* 52: 41–49.

Meunier, M., Bachevalier, J., Mishkin, M., and Murray, E. A. (1993) Effects on visual recognition of combined and separate ablations of the entorhinal and perirhinal cortex in rhesus monkeys. *J. Neruosci.* 13: 5418–5432.

Miller, E. K. (2000) The prefrontal cortex and cognitive control. *Nature Rev. Neurosci.* 1: 59–65.

Miller, E. K., Li, L., and Desimone, R. (1991) A neural mechanism for working and recognition memory in inferior temporal cortex. *Science* 254: 1377–1379.

Miller, E. K., Erickson, C. A., and Desimone, R. (1996) Neural mechanisms of visual working memory in prefrontal cortex of the macaque. *J. Neurosci.* 16(16): 5154–5167.

Miyashita, Y., and Chang, H. S. (1988) Neuronal correlate of pictorial short-term memory in the primate temporal cortex. *Nature* 331: 68–70.

Morris, R. G. M., Garrud, P., Rawlins, J. P., and O'Keefe, J. (1982) Place navigation impaired in rats with hippocampal lesions. *Nature* 297: 681–683.

Muller, R. U., Bostock, E., Taube, J. S., and Kubie, J. L. (1994) On the directional firing properties of hippocampal place cells. *J. Neurosci.* 14: 7235–7251.

Murray, E. A., and Bussey, T. J. (1999) Perceptual-mnemonic functions of the perirhinal cortex. *Trends Cognitive Sci.* 3: 142–151.

Murray, E. A., and Mishkin, M. (1998) Object recognition and location memory in monkeys with excitotoxic lesions of the amygdala and hippocampus. *J. Neurosci.* 18(16): 6568–6582.

Otto, T., and Eichenbaum, H. (1992) Complementary roles of orbital prefrontal cortex and the perirhinal-entorhinal cortices in an odor-guided delayed non-matching-to-sample task. *Behav. Neurosci.* 106: 763–776.

Perrett, D. I., Rolls, E. T., and Caan, W. (1982) Visual neurones responsive to faces in the monkey temporal cortex. *Exp. Brain Res.* 47: 329–342.

Ramus, S. J., and Eichenbaum, H. (2000) Neural correlates of olfactory recognition memory in the rat orbitofrontal cortex. *J. Neurosci.* 20: 8199–8208.

Rampon, C., Tang, Y.-P., Goodhouse, J., Shimizu, E., Kyin, M., and Tsien, J. (2000) Enrichment induces structural changes and recovery from non-spatial memory deficits in CA1 NMDAR1-knockout mice. *Nature Neurosci.* 3: 238–244.

Schacter, D. L., and Tulving, E. (1994) What are the memory systems of 1994? In D. L. Schacter and E. Tulving, eds. *Memory Systems 1994*. Cambridge, Mass.: MIT Press, pp. 1–38.

Scoville, W. B., and Milner, B. (1957) Loss of recent memory after bilateral hippocampal lesions. *J. Neurol. Neurosurg. Psychiat.* 20: 11–21.

Squire, L. (1992) Memory and the hippocampus: A synthesis from findings with rats, monkeys, and humans. *Psychol. Rev.* 99(2): 195–231.

Squire, L. R., and Zola, S. M. (1998) Episodic memory, semantic memory and amnesia. *Hippocampus* 8: 205–211.

Suzuki, W. A. (1996) Neuroanatomy of the monkey entorhinal, perirhinal, and parahippocampal cortices: Organization of cortical inputs and interconnections with amygdala and striatum. *Seminars Neurosci.* 8: 3–12.

Suzuki, W., and Eichenbaum, H. (2000) The neurophysiology of memory. *Ann. N. Y. Acad. Sci.* 911: 175–191.

Tanaka, K. (1993) Neuronal mechanisms of object recognition. *Science* 262: 685–688.

Vargha-Khadem, F., Gadin, D. G., Watkins, K. E., Connelly, A., Van Paesschen, W., and Mishkin, M. (1997) Differential effects of early hippocampal pathology on episodic and semantic memory. *Science* 277: 376–380.

Wan, H., Aggleton, J. P., and Malcolm, W. B. (1999) Different contributions of the hippocampus and perirhinal cortex to recognition memory. *J. Neurosci.* 19: 1142–1148.

Wiener, S. I., Paul, C. A., and Eichenbaum, H. (1989) Spatial and behavioral correlates of hippocampal neuronal activity. *J. Neurosci.* 9: 2737–2763.

Wood, E., Dudchenko, P. A., and Eichenbaum, H. (1999) The global record of memory in hippocampal neuronal activity. *Nature* 397: 613–616.

Wood, E., Dudchenko, P., Robitsek, J. R., and Eichenbaum, H. (2000) Hippocampal neurons encode information about different types of memory episodes occurring in the same location. *Neuron* 27: 623–633.

Young, B. J., Otto, T., Fox, G. D., and Eichenbaum, H. (1997) Memory representation within the parahippocampal region. *J. Neurosci.* 17: 5183–5195.

Zola, S. M., Squire, L. R., Teng, E., Stefanacci, L., Buffalo, E. A., and Clark, R. E. (2000) Impaired recognition memory in monkeys after damage limited to the hippocampal region. *J. Neurosci.* 20: 451–463.

Zola-Morgan, S., Squire, L. R., Amaral, D. G., and Suzuki, W. (1989) Lesions of perirhinal and parahippocampal cortex that spare the amygdala and the hippocampal formation produce severe memory impairment. *J. Neurosci.* 9: 4355–4370.

6 Cognitive Processes in Replacement Brain Parts: A Code for All Reasons

Robert Hampson, John Simeral, and Sam A. Deadwyler

There are very few topics that are more provocative in modern neurobiology than the notion that the nervous system not only possesses enough plasticity to repair itself, but that when it cannot, such repair can be accomplished by replacing cells or structures with manmade devices. The theme of this book addresses the feasibility of replacement specifically with reference to the "substitution" of missing cells or even entire brain regions, with neural "components" manufactured and programmed according to specification. This contrasts with more traditional approaches to the recovery of neural function in that such repair is not effected by stimulating neurons to either regenerate or grow new connections (i.e., through administration of growth factors). Rather, this theme takes a more or less "mechanical" perspective, confronting the issue of whether a missing a cellular element in a neuronal circuit (i.e., one that cannot be reestablished neurally), can be replaced by a synthetic component.

Neural Function Is What Must Be Repaired

It is not by chance that neurons evolved the way they did; they were designed by nature to transmit information, and they accomplish this in a superb manner. What this entails in the simplest of circumstances is the neuron detecting a change on one part of its surface and then transmitting that information to another part. As an extension of this basic operation, a connection formed between two of these units would provide the means of transmitting the information over large distances, depending upon the number of units serially connected and the ability of each unit to regenerate the signal at each connection. From this basic premise we know that it is possible for neural systems not only to pass on information but also through these connections to perform elaborate computations. The possibility exists that we may never be capable of understanding some of these computational processes, which are performed at relatively high speeds and completely without our awareness. Perhaps the best we can hope for in this respect is to relate the information processed by these networks to a functional outcome, a movement, a visceral reaction, or a verbal report. The issue of replacing brain parts therefore is reduced to the challenge of making a device or devices that perform similar detectable or observable "functions" given that the same information is supplied.

Potential Approaches: Duplication versus Simulation

This mission can be addressed with different degrees of certitude, depending upon the system in which the neural components are to be replaced. "Repairing" a limb so that it can touch a keyboard or press a button may be somewhat easier than a repair to recover one's golf swing. Can recovery be effected by substitution with lots of the same types of devices (neurons) all of which perform similarly with respect to eventually generating a useful code, or must certain devices perform one type of computation and others different sets of operations on the same data?

In the case of moving a limb from point A to point B, it might be appropriate to build a device that simply duplicates the set of commands from the replacement "neurons" in the motor cortex to the motor neuron pool innervating the appropriate muscles for moving the arm. However, as the functions that the replacement neurons perform become more complex (i.e., initiating the pattern of impulses to the muscles during a golf swing), the number of interactions and units within the device (interneurons, higher-order connections, etc.) make straightforward "duplication" of biological neurons much less feasible as a means of repair.

A different approach would be to "simulate" the movements in a golf swing by using an algorithm that initiates this action in a way that is different from that of normal neural connections. This "prosthetic" device would solve the problem externally, bypassing the neural systems involved in the computations and substituting a real-time computer-based program to "drive" or activate the muscles in a particular pattern (cf. Chapin et al., 1999; Nicolelis, 2001). While this approach may be feasible in many applications that are indeed more complex than simply moving a limb, such as walking upstairs or getting into a wheelchair, it is still rather unlikely that in our example a person would ever "break a hundred" on the golf course using this approach.

Component Requirements: Size and Computational Power

The two approaches described above (duplication and prosthetics) lack appeal because it is clear that neither can restore the richness and fluidity of movement inherent in the original system. For that matter, is it reasonable, given our current state of knowledge, to expect a damaged neural system to be fully repaired? This outcome requires components that would simulate the function of damaged neurons in the circuit but would not require an external prosthetic "loop" to accomplish movement.

Could the capacity to transmit the necessary information to the various stages in the circuit be contained in a replacement component? In order for this to happen, two major problems must be solved. First, a device has to be built that can perform real-time computations within physical dimensions that allow implantation in the central nervous system (CNS). Second, the device must contain the appropriate code for translating information between the units that it replaces. In this chapter we discuss the second issue, namely, what codes might be required for replacement devices to work efficiently.

We have obtained some idea of these requirements from recordings of populations of neurons and assessing how information is "packaged" within these populations and how ensembles encode information during the performance of complex tasks that require moment-to-moment processing of information on a trial-by-trial basis. In the following sections we provide a list of computational rules we believe are critical for translating information between replacement components that interact with existing biological neurons. To accomplish this, it is reasonable that we explore methods of condensing the computational operations required by such units into a format that mimics the functional characteristics of the elements being replaced.

Ensemble versus Functional Codes: Are They Different?

It is obvious that the type of code that will have to be imbedded in a replaceable brain part that participates in cognitive processing will depend upon the role the damaged area played in transmitting information from one region to the next. At the individual neuron level, encoding of relevant events seems to be a feature of cortical neurons, while modulation of firing rate is more associated with encoding of sensory events and motor responses (Carpenter et al., 1999; Christensen, 2000; Furukawa, 2000; Singer, 2000; Freedman et al., 2001). The information encoded by neurons is a function of the divergence or convergence of their respective synaptic inputs (Miller, 2000), and the timing of those inputs, as in the mechanisms involved in synaptic enhancement (van Rossum et al., 2000).

Cortical neurons by definition receive inputs that have been heavily "filtered" with respect to other relays within their particular circuits. Thus encoding by cortical neurons may be different at each stage, even though the neurons are part of a common circuit. It is also possible that the codes that individual neurons carry may be "read" not only by the next set of neurons in the circuit, but may be a part of a larger, more complex code transmitted by many different neurons that encode only single "components" of an overall pattern (Bell and Sejnowski, 1997; Deadwyler and Hampson, 1995; Laubach et al., 1999). In this case, information is transmitted as a "population code" in which individual neuronal activity does not reflect the functional code within the total ensemble. This is true of even the simplest convergent networks, such as those that represent "face cells" in the visual system (Rolls, 2000) or ensembles that process "intention vectors" in the motor system (Schwartz, 1999; Georgopoulos, 1999). In each of these cases it is the *pattern* of activation that is critical to the representation of information.

Although it is not necessary that such encoding have emergent properties, it is necessary that the transferred pattern be precise enough to trigger the next set of neurons tuned to read that pattern. In other words, the code that is utilized within the population has to have a functional basis with respect to how it preserves information from its input as representative of the outside world. It is not difficult to understand, given the necessary degree of resolution, that the functional "links" between structures using such codes are often better achieved by population rather than single neural codes. In the case of cortical neurons, this is probably the only way to encode complex information relevant to cognitive processes.

Cognitive Neural Codes Are Dichotomies of Referent Information

Feasible encoding for replacement brain parts will require an extraction of features encoded at the neuronal as well as the population level. Codes can be extracted from single neurons only by analyses of individual spike trains, which requires detailed temporal characterization to determine whether increased or decreased rates are significant. A high degree of control over situational variables is necessary to "discover" the features that cause a change in firing rate. Codes can also be extracted from neural populations by statistical procedures that identify sources of variances in firing across neurons within a given set of circumstances. These sources need not be identified at the individual neuron level since a given component of the variance might reflect a pattern of firing that is only represented by several neurons firing simultaneously.

Once the sources of variance have been identified, the next step is to determine how the underlying neuronal population contributes to those variances. Since a particular component of variance can arise from several different underlying neuronal firing patterns (Deadwyler et al., 1996), finding the factors responsible may not be a trivial task. First, there will be at least some neurons that encode the input features to the ensemble, especially in cases where the identified source(s) reflect prominent dimensions of the stimulus or task (i.e., direction or location and time or phase differences). However, other components of the ensemble may reflect interactions between dimensions, such as the occurrence of a particular response at a particular time in a particular direction. Because there could be more than one way in which the population could encode such information, it is necessary to understand how individual neurons fire with respect to relevant dimensional features of the task.

The three-dimensional (3-D) ensemble histogram in figure 6.1 shows 24 neurons recorded from the rat dorsal hippocampus during performance of a delayed

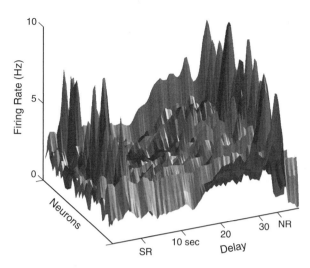

Figure 6.1
Ensemble of neurons recorded from the rat hippocampus during performance of a delayed–nonmatch-to-sample (DNMS) task (Deadwyler et al., 1996). The three-dimensional graph shows individual neurons (horizontal axis at left), versus time during a DNMS trial. The firing rate is depicted by vertical deflection. The mean firing over 100 trials is shown for 24 neurons. The phases of the DNMS trial are SR, response on the sample lever; NR, response on the nonmatch lever. The seconds indicate the delay interval after the sample response. Note the diversity in individual neuron responses at the DNMS events.

nonmatch-to-sample (DNMS) task (Deadwyler et al., 1996). Each neuron responds with an increased firing rate to different features or events within the trial. No single neuron is capable of encoding the total information in the task, nor does straightforward examination of the ensemble firing rate lead to derivation of the encoded information, since each neuron does not always fire during all trials. However, by combining statistical extraction methods applied to the total population of recorded neurons with categorization of individual cell types, the nature of the encoding process is gradually revealed. Figure 6.2 illustrates the extraction of the largest variance component, or discriminant function (DF1), which differentially represents the phase of the DNMS task. The 3-D histograms illustrate several neurons with either sample or nonmatch phase selectivity. The trials were divided according to whether the sample response was to the left (left trial) or right lever (right trial), but there was no distinction in phase responses of these neurons with respect to position. The raster diagram at the top right shows a single, nonmatch, cell with elevated firing only at the nonmatch response, irrespective of response position. This encoding of the DNMS phase by single neurons underlies the differential encoding of the task phase by the ensemble, as shown by the discriminant scores at the bottom right.

Further allocation of variance revealed a complementary set of neurons that encoded response position irrespective of DNMS phase. Figure 6.3 illustrates these

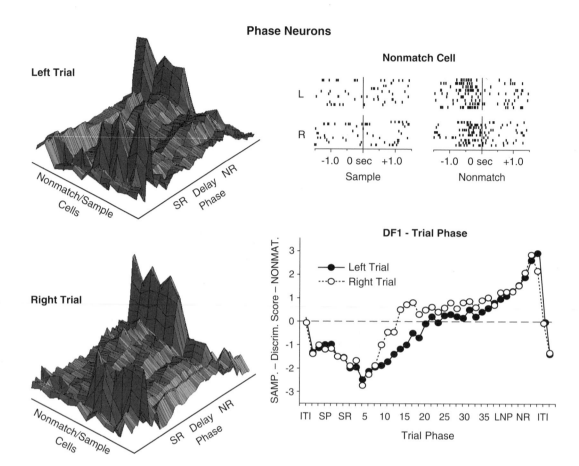

Figure 6.2
Derivation of the source of variance in a DNMS task phase. Ensembles of 10–16 neurons were recorded from the rat hippocampus and analyzed via canonical discriminant analysis (Deadwyler et al., 1996; Hampson et al., 1996). The greatest percent of variance (42%) was contributed by a discriminant function (DF1) that differentiated the sample from the nonmatch phase. The graph at the bottom right shows the maximum separation of discriminant scores for DF1 at the sample response (SR) and nonmatch response (NR) events, with scores near zero during intertrial interval (ITI), delay, and last nosepoke during the delay (LNP). There was no significant difference in firing at left (left trial) or right (right trial) lever positions. The three-dimensional histograms at the left depict the firing of 12 neurons, 6 sample (toward the lower right) and 6 nonmatch (toward the upper left). Note that the same neurons were active during sample or nonmatch phases on both trial types. The rastergrams (top right) show the activity of a single nonmatch cell. The trials are represented by rows, with each dot indicating a single action recorded potential. Firing is shown for ±1.5 s around sample and nonmatch responses on the left (L) and right (R) levers.

"position neurons" identified by the second discriminant function (DF2). Note that the same neurons were active during the sample phase of one trial, but also during phase of the other. Since the animals were required to "nonmatch," responses were necessarily at the position opposite to the sample; thus, "right position" cells would fire during the sample phase of a right trial, as well as during the nonmatch phase of a left trial. The single trial rasters at the top right show the firing of a single left position cell during both sample and nonmatch responses at the left, but not the right, position. The discriminant scores therefore also selectively reflected ensemble encoding of response position in the DNMS task.

Note that the variance sources contributing to this ensemble activity clearly encoded information consistent with the features or events of the DNMS task. This is not a necessary outcome of the discriminant analysis because there may be sources of variance encoding other sensory, attentional, or motivational features of the task. However, in each case, once a source of variance is identified, it should be possible to identify single neurons that contribute to that variance, and hence demonstrate the same encoding features. If there are variance components that cannot be accounted for by the identification of individual cell types responding during the task, it is likely that some encoded features of the task are "out of control," suggesting an element of the experiment that the animal responds or attends to that is not controlled by the intended task variables. The existence of such unexplained components can be a helpful indicator of the task-relevant firing correlates within a particular behavioral paradigm.

Deciphering the Code

When neurons interact, they inevitably form multiple contacts, making an analysis of functional characteristics of the network at the level of reconstructing individual synapses (weights) difficult, if not impossible. Another approach is to assume that the individual connections themselves are not important and let an artificial neural net "settle" into the state defined by the weights of the synaptic inputs that develop as the input patterns are fed into the net. The problem is that certain input patterns may predominate that are in fact irrelevant to information a prosthetic network is required to process. Therefore, it cannot be assumed that the network will process the information necessary to perform the task unless some preassessment is utilized to limit the manner in which information is to be dichotomized.

The identification of neurons that encode different features of a task which comprise a neural network is diagrammed in figure 6.4. Inputs to the network consist of the salient sensory features of the task, such as phase and position, as well as other features not yet determined. If the network is allowed to settle into a "winner-take-all" state, it is inevitable that outputs of the net would take that form of combi-

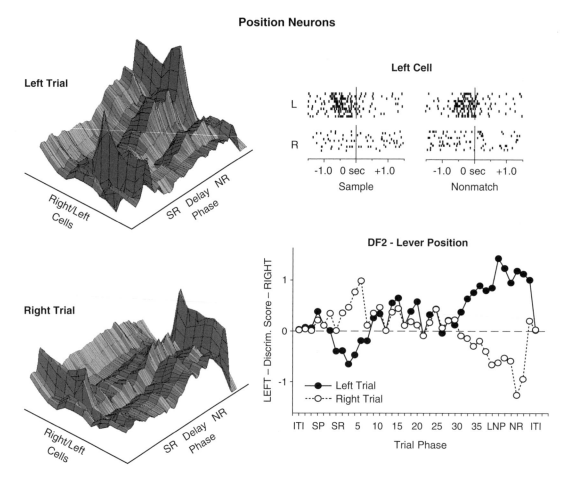

Figure 6.3
Derivation of source of variance in DNMS response position. The second largest source of variance (15%) discriminated the left from right response position. The discriminant scores at the bottom right indicate a positive score for right and a negative score for left sample responses; however, on the same trial, the scores reversed, since responses during the nonmatch phase were at the *opposite* position. The 3-D histograms at left show the same 12 neurons, 6 left (toward lower right on cell axis) and 6 right (toward upper right on cell axis) encoded reciprocally on left and right trials, irrespective of DNMS phase (see figure 2). The rastergrams indicate the firing of a single left position cell.

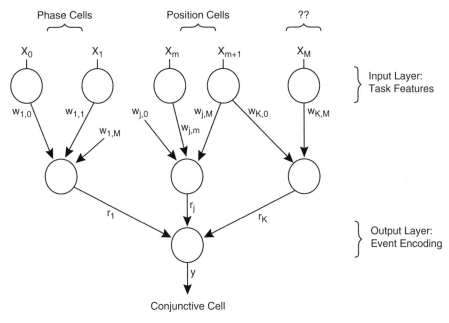

Figure 6.4
Example of neural network encoding DNMS task features. The network is diagrammed as a three-layer perceptron, with the phase and position encoding cells in the input layer. Additional unspecified task features can be input as indicated by "??." Not all neurons encoding task features would be active at a given time, since several features would be incompatible (e.g., a response cannot be left and right at the same time). However, a convergence of inputs onto hidden and output layers would produce neurons that selectively encode specific combinations or "conjunctions" of task features. For example, a convergence of sample and right features would produce a "conjunctive" neuron that encoded the specific right sample event of the DNMS task.

nations or "conjunctions" of these features. The more a network receives broad descriptive inputs, the more it is capable of encoding discrete behavioral events. Multiple parallel networks would allow for a whole population of neurons capable of encoding all relevant events within a given task or behavioral context. Figure 6.5 illustrates these "conjunctive" neurons recorded from the rat hippocampus as described earlier. Individual neurons were identified that encoded single DNMS events that were combinations of task phase and response position (e.g., left non-match as illustrated by the rastergrams at the right). Note that these neurons were not identified by one distinct source of variance, since conjunctive neurons are influenced equally by identified phase and position components. Thus conjunctive neurons most likely represent the operation of a network (figure 6.4), which generates event encoding within a population of neurons by extended processing of other features already encoded by the population.

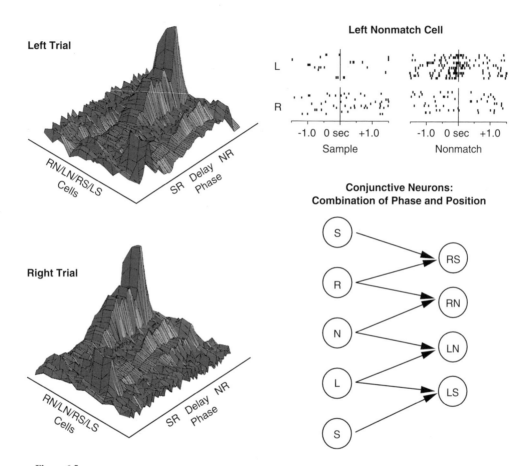

Figure 6.5

Conjunctive neurons recorded from the rat hippocampus. Neurons encoding discrete events were not identified by a separate source of variance, but contributed to the encoding derived by DF1 and DF2. The three-dimensional (3-D) histograms depict 12 neurons, 3 each of right nonmatch (RN), left nonmatch (LN), right sample (RS), and left sample (LS) plotted left to right on the cell axis. Note that none of the neurons fires in more than one trial or phase. The rastergrams show an example of a left nonmatch cell that does not fire on any sample or right position response. The schematic at the bottom right depicts how conjunctive firing can result from a convergence of inputs from phase (sample, S or nonmatch, N) and position (left, L and right, R) neurons.

The types of encoding by populations or neurons described here operate according to what can be considered relatively straightforward rules. In the hippocampus, many encoding schemes reflect the categorization of stimuli into representations of task-relevant features (Deadwyler and Hampson, 1995; Deadwyler et al., 1996; Hampson and Deadwyler, 2001). This can be verified by reclassification procedures that score the relevance of the encoding on a trial-by-trial basis (Deadwyler and Hampson, 1997; Hampson and Deadwyler, 1999). One important feature of this scheme is that the encoded task-dependent features are "incompatible" temporally and spatially. For instance, the more specific the code (i.e., firing that occurs only if there is a combined or conjunctive set of elements), the more likely that encoding will be incompatible with a different conjunctive code in another set of neurons.

An extension of the above are the "trial-type" neurons shown in figure 6.6. These neurons appear to combine the codes of two distinct types of conjunctive neurons to represent two associated behavioral responses. The codes are spatially incompatible, since the response obviously cannot be on the left and right levers at the same time. Hence the codes are also temporally incompatible (i.e., sample versus nonmatch phase). However, these combinations of events represent two compatible responses that can occur within a single DNMS trial. This code corresponds to a third source of variance that discriminated between the two possible trial types in the task. Thus, a left sample response is paired with a right nonmatch response (left trial), and a right sample response is paired with a left nonmatch response (right trial).

The presence of incompatible codes within a population provides a means of ensuring that only certain cells will be active at the appropriate times. Ensemble firing is unique in that firing across the ensemble is "sculpted" out in a spatiotemporal manner via sets of conjunctive elements tuned to particular combinations of task-relevant events. Therefore the ensemble, unlike individual neurons, must continually change its activity to reflect the change in cognitive or behavioral context, which can be done by continuously activating different sets of conjunctive neurons (figures 6.1 and 6.4).

This is illustrated in hippocampal neurons by the transition from "sample" to "nonmatch" phase firing during performance of the DNMS task in which the state of the ensemble completely changes (see figure 6.1). There are many ways in which this transition could take place, but in the hippocampus it occurs in a relatively straightforward manner. After the neurons that encode the sample event produce a peak discharge, they revert to background firing levels for approximately 5–10 s. Since hippocampal neurons are not firing during this time, they cannot "represent" information during that time of the trial. The code must therefore be present in some other brain region in a set of neurons that are active during this period. We have shown that the subiculum is a likely candidate (Hampson and Deadwyler, 2000). After 15 s on long-delay trials, firing resumes in the hippocampal ensemble,

Trial-Type Neurons

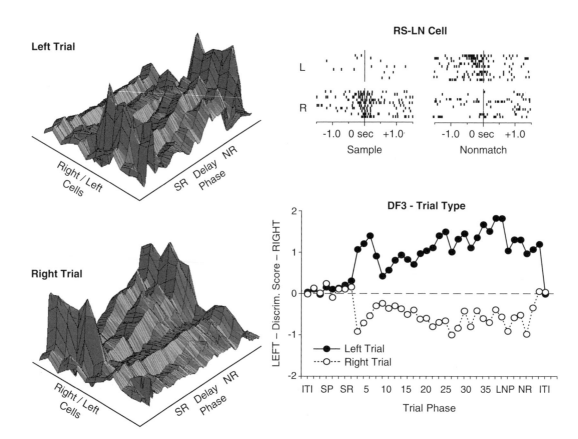

Figure 6.6
Variance associated with type of DNMS trial. The third largest source of variance (11%) was consistent across trials that were initiated with a given sample lever. Hence, discriminant scores (bottom right) remained positive on left trials, and negative on right trials. Specific hippocampal neurons were identified that encoded this discrimination, firing on both responses of right trials (right sample and left nonmatch) or left trials (left sample and right nonmatch). The 3-D histograms depict the same 12 neurons, 6 left trial (toward lower right on cell axis) and 6 right trial (toward upper left on cell axis) on left and right trials. Note that the same neurons are active in both sample and nonmatch phases, but only for a given trial type. The rastergrams (*top right*) show that firing for a given neuron is incompatible with respect to a single feature of the DNMS task (i.e., phase or position), but occurs at separate times. Trial-type neurons thus represent a further convergence of input from conjunctive neurons.

but in a completely different set of neurons. Firing in this set of neurons increases until the occurrence of the nonmatch response, at which point the nonmatch response is executed. Since this transition between sets of neurons within the ensemble occurs spontaneously, it could reflect a difference in input patterns to different cells, or triggering of a principal set of conjunctive cells within the ensemble by the initial sample phase firing.

Programming Replacement Brain Parts

Since functional neuronal codes are the essence of useful information to be programmed into replacement brain parts, replacement elements will have to provide the missing features of the population code. One approach would be to allow the replacement device to respond to the input pattern in a manner dictated by a neural network, with "synaptic weights" being determined by connectivity and input patterns (figure 6.7). However, in many brain regions the pattern of inputs will have already been "filtered" in some manner, and the dichotomy of information that the network parcels may not be appropriate for that stage of processing. The network diagrammed in figure 6.7 would be appropriate for simulating the phase, position, conjunctive, and trial-type neurons recorded in the hippocampus, as shown earlier. Allowing additional inputs to represent features not yet identified in the task would provide a measure of flexibility to the network. However, if the network or algorithm in effect at a particular processing stage is not tuned to extract the same rank order of firing variances as the original population, what is encoded from the same inputs may not be compatible as a useful behavioral correlate. It would therefore be valuable to know the categorization principles used by the population of neurons that are to be replaced (figure 6.7). Programming the replacement parts to derive those features would avoid problems associated with deriving inappropriate features by limiting computation to "functionally" relevant codes.

Clearly the types of categorization of neuronal firing (conjunctive neurons) are different within different structures. The approach described here has marked advantages for providing "customized" sets of networks for different brain regions by using statistical evaluations to determine which factors in specific neural populations are the most relevant. It is therefore possible to limit categorization within replacement devices to a smaller set of features than would be necessary if the population variances were not known. By tuning such replacement networks to recognize features extracted by statistical assessment of intact, i.e., remaining, populations, the important information categories would be maintained and recognized at the appropriate stages of processing.

This approach need not eliminate the ability of the replacement network to organize differentially (i.e., to change the categorization rules) when the input patterns

Neural Network for Trial Encoding

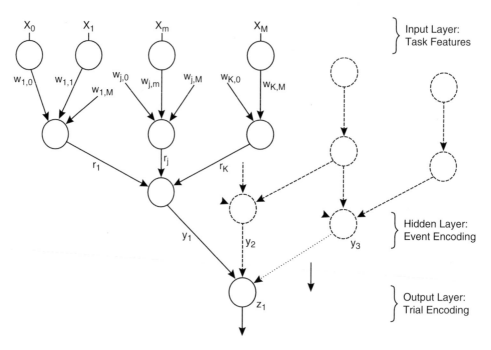

Figure 6.7
Schematic for a neural network that encodes DNMS trial information. The network is built from multiple parallel copies of the three-layer model shown in figure 6.4. Each copy of the smaller model produces a single conjunctive neuron. Multiple conjunctive neurons then project to a trial-type neuron. Note that only three parallel networks are shown although an actual network would most likely consist of thousands of input neurons (X_n) and hundreds of parallel sheets of event encoding neurons (Y_n), converging on a relatively sparse number of trial-encoding neurons (Z_n). A complex network is thus formed, with task features on the input layer, discrete task events encoded by hidden layers, and encoding of trials or complex task correlates on the output layer.

differ; it merely requires the network to represent features along dimensional lines and to ignore computed consequences that fall outside a given categorization framework. The latter facet is important because it retains the flexibility of the replacement network to alter its weighting of representations within the set of appropriate task dimensions. As an example, two major sources of variance within a population code for arm movement might be location and direction. For a given circumstance, moving the arm from location x to y defines a particular trajectory (i.e., for removing one's hat). Neurons in the motor cortex will encode this so that the peak firing within the population occurs as the arm is moved along this trajectory. However, if in another context the arm is to be moved in a different trajectory, the firing variances across the population may differ with respect to speed and directional firing, but the two categories to which the neurons respond (location and direction) will not differ. Thus the same population can compute trajectories within different contexts, but the circumstance of having the replacement network inadvertently encode an irrelevant feature (i.e., the type of hat that is taken off) is avoided.

What Do the Codes Mean?

The spatiotemporal patterns generated within ensembles across time would appear to incorporate all the necessary components of the code if there is a high correlation with behavior. However, this is not necessarily the case. Discriminant analyses such as principal components, independent components, or even canonical types will extract whatever sources of variance are present in the data, not necessarily those that are task related. This provides a good check on the appropriateness of the paradigm, but it also indicates to what degree a given code reflects task-relevant information. When there are sources of variance that are unaccounted for, it is likely that neurons within the ensemble are either categorizing the task-specific information in a different manner or are "dimensionalizing" the task in a different way.

In some cases information will be revealed in the discriminant analysis by the presence of components that are not obviously directly related to the behavioral outcomes. For instance, the presence of "trial-type" cells in the hippocampus (figure 6.5) reflects firing to one set of events in the sample phase (left-sample) and another set in the nonmatch phase (right-nonmatch). By definition these cells cannot represent or encode a single feature of the task within the trial since they fire equivalently to conjunctions of events. However, these same cells do not fire when the opposite trial type is present, even though the animal responds to the same levers as before, *but in a different sequence* (i.e., right sample-left nonmatch). This differential firing of neurons with respect to coded type of trial suggests an extended, hierarchical set of connections between conjunctive neurons to provide a level of code signifying a completely abstracted dimension.

The New Prosthetics

The advent of population recording has provided a means of establishing a new approach to the design of neural prostheses. Recent breakthroughs in this area by Chapin, Nicolelis, Schwartz, and others (Georgopoulos, 1994; Chapin et al., 1999; Nicolelis, 2001; Wessberg, 2000; Georgopoulos, 1999; Isaacs, 2000) have provided the first concrete examples of how population recording methods can have profound implications for rehabilitation of peripheral neural damage limbs and, potentially, other neural functions. The approach utilizes the ability to extract population codes for particular movements from the motor and sensory cortices that provide the basis for algorithms that can be applied to devices that mimic limb movements. It thus bypasses the necessity for the neuronal code to be translated into specific "instructions" to move individual muscles, while preserving the functional consequences of the movements in terms of intent and direction. Such algorithms derived from population firing code(s) are sufficiently explicit to allow incorporation into devices that operate in the real world, so that a person could initiate a movement by "thinking" it instead of having to initiate the action physically (Nicolelis, 2001). By successfully closing the "loop" between the outcome of the movement and the neural activity that generates it, the procedure provides a means of translating neural codes into actions.

The possibilities of these new and exciting findings for rehabilitation and neural prostheses are obvious; however, they also have significance in the context of replaceable brain parts. The codes that are utilized to generate algorithms for a particular action could also be used to "teach" or "train" replacement brain parts. For instance, an algorithm generated from the population code to move an object may also be used as a basis for training an implanted device to activate the muscles normally responsible for a particular movement. This essentially amounts to using one population code to train another population of artificial neurons. An encouraging outcome of the work in neural prosthetics as it relates to replacement brain parts is the discovery that relatively small number of recorded neurons are needed to construct successful algorithms. If the effective code can be extracted from as few as 24 simultaneously recorded neurons (Schwartz, 2000), it indicates that the task is being accomplished by the method cited earlier, namely, a broad categorization of neurons differentially "tuned" to fire to conjunctions of events.

The relatively small sample of neurons required to predict events with a high degree of accuracy suggests that the underlying means of partitioning information in such networks is through segregation into functional categories. This is supported by the fact that the most successful algorithms derived from population recordings perform a principal components analysis extraction as the first step in modeling the online process. The sources of variance in the population are therefore identified, and as a result the critical firing patterns of neurons for performing the task can be detected within the ensemble.

Summary

In summary, it can be stated that replacement brain parts need not mimic or process information in exactly the same manner as the original circuits. However, one thing is clear: Whatever their means of computation, the functional codes that are generated in those devices need to be compatible with the ensembles they represent are a component and with the behavior or cognitive processes they support. It is unlikely that replacement processes as discussed here will provide the same degree of flexibility or accuracy of the original networks. However, there is no reason to assume that algorithms developed to replicate the types of categorization of sensory and behavioral events present in the original population will not go much further than what is currently available to provide recovery of critical functions that are lost as a result of injury or disease.

Acknowledgment

This work was supported by DARPA National Institutes of Health grants DA03502 and DA00119 to S.A.D. and MH61397 to R.E.H. The authors thank Terence Bunn, Erica Jordan, Joanne Konstantopoulos, and John Simeral for technical support.

References

Bell, A. J., and Sejnowski, T. J. (1997) The "independent components" of natural scenes are edge filters. *Vision Res.* 37: 3327–3338.

Carpenter, A. F., Georgopoulos, A., and Pellizzer, G. (1999) Motor cortical encoding of serial order in a context-recall task. *Science* 283: 1752.

Chapin, J. K., Moxon, K. A., Markowitz, R. S., and Nicolelis, M. A. (1999) Real-time control of a robot arm using simultaneously recorded neurons in the motor cortex. *Nature Neurosci.* 2: 664–670.

Christensen, T. A. (2000) Multi-unit recordings reveal context-dependent modulation of synchrony in odor-specific neural ensembles. *Nature Neurosci.* 3: 927–931.

Deadwyler, S. A., and Hampson, R. E. (1995) Ensemble activity and behavior: What's the code? *Science* 270: 1316–1318.

Deadwyler, S. A., and Hampson, R. E. (1997) The significance of neural ensemble codes during behavior and cognition. In W. M. Cowan, E. M. Shooter, C. F. Stevens, and R. F. Thompson, eds. *Annual Review of Neuroscience*, vol. 20. Palo Alto, Calif.: Annual Reviews, pp. 217–244.

Deadwyler, S. A., Bunn, T., and Hampson, R. E. (1996) Hippocampal ensemble activity during spatial delayed-nonmatch-to-sample performance in rats. *J. Neurosci.* 16: 354–372.

Freedman, D. J., Riesenhuber, M., Poggio, T., and Miller, E. K. (2001) Categorical representation of visual stimuli in the primate prefrontal cortex. *Science* 291: 312–316.

Furukawa, S. (2000) Coding of sound-source location by ensembles of cortical neurons. *J. Neurosci.* 20: 1216–1228.

Georgopoulos, A. P. (1994) Population activity in the control of movement. *Int. Rev. Neurobiol.* 37: 103–119; discussion.

Georgopoulos, A. P. (1999) Neural coding of finger and wrist movements. *J. Comput. Neurosci.* 6: 279–288.

Hampson, R. E., and Deadwyler, S. A. (1999) Strength of hippocampal ensemble encoding predicts behavioral success in rats performing a delayed-nonmatch-to-sample task. *Soc. Neurosci. Abstr.* 25: 1385.

Hampson, R. E., and Deadwyler, S. A. (2000) Differential information processing by hippocampal and subicular neurons. In M. P. Witter, ed., *The Parahippocampal Region: Special Supplement to the Annals of the New York Academy of Sciences.* New York: New York Academy of Sciences.

Hampson, R. E., and Deadwyler, S. A. (2001) What ensemble recordings reveal about functional hippocampal cell encoding. In M. A. L. Nicolelis, ed., *Population Coding of Neural Activity: Progress in Brain Research.* 130: 345–357.

Isaacs, R. E. (2000) Work toward real-time control of a cortical neural prothesis. *IEEE Trans. Rehabil. Eng.* 8: 196–198.

Laubach, M., Shuler, M., and Nicolelis, M. A. (1999) Independent component analyses for quantifying neuronal ensemble interactions. *J. Neurosci. Meth.* 94: 141–154.

Miller, E. K. (2000) The prefrontal cortex and cognitive control. *Nat. Rev. Neurosci.* 1: 59–65.

Nicolelis, M. A. (2001) Actions from thoughts. *Nature* 409 Suppl: 403–407.

Rolls, E. T. (2000) Functions of the primate temporal lobe cortical visual areas in invariant visual object and face recognition. *Neuron* 27: 205–218.

Schwartz, A. B. (1999) Motor cortical activity during drawing movements: Population representation during lemniscate tracing. *J. Neurophysiol.* 82: 2705–2718.

Schwartz, A. B. (2000) Arm trajectory and representation of movement processing in motor cortical activity. *Eur. J. Neurosci.* 12: 1851–1856.

Singer, W. (2000) Why use more than one electrode at a time? In *New Technologies for the Life Sciences— A Trends Guide*. Amsterdam: Elsevier, pp. 12–17.

van Rossum, M. C. W., Bi, G. Q., and Turrigiano, G. G. (2000) Stable Hebbian learning from spike timing-dependent plasticity. *J. Neurosci.* 20: 8812–8821.

Wessberg, J. (2000) Real-time prediction of hand trajectory by ensembles of cortical neurons in primates. *Nature* 408: 361–365.

7 Mathematical Modeling as a Basic Tool for Neuromimetic Circuits

Gilbert A. Chauvet, P. Chauvet, and Theodore W. Berger

A Mathematical Approach versus an Analogical or Computational Approach

The analysis of the nervous system, or any part of it, as an integrated system requires a mathematical formalization that itself calls for an appropriate representation. This raises two basic questions: First, why do we need a mathematical formalization? Second, what kind of representation should we use and which techniques are best adapted for the integrated solution of the problem posed? Finally, in the case of neuromimetic circuits, would it be better to use an analogical, that is, a computational method, or a mathematical method?

In addition to the rigorous nature of mathematics, based on definitions commonly accepted by all members of the scientific community, the power of the derived propositions, and quantitative physical laws, a mathematical model incorporates relationships among state variables, which are the observables describing the elementary mechanisms of a system. Each of these mechanisms is mathematically described as a set of differential or algebraic equations, and the mathematical integration of these sets will provide the global solution of the observed phenomenon resulting from the mechanisms. Mathematical modeling thus has two advantages. First, it simplifies the behavior of a system that is experimentally observed over time and space. Second, it numerically reveals the consequences of some constraints that are difficult to observe experimentally, for example, the removal of couplings between subsystems.

Mathematical modeling corresponds to a certain reality; that is, the complicated integration of known mechanisms with physical, chemical, or other constraints (Koch and Laurent, 1999). Equations show how the mechanisms operate in time and space, and, what is crucial in this approach, a mathematical development based on these mechanisms leads to nonobvious, specific natural laws. As will be shown in the following sections, "emerging" laws may appear in an appropriate representation, which in the present case corresponds to a hierarchical representation. Because of the generally complicated mathematical treatment required by complex equations, the final step will be the numerical resolution of these equations on a computer. We may observe that this resolution, based on the rigorous methods of numerical analysis, occurs only in the terminal phase of the modeling process. This approach is rather different from the computational approach, in which the numerical resolution is made a priori by considering "analogical" neurons generally represented by resistive-inductive-capacitive (RLC) circuits (Bower and Beeman, 1995). In the best case, these neurons correspond to a preliminary discretization of space. If each neuron is an elementary circuit, then discretization is done at each point in space where a given neuron exists. In contrast, with mathematical modeling, the resolution of equations is carried out in a continuous space, and discretization does not depend on the position of neurons, only on the mathematical constraints of resolution. In simple cases, the two techniques may give the same results. However, as we will see, with more complicated models, only the mathematical approach is appropriate.

Indeed, mathematical modeling does more than establish relationships between observables. In a correctly adapted representation, not only simplifications, but also a certain type of organization, a functional order, may appear. Let us consider an example. Determining the space, that is, the eigenvectors, in which a matrix is transformed into a diagonal matrix (in which only the diagonal numbers, the eigenvalues, are not null) puts the response of the system in a direct relationship to the input. By using this mathematical transformation, the state variables are kept distinct. There is a decoupling in the subsystems, each of them being represented by a single state variable. Similarly, when the matrix is reduced to diagonal blocks, several state variables describe the subsystem. Their number corresponds to the size of the submatrix. As we see in this simple case, the new representation has led to new properties for the couplings between subsystems. More generally, with this type of representation we may obtain a new interpretation and discover new properties specific to the phenomenon observed. Of course, the objective is to obtain the correct and appropriate representation that will lead to interesting new, coherent, "emerging" laws for the working of the system.

We have chosen hierarchical structural and functional representations, which provide new laws for the functional organization of biological systems. In this chapter we propose to present a "light" version of this theory by means of the basic concepts and some elements of the formalism. Because the formulation calls for complex mathematical techniques, the equations have been grouped in appendices. Here, the interested reader will find part of the mathematical reasoning behind the theory. Two kinds of neural networks, artificial and real, will be presented first, followed by the theoretical framework. The method will then be applied to the cerebellum and the hippocampus. In the concluding section, we discuss the technique appropriate for neuromimetic circuits.

What Is an Artificial Neural Network?

The field of artificial neural networks has been extensively developed in the past few years. Each artificial neuron is a mathematical entity possessing two properties: (1) the output Y is the sum of the inputs X_i, weighted by the synaptic efficacies μ_i; and (2) the variation of the synaptic efficacy is proportional to the input signal X_i and the output signal Y. In the case of a network of n neurons connected to a given neuron, these properties are mathematically represented by a nonlinear dynamic system:

$$Y = F\left[\sum_{i=1}^{n} \mu_i X_i\right]$$

$$\frac{d\mu_i}{dt} = \alpha_i X_i Y, \quad i = 1, \ldots, n,$$

(7.1)

where F is a nonlinear, given, bounded function. The second equation of this system is known as the learning rule of the neural network.

With a given connectivity between neurons, the problem is to determine the mathematical properties of the network related to the learning and memorization of patterns. In fact, several characteristics of neural networks play an important role in learning and memorization: the number of neural layers in the network, particularly the inner or "hidden" layers, the number of neurons per layer, and the learning rule. Since the construction of the "perceptron" by Rosenblatt in the 1950s, various other neural networks have been developed, such as Hopfield's supervised network (Hopfield, 1982) with its internal dynamics, and Kohonen's nonsupervised, self-organizing network with its feedback and feedforward loops (Kohonen, 1978). All these networks possess specific mathematical properties that unfortunately do not correspond to biological reality.

Another difficulty arises from the nonlinearity of the mathematical systems and the impossibility of finding an analytical solution for a dynamic system involving synaptic weighting. The true complexity of the problem will be readily appreciated when we consider that the artificial neuron and its corresponding network are extremely simple compared with the real neuron surrounded by nervous tissue.

What Is a Real Neural Network?

From the biological point of view, the complexity of the phenomena involved is essentially the same whether we consider a real, isolated neuron or a network of artificial neurons. This idea stimulated the search for a representation incorporating the properties of a real neural network (G. A. Chauvet, 1993a). Over the past few years, much headway has been made in the mathematical description of a real biological system. The hierarchical organization of biological structural units from the cellular to the organismal levels (cell organelles, nuclei, neurons, synapses, neural groups, nervous tissue, and cerebral organs), naturally suggested a hierarchical representation of a system. However, the hierarchical aspect of the corresponding functional organization is far from evident. The novel three-dimensional representation of a biological system that one of us has proposed (G. A. Chauvet, 1996a), with axes for space scales, time scales, and structural units, allows visualization of the coupling between the structural and functional organizations. This representation is based essentially on the determination of the time scales of the dynamic systems describing physiological functions. This functional hierarchy is useful for determining the physiological functions associated with nervous structures. In the case of real neural networks, there are at least two physiological functions: the propagation of membrane potential on a time scale on the order of milliseconds, and the modification of synaptic efficacy on a time scale on the order of seconds or even hours. Thus, the functional order has its origin in a functional hierarchy that is evidently a manifestation of molecular mechanisms.

Typically, the artificial neural networks generally studied have several neuron layers. Figure 7.1 shows a hierarchical neural network. The structure-function relationship is more evident in this representation than in any other one. The hierarchical network is fundamentally different and, in particular, possesses specific emergent properties, that is, properties that appear at a higher level in a new structure. An im-

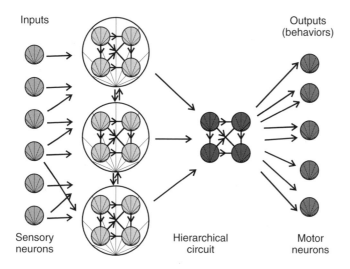

Figure 7.1
Hierarchical neural network. Properties emerge from a lower level and appear at a higher level inside a new structure. This new structure is called a functional unit if, and only if, it has a specific function.

portant advantage of the hierarchical representation is that it offers a rigorous approach to the notion of a functional unit that may now be defined as a structural unit with a specific function at a higher level of organization (G. A. Chauvet and Chauvet, 1999).

The functional unit, possessing its own time scale, incorporates a new function that can be derived mathematically from the lower levels of organization in a biological system. For example, a neuromimetic circuit may be considered as a functional unit.

Hierarchical Representation of a Biological Theory of Functional Organization

Functional Interactions

In the course of our work on physiological models, ranging from the molecular to the organismal levels (G. A. Chauvet, 1996b), some novel ideas specific to the study of biology have been introduced, in particular the concepts of nonsymmetric and nonlocal functional interactions in hierarchical space. These basic concepts emerged from a bottom-up approach to living systems; that is, from a systematic study of isolated physiological functions, followed by the integration of these functions at the level of the organism. A significant consequence of this theory is that living organisms can be given not only a double organizational representation that is simultaneously structural and functional but also a double mathematical representation that is simultaneously geometric and topological.

What exactly is a physiological function? We may compare it to a mathematical function in the sense that the action of one structure on another results in a certain product. The physiological function would then be the action (the application, in mathematical terms) and the product would be the result of the function (the value of the function, in mathematical terms) that is often identified with the physiological function itself. Although this definition is general, it is unfortunately not operational. It is relatively easy to describe particular physiological functions such as vision, digestion, memorization, and so on, but it is far more difficult to give an operational definition of a physiological function in general. One possibility may be to define a physiological function in terms of a combinatorial set of functional interactions between structures. Such functional interactions are evidently specific since they describe the action (whatever its nature) of one structure on another or, more precisely, the action of a source on a sink, after the action has undergone a transformation in the source. This action clearly possesses the property of nonsymmetry. In addition, it has another important property, that of nonlocality, a notion somewhat more difficult to appreciate since it stems from the structural hierarchy of the system (G. A. Chauvet, 1993c); that is, certain structures are included in others.

This may be explained as follows: (1) From a mathematical point of view, in a continuous representation, the action of one structure on another is necessarily the action of one point on another. This does not correspond to the action of one cell on another in physical space since a cell contains regions with specialized functions and therefore cannot be reduced to a point. (2) The interaction between one structure and another has to operate across other structures, which we have called structural discontinuities, within which the processes follow a different course. Thus, other levels of organisation in the hierarchical system contribute to the working of a given structure at a given level in the hierarchy. This is nonlocality, which is due to the choice of the representation, here a hierarchical representation. Equations that represent processes have then a different structure and must include nonlocal terms.

The same reasoning applies to the dynamic processes of functional interactions operating, for example, between neural groups or between endocrine glands. In more general terms, this can be extended to the entire activity of the organism, provided that all the functional interactions involved are correctly represented. We may then formulate a hierarchical theory of functional organization as follows: In a multiple-level hierarchical system, each functional interaction is described by the transport of an activating and/or inhibiting signal (in the form of an action potential, a hormone, or some other type of interaction) between a source and a sink, and each physiological function results from a combination of such interactions. This idea can be conveniently expressed in terms of a field theory according to which an operator transmits an interaction at a certain rate from a source to a sink situated in the space of units, with the source and the sink each being reduced to a point. This representation constitutes the basis for the definition of a physiological function as the overall behavior of a group of structural units within a hierarchical system.

From a mathematical point of view, a functional interaction is defined as the interaction between two of the p structural units u_i and u_j $(i, j = 1, p)$ of a formal biological system (FBS). One of the units, for example, the source u_i, emits a signal that acts on the other, the sink u_j, which in turn emits a substance after an eventual transformation (figure 7.2). This interaction, called an elementary function, is represented by ψ_{ij} and constitutes an element of the mathematical graph representing the organization of the formal biological system (O-FBS). The dynamics of the functional interactions are then described by a system of equations of the type:

$$\dot{\psi}_{ij} = f_{ij}(\psi_{12}, \psi_{13}, \ldots; \rho_1, \rho_2, \ldots), \quad i, j = 1, \ldots, p, \tag{7.2}$$

where the ρs are specific physical or geometric parameters.

The structural unit is defined as the set of anatomical or physical elements intervening in the physiological function.

Thus, from a functional point of view, a system made up of a set of elements, such as molecules, cellular organelles, cells, tissues, and organs, is represented by functional interactions and structural units. This structural hierarchy is shown in figure 7.3.

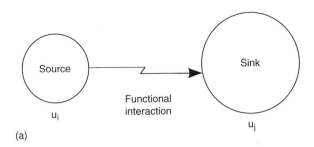

(a)

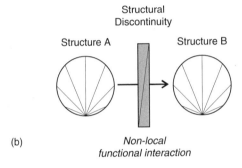

(b)

Figure 7.2
(*a*) Nonsymmetric functional interaction. (*b*) The interaction between structures A and B occurs through a structural discontinuity at a lower level (after G. A. Chauvet, 1996a, vol. II, p. 452).

Structural Discontinuities Functional interactions may be identified by the presence of structural discontinuities. Suppose we have two structural units separated by a structural discontinuity. The interaction is propagated from one unit to the other across the discontinuity, which could, for example, be a membrane allowing active transport. The membrane is at a lower level in the structural hierarchy than the two interacting units. From the point of view of the dynamics of the functional interaction, we may say that this interaction consists of a certain physiological process operating in the two units [located at r' and r in the space of units, that is, the r-space, referred to as $r'(x', y', z')$ and $r(x, y, z)$ in the physical three-dimensional space], with a different physiological process being executed at a lower level in the structural discontinuity. Such a functional interaction may be represented in the form of a diagram, as shown in figure 7.4. The equation governing the transport of the interaction applies to a continuous medium and explains why the equation for the process is different at the lower level of organization. This observation constitutes the basis of a new formalism (G. A. Chauvet, 1999, 2002) involving what we have called structural propagators (S-propagators) as described later (see also appendix A).

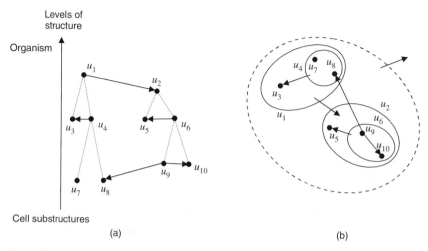

Figure 7.3
Each hierarchical level is composed of structural units on the same space scale. The hierarchical system is viewed (*a*) as an arborescence and (*b*) as a set of inclusions. Functional interactions are directed from sources to sinks.

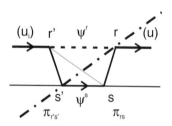

Figure 7.4
A diagrammatic representation of the propagation of a functional interaction through a structural discontinuity (1) at the higher level l (r-level) in the unit u_i [volume (V_i) of figure 7.5], (2) then according to a new functional interaction ψ^s at the lower level l-1 (s-level) inside the structural discontinuity, and (3) at the higher level l (r-level) in the unit u (volume V).

A Three-Dimensional Representation of a Biological System

A physiological function may be represented by a mathematical graph in which the nodes correspond to the structural units and the edges correspond to the oriented, nonsymmetric interactions. All physiological functions are intricately linked in a hierarchical fashion. They are linked relatively to space, which is evident, but also to time, which represents the decoupling of physiological functions with respect to time. Probably the best way to realize this aspect of the hierarchy is to consider the intricate time loops of the algorithm that represents the working of the function. We

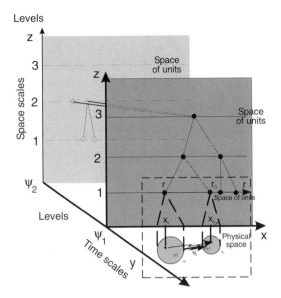

Figure 7.5
Relation between structural and functional organizations. Functions defined by their time scales are shown on the y-axis, and structures defined by their space scales are shown on the z-axis. At each of these levels, structural units belonging to a given space scale for a given time scale are shown on the x-axis. It should be noted that in this formal representation, the distances in natural space have no meaning (after G. A. Chauvet, 1999).

have therefore to consider not only the structural hierarchy but also the functional hierarchy of the system. Then, each level of the functional organization will correspond to a particular physiological function, that is, a process that occurs on a certain time scale. How do we define these two types of hierarchy? It is convenient to consider the structural hierarchy as being organized along the space scales of a physiological process while the functional hierarchy is organized according to the corresponding time scales. Moreover, it offers the advantage of clearly separating the structural and functional organizations, that is, the structure and the function of the biological system studied.

This "separation" may be viewed as follows. Using axes for the space scales, the time scales, and the space of structural units, we have a three-dimensional representation of a physiological function (figure 7.5), showing:

• the structural units in space for a given function and the hierarchical organization of physiological functions for a given space scale

• the integration of physiological functions

The identification of the couplings between the functions requires determination of the functional interactions at the different hierarchical levels involved. For example, the interactions at the molecular level between angiotensin and renin will be situated at the lowest level of the hierarchical organization representing blood circulation, and will themselves be coupled with the neural network. This complex task can only be undertaken using the highly abstract and technically advanced mathematical methods presented next.

Fields and Functional Interactions

With the theoretical hierarchical framework described here, we can represent a physiological process, expressed by functional interactions related to the geometry of the structure, in terms of the transport of a field variable submitted to the action of a field operator. Let $\psi^r(r, t)$ be the field variable defined in the r-space, e.g., the membrane potential, and let H be the field operator that depends on ψ^r and on successive derivatives $\psi^{r,(n)}$ with respect to time and space coordinates. The general form of the field equation is given by:

$$[H(\psi^r, \psi^{r,(n)}, n = 1, 2, \ldots)\psi^r](r, t) = \Gamma(r, t), \tag{7.3}$$

where Γ is the source term. In this equation, H describes the propagation of the field variable ψ from r' to r, and the local transformation in r is represented by $\Gamma(r, t)$. Since the operator acts from one point in space on another, it must take into account the distance between these two points, and thus include an interaction operator. More generally, the influence of the location of the points, that is, the role of geometry on the dynamical processes, may be studied by means of a field theory. The dynamical processes that express the behavior of the related functional interactions occur continuously in space and time with a finite velocity. Thus, what is observed at point (r, t) results from what was emitted at point (r', t'), where $t' = t - \|r' - r\|/v_r$ and v_r is the velocity of the interaction.

The finite value of the velocity v_r of the transport of the interaction, that is, the transport of molecules, potentials, currents, or parametric effects, depending on the elementary physiological function, has a major effect on the behavior of the biological system. This is particularly true of the delay in the response between units. These effects are included directly in the field interaction operator. Let us now determine the specific operator that describes a physiological mechanism.

S-Propagator Formalism

The S-propagator formalism describes the dynamics in the structural organization. The units u_i and u are assumed to be at level r in the structural organization (space scale κ), and at level T in the functional organization (time scale T) (figure 7.6). The couple (κ, T) in the 3-D representation (figure 7.7) defines the organization of the physiological function ψ^r. There is a structural discontinuity between the two units. Because of the hierarchy, u_i and u are associated with a nonlocal functional

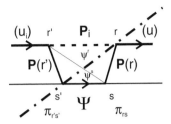

Figure 7.6
Physiological interpretation of the generation of the field variable. Propagation of the field variable ψ^r (S-operator $\mathbf{P}_i$) inside the hierarchical structural organization in u_i from r' to s' [trans-propagator $\mathbf{P}(r')$], propagation in the s-level (field variable ψ^s, in-propagator Ψ), and propagation of the field variable ψ^r inside the hierarchical structural organization in u from s to r [trans-propagator $\mathbf{P}(r)$]. The denomination of the propagators stands for trans-levels or inside levels. The dynamics at the r-level result from the dynamics at all the lower levels.

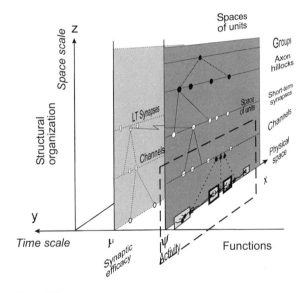

Figure 7.7
Three-dimensional representation of the nervous tissue that is a particular case of the biological system shown in figure 7.5. Two physiological functions are presented: activity and synaptic modulation.

interaction represented by the field $\psi^r(r,t)$, where $r(x,y,z)$ is the coordinate in the space of units, itself depending on coordinates (x,y,z) in the physical space. Using operators, the local time variation may be expressed as

$$\mathsf{H}\psi^r = \Gamma \quad \text{with} \quad \mathsf{H} = \frac{\partial}{\partial t} - D\nabla^2 - \mathsf{H}_I, \tag{7.4}$$

where H_I is the nonlocal operator. What are these operators? As shown in figure 7.4, in going from u_i at r' to u at r, the functional interaction must cross the structural discontinuity at the lower level, that is, it must use processes "outside" the level.

In appendix A, the S-propagator formalism has been summarized that leads from Eq. (7.4) to the local time and nonlocal space equation (hierarchical field equation) (A.8) for the dynamics of the field variable ψ^r:

$$\frac{\partial \psi^r}{\partial t}(r,t) = \nabla_r[D^r \nabla_r \psi^r(r,t)]$$

$$+ \int_{D_r(r)} \rho^r(r') \mathbf{P\Psi}(r)\mathbf{P}(r')\psi^r\left[r', t - \frac{d(r',r)}{v^r}\right] dr' + \Gamma_r(r,t), \tag{7.5}$$

where the sumation is on the domain $D_r(r)$ of the u-units connected with the units at r. Here, D^r need not be constant because the medium may not be heterogeneous, in which case the term may be space dependent. The time scale is T and $d(r',r)$ is the distance between r' and r in the space of units u. The S-propagator describes the functional action of u' at r' onto u at r per unit of time, because the field variable ψ^r is emitted by u' at r' and is transported to u at r. Locally, the field variable depends on the lower levels and is under three influences, which are shown by the three terms in Eq. (7.5): the first is a local process of diffusion between units through the extra-unit space, that is, transport through the medium in which the units are located, as defined by the diffusion constant D^r; the second term is the S-propagator $\mathbf{P\Psi}(r)\mathbf{P}(r') \equiv \mathbf{P}_i[\psi^s] = \mathbf{P\Psi P}_i$ represents the transport of the field variable through "homogeneous" structures at the lower level inside u_i or u, that is, structures that are homogeneous relative to the processes in a medium with locally identical properties, without structural discontinuities; and the third term is the generation of the field variable at r as a result of local processes in physical space, represented by the source term Γ_r, and possibly due to the higher levels.

Finally, the determination of the dynamics of physiological functions results from the determination of the propagators $\mathbf{P}$ in the Eq. (7.5). This is shown in appendix A, where the linear case is explicated. In the next section, this formalism is used for the dynamics of the nervous system. These results are valid whatever the level of organization. Because the same formalism applies to each level of the hierarchy, it provides a tool for the rigorous study of coupled biological systems in terms of elementary mechanisms. As shown in the next section, the mechanisms included in Eq. (7.5) provide the neural field equations.

Neural Field Equations Based on S-Propagators

Let us describe the neural network based on the hierarchical 3-D representation in figure 7.5. There are two different time scales corresponding to the two following functions: activity (milliseconds) and synaptic modulation (seconds). For each of them, the structural hierarchy is given in terms of neurons (axon hillocks), synapses, and channels (figure 7.7). Functional interactions are for activity, the membrane potential ψ that propagates from one neuron at r' to another at r and for synaptic modulation, the postsynaptic potential Φ at s, or equivalently, synaptic efficacy μ. Let the density of neurons at r be $\rho(r)$ and the density connectivity between the neurons at r' and the synapses at s' be $\pi_{r's'}$. For synapses at s in neurons at r, the density connectivity π_{rs} is determined by the connectivity in the postsynaptic neuron between spines and soma where the membrane potential is measured. The diagram corresponding to figure 7.4 is given in figure 7.8. A similar hierarchical structure in the synapses in which the channels are distributed leads to a similar field equation for the functional interaction at this level, say γ, given the anatomy of the system.

Operators are determined by the explicit analytical relationship between input and output: $\mathbf{P}(r')$ applies to ψ; that is, it transforms the action potential ψ into the postsynaptic potential ϕ using the synaptic efficacy σ in the activity time scale. The structure of the field equation is such that these operators correspond to an input-output block model, that is, a nonlinear transfer function. $\mathbf{P\Psi}(r)$ applied to postsynaptic potentials ϕ, and then integrated over all the pathways gives rise to the membrane potential at r. The same method applies to the synapses. These operators may be developed as in Eq. (A.9) in appendix A. The neural field equations derived using the S-propagator formalism for the ψ-field at (r, t) in the time scale $\{T\}$, and with the unknown factor $K(s', s, \delta)$ (in case of linearity for the propagators $\mathbf{P}$) for the ϕ-field equation at (s, t) in the time scale $\{t\}$, are given by Eq. (A.10):

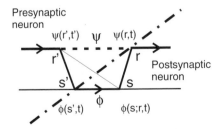

Figure 7.8
Diagram given in figure 7.4 for nervous tissue.

In time scale $\{T\}$ for activity (membrane potential):

$$\frac{\partial \psi}{\partial t}(r, t) = \nabla_r[D'\nabla_r\psi(r, t)] + \int_{D_r(r)} \int_{D_s(r', r)} \int_{D_s(r)} \rho(r')\pi_{r's'}\pi_{rs}$$

$$P_{s', s}[\gamma]\sigma(r', s')A(s)\psi\left[r', t - \frac{d(r', r)}{v_r}\right] dr' \, ds \, ds' + \Gamma_r(r, t)$$

(7.6)

In time scale $\{t\}$ for synaptic modulation (postsynaptic potential):

$$\frac{\partial \phi}{\partial t}(s, t) = \nabla_s[D^s\nabla_s\phi(s, t)] + \int_{D_s(s)} \rho^s(s')\mathbf{P}\Phi(s)\mathbf{P}(s')\phi(s', t') \, ds' + \Gamma_s[s(r), t],$$

(7.7)

where ϕ is a function of ψ, so that synaptic efficacy μ is given by the local internal dynamics of synapses, that is, another coupled system of equations that represents the dynamics in the other levels of structural organization. The kernel $K(s', s, \delta)$ in Eq. (A.9) describes the nonlocal dynamics between synapses, and the coefficient A describes passive propagation along the postsynaptic neurons' dendrites.

Each of these equations corresponds to a level of functional organization. Equation (7.6) corresponds to activity (with a time scale on the order of a millisecond) and Eq. (7.7) to synaptic modulation (with a time scale ranging from seconds to hours). These two levels of functional organization are coupled by a relationship, for example:

$$\forall t \in [t_i, t_i + \Delta t]: \sigma(t) = \sigma(t_i) = \mu(t_i) \quad \text{or} \quad \langle\sigma(t)\rangle_{\Delta t}(t_i) = \mu(t_i),$$

(7.8)

where Δt is the time unit defined experimentally and $\langle\sigma(t)\rangle$ denotes the average value of $\sigma(t)$ taken over this time interval.

The ideas and some parts of the formalism presented here may now be applied to the cerebellum to obtain an interpretation of the coordination of movement (considered as the "intelligence" of movement), and to the hippocampus.

Application of the Formalism

The Cerebellum and the Coordination of Movement

Clinical studies have established that the coordination of movement depends on specific circuits in the cerebellar cortex and on highly organized interactions among several nuclei in the brain (Thompson, 1986, 1990). Over the past few years, the adaptive control of movement has been extensively investigated through mathematical studies of artificial as well as biological neural networks (Barto et al., 1999; Houk et al., 1991). Much effort has gone into determining the mechanisms of pattern learning and recall; in other words, toward defining the conditions of stability in dynamic systems.

The cerebellar cortex is a network of networks. An element of the cerebellar cortex, called the Purkinje unit, consists of five types of cell: the Purkinje cell, which has the largest number of dendrites; the granular cells; the Golgi cell; and the basket and stellar cells. The geometry of the cortex allows us to define (approximately) a Purkinje unit. Consider a granular cell (gc) belonging to the unit containing the nearest Purkinje cell it is in contact with. Then (gc) may be considered to belong to a specific unit labeled k if the following conditions are satisfied: (gc) synapses with at least one Purkinje cell of unit k, the distance between (gc) and the Purkinje cells is the smallest distance between (gc) and any Purkinje cell it is in contact with outside the unit, and (gc) synapses with at least one Golgi cell of unit k. The basket and stellar cells included in the unit are those that are in contact with the Purkinje cell of unit k. This unit may be divided into two subsystems, the granular cell subsystem (GCS), that is, the neural network composed of granular cells (figure 7.9a), and the Purkinje cell subsystem (PCS) (figure 7.9b). The Purkinje unit, which is the repeating unit of the cerebellar cortex, is thus the basic element of a hierarchical network.

Obviously, this geometric definition is somewhat incomplete. We know that the function of the cerebellar cortex is the learning and recall of spatiotemporal patterns (Thompson, 1994). Therefore, a satisfactory transformation of the cerebellum would

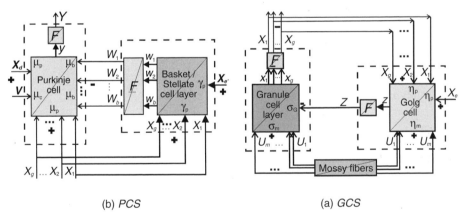

(b) PCS   (a) GCS

Figure 7.9
(a) The granule cell subsystem is composed of the granule cell layer and the Golgi cell. Inputs come from the mossy fibers and are denoted as U_i. Outputs are denoted as X_i. Output from the Golgi cell is Z. The nonlinear transformation is F, and for signals before transformation, lower-case letters are used (e.g., z and x_i). The two other inputs for the Golgi cell are V (climbing fiber) and X_e, the "external context" that comes from other Purkinje units. (b) The Purkinje cell subsystem is composed of a Purkinje cell and the basket and stellate cell layer connected with the Purkinje cell. Inputs are the outputs X_i of the granule cell subsystem (on the right). There are three other inputs: $X_{e'}$ and X_d from the other Purkinje units (the "external context" for the basket cells and the Purkinje cell), and V carried along the climbing fiber. The output of the system is Y. The nonlinear transformation is F. Lower-case letters (e.g., z and x_i) identify activities before transformation (after P. Chauvet and G. A. Chauvet, 1999).

require that the output of the system remain within physiological limits and that the modifiable synaptic weights be asymptotically stable to ensure the learning process. The conditions necessary for the stability of the observed function call for adequate values of geometric and physiological parameters, that is, the number of cells involved, the value of the synaptic weighting, and so on. These conditions thus contribute to the determination of the Purkinje unit.

Using the earlier definition of a functional unit, the Purkinje unit associated with the deep cerebellar nuclei, that is, the local circuit composed of one Purkinje cell and its associated cells, can be considered as the functional unit of the cerebellar cortex. This is supported by the following arguments:

• The definition of a Purkinje unit is geometric as well as functional. A set of Purkinje units corresponds to a microzone (Ito, 1984), although it should be noted that the definition of the microzone is not based on mathematical criteria.

• The stability of the function, which takes into account the internal dynamics that are due to the time lag in the propagation within the unit and between two units (P. Chauvet and Chauvet, 1995), determines the conditions for the definition of the structural unit.

• Variational learning rules (VLRs) (G. A. Chauvet, 1995) deduced from neural learning rules apply to Purkinje units and govern the coordination of movement through excitatory and inhibitory interactions among the units. The hypothesis of synaptic plasticity, applied to granular cells, reveals a wide range of learning behaviour. The same learning rules probably apply during the developmental period as well as in adult life to ensure the convergence of signals carried by the climbing fibers of the cerebellar cortex.

• The coupling between units increases the overall stability of the system, in agreement with the general theory (G. A. Chauvet, 1993b).

Appendix B lists various structures of the cerebellum and the corresponding functions, with their mathematically derived properties.

The Network of Purkinje Units   Let us now consider the hierarchical network of Purkinje units in which each unit is itself a neural network as defined earlier. The interactions among the Purkinje units lead to new learning rules governing the coordination of movement on the basis of the external context. Here we refer to the learning mechanisms associated with circuits adjacent to the local circuit corresponding to the individual Purkinje unit. These rules, which we have called variational learning rules, allow the learning of patterns associated with the "unlearning" of those of the context. The "unlearned" patterns are transformed in the local circuits belonging to the external context. Basically, the dynamics of the coordination may be explained by the hierarchy of the system of Purkinje units and by the granular cell subsystem associated with a Golgi cell. The learning rules then emerge at a higher level of Purkinje units, if certain conditions are satisfied [see Eqs. (C.1) and (C.2) in appendix C].

Applied to Purkinje units, these learning rules give the model a predictive value, at least from a qualitative point of view. For example, it is sufficient to know the sense of the variation in cerebellar inputs to be able to determine the sense of the variation in the synaptic efficacies and the outputs. In the learning phase, the outputs and the modifiable synaptic weights are given by the solutions of algebraic nonlinear equations coupled with integral-differential nonlinear equations. Here again, the conditions of stability found [see Eqs. (B.1), (B.5), and (B.6) in appendix B] are confirmed by the field equations. The Purkinje network, because of its hierarchical nature, may thus be conveniently investigated on a mathematical basis. This is the preliminary condition necessary to implement the coordination of movement on a computer.

The mathematical conditions for the stability of the network have been determined by means of a Lyapunov function (P. Chauvet, 1993). Using the properties of interconnected neurons described earlier, the equations for coupled units, indexed (l), are given by:

$$\mathbf{X}^{(l)}(t) = -\mathbf{G}^{(l)}\mathbf{X}^{(l)}(t - T_G) + \mathbf{X}_0^{(l)} + \mathbf{S}^{(l)}\mathbf{U} - \boldsymbol{\eta}_c^{(l)} V^{(l)} - \mathbf{X}_{ext}^{(l)}(t)$$

$$Y^{(l)}(t) = Y_0^{(l)} + {}^t\boldsymbol{\mu}_p^{(l)}\mathbf{X}^{(l)}(t) - {}^t\boldsymbol{\gamma}_{\mathbf{p}}^{(l)}\mathbf{X}^{(l)}(t - T_p) + \boldsymbol{\mu}_c^{(l)} V^{(l)} + Y_{ext}^{(l)}(t)$$

(7.9)

in which the notations [e.g., $\mathbf{X}^{(l)} = (x_1, \ldots, x_g)$] correspond to those of figures 7.9.

The hierarchical approach thus leads to the emergence of new properties at the higher level. It should be noted that the learning rules have been mathematically deduced from the natural rules operating at the neuronal level. This is a good illustration of the effects of the cerebellar hierarchical organization on its function, which has been shown to be the "intelligence of movement" (G. A. Chauvet, 2003). In this approach, intelligence of movement corresponds to the combination of the activities of a set of Purkinje units. Figure 7.10 is a three-dimensional representation of this physiological function. Defined on the basis of the contexts created by functional units, coordination of movement is clearly a physiological function that can be implemented on a computer. The n-level field theory also may be used to better characterize these results because of the delays involved in the propagation between any two neurons (Daya and Chauvet, 1999). Let us now examine the example of the hippocampus.

The Hippocampus and Learning and Memory
The properties of the hippocampus have been mainly explored through experiments with synaptically evoked population activity. Presynaptic neurons were stimulated for various intensities and the extracellular field potential (EFP) recorded at various

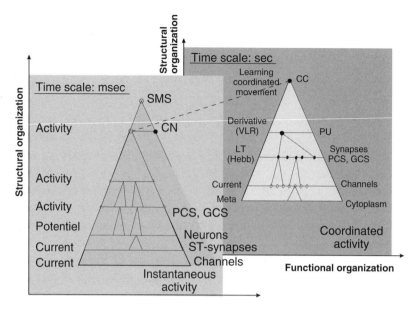

Figure 7.10
Intelligence of movement and the organization of the cerebellar cortex. For each function (activity or coordination of movement, i.e., variational learning rules) determined by a specific time scale, there is a structural hierarchical organization with its own structures. For each "pyramid," the functional interactions are shown on the left with the corresponding structural units on the right (after G. A. Chauvet and P. Chauvet, in *Advances in Synaptic Plasticity*, M. Baudry, J. L. Davis, and R. F. Thompson, eds., MIT Press, Cambridge, Mass., chap. 12, pp. 277–298, 1999).

locations (Yeckel and Berger, 1998; Berger and Bassett, 1992). These EFPs are the images of the variation in time of the fields at the corresponding points in the space.

The extracellular wave form can be viewed as the image of the number of synapses that create an extracellular potential at a given time, that is, in relation to the number of micropotentials created by the corresponding synapses at one point of the extracellular space. Specifically, we may interpret an EFP wave form as resulting from two processes: firing of stimulated neurons when the membrane potential ψ (the value of the field variable) is over threshold, and synaptic activation that results from all the ionic current variations in the recorded volume of granule cells. The first process is completely determined by the resolution of the field equation [Eqs. (7.6) and (7.7)]. The second process reflects the time distribution of the summed excitatory postsynaptic potential (EPSP) in this volume, owing to the large number of causes, such as the orientation of currents in space, the location of dendrites and synapses, and the distance between the synapse and the recording electrode. Because of these independent influences on the extracellular potential measured at a distance, the central limit theorem in the theory of probability establishes that this sum is a Gaussian variable. Thus, we have a statistical interpretation of the extracellular wave form, confirmed by the observed wave forms (G. A. Chauvet and Berger, 1996). Appendix D summarizes the specific statistical method based on the meaning of the field variables that allows the deduction of the EFP behavior of a population of neurons from the fields at all levels.

Because the state of a synapse is defined by two field variables, the postsynaptic potential ϕ (short time scale) and the synaptic efficacy μ (long time scale), the theoretical results shown in appendix D apply. We have considered the distribution function of the state variables f as the new time distribution function defined by $F(t; \psi, \mu) = N^*(t)/N(t)$ where $N^*(t)$ is the sum of the micropotentials created by the activated synapses at time t [$N(t)$ is the number of synapses in the considered volume]. Therefore, $F(\psi, \mu, t)$ will be interpreted as the time distribution of the micropotentials v_e created by the activated synapses. This method provides a means to define the relation between the intracellular and the extracellular potentials using new parameters at the level of the neuronal population having a physiological interpretation.

Following appendix D, the time distribution function of micropotentials includes three kinds of variations representing: (1) the fraction $Q(t)$ of synapses that modify their state as a consequence of an external stimulus; (2) the modification of the internal state of the cell and the corresponding synaptic states, either as a consequence of stimulation that leads to firing (feedback from the action potential to the emitting cell) or a spontaneous "relaxation," that is, a modification of potential without external stimulation but with internal modification $\phi(\psi)$ (such as from a voltage-dependent conductance); and (3) any long-term variation in synaptic efficacy. This sum can be written as Eq. (D.3):

$$dF(t; \psi, \mu) = Q(t)F \, dt + (dF)_\psi + (dF)_\mu, \qquad (7.10)$$

where the relationship $\phi(\psi)$ is included. This equation joined to the field equations (7.6) and (7.7) gives an expression of ϕ, μ, and F, that is, it determines the global intracellular potential. The numerical simulations given in figure 7.11 show the role of the macroscopic parameters that describe synaptic activation and the propagation of activity for a given intensity.

Conclusion

The models described here are based on a general theory incorporating new concepts: Any biological system may be represented as a combinatorial set of nonsymmetric and nonlocal functional interactions in a specific, hierarchical representation, in which the structures are distributed along space scales, and functions along time scales. What leads to this theoretical framework?

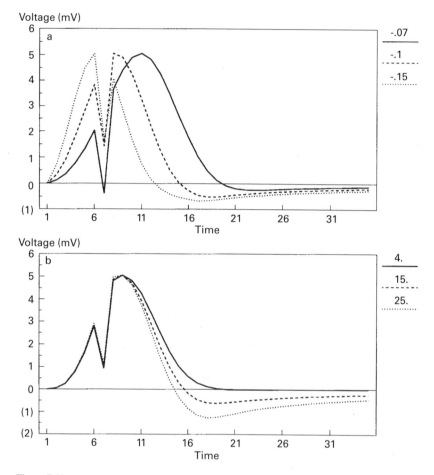

Figure 7.11
Extracellular field potential wave forms obtained by numerical simulation for three values of the parameter included in the model. (*a*) Effect of the parameter $Q(t)$, which represents the fraction of synapses that modify their state as a consequence of an external stimulus. (*b*) Effect of the source of the field equation, represented by a firing coefficient (after G. A. Chauvet and T. W. Berger, in *Neurobiology*, V. Torre and F. Conti, eds., Plenum, New York, 1996).

Applied to the nervous tissue, elementary physiological mechanisms, such as synaptic molecular mechanisms, can be integrated at the level of a neuron, and neuronal mechanisms at the level of the neural network. The crucial point is that the integration leads to new functional laws that can be simulated with a computer, using the techniques of numerical analysis, and tested through specific experiments. This kind of approach seems to be a necessary condition for the mimesis of a physiological function by a neural prosthesis.

The theory proposed has been illustrated here by two examples: the cerebellum and the hippocampus. First, the hierarchical organization of the cerebellum, proved mathematically from the functional point of view, has led to the concept of the functional unit. New learning rules have been shown to appear at the higher levels of functional organization [Eqs. (C.3) and (C.4)], together with the necessary stability of the dynamics that are demonstrably related to the hierarchy. We thus have, on one hand, the functional hierarchy created by time scales [conditions (B.2)] and on the other, the structural hierarchy created by space scales [conditions (B.5)]. Since the conditions of stability originate in the nature of the hierarchy, the functional unit, that is, the structure that has the desired function at a higher level, may be derived.

Thus, the mathematical model appears to reveal properties that would not be apparent without formalization (G. A. Chauvet, 2002). This approach, which consists of making a profound mathematical study before using numerical computation, is very different from the usual computational approach, which to a certain extent could be considered as being analogical.

In the case of neural prostheses, the implant must simulate the physiological function of the neural network it replaces. Thus, functional integration must result from the working of the implant, given that the neural network, which is hierarchical, integrates the function of a large number of elements, for example, activity (P. Chauvet and Chauvet, 2002). Moreover, the input of the system is a spatiotemporal pattern, as is its output. The model must therefore be able to realize the spatiotemporal function that results in collective activity. This is the case of the cerebellar cortex, where each element is itself a neural network. We have shown that the functional unit is the Purkinje domain, an ensemble of Purkinje units associated with neurons of the deep cerebellar nucleus. We now know how to simulate, by means of a mathematical algorithm, the learning and memorization of the coordination of movements by an ensemble of Purkinje domains.

In the same way, the cognitive function of the hippocampus must be a product of the collective activity of its intrinsic neurons. The information represented in this collective activity can only be understood if we consider the spatiotemporal distribution of active cells, given the complexity of the representations for any one set of conditions and the fact that the information represented in the activity of hippocampal neurons changes dynamically according to the environmental conditions. In the two cases we have considered in this chapter, it is clear that developing a model of the coordination of movement by the cerebellum, or the learning and memory functions of the hippocampus, will allow cognitive operations to be related to the spatiotemporal distribution of activity in the cerebellum or hippocampus and the specific molecular mechanisms of synaptic plasticity.

Would it be possible to make these transformations, which lead to the simulation of cognitive functions, by using an "analogical" approach? We do not think so, for at least two reasons. First, the size of the neuromimetic network would be immense, since it has to correspond strictly to the number of elements of the real network. Second, and more fundamentally, the specific functions provided by the global, nonlocal integration of structures would not be obtained. We have seen the example of the hippocampus, for which a statistical interpretation was needed. However, it is clear that the implementation of the algorithm will have to be of an analogical, non-numerical nature because of the necessarily adaptive nature of the learning and memory system.

Appendix A: Structural Propagators

In the most general case, the biological system is assumed to have:

• n levels of structural organization denoted as $r, s, c \ldots$ from the highest to the lowest (equivalent to $n, n - 1, \ldots 1$) indicating r-space, s-space, etc.;

• each level, except the lowest, represents a structural discontinuity;

• only one time scale for all the levels.

Phenomena are observed at the highest level, which means:

• The functional interaction ψ^r traverses levels successively from the highest to the lowest.

• At each level, the interaction cannot go directly from one point to another without traversing the lower levels because each level represents a discontinuity; thus, at each level, except the lowest, the field equation is nonlocal.

• At the lowest level (molecular level), the field equation is local (reaction-diffusion type).

In terms of operators, the local time variation may be expressed as

$$\mathscr{H}\psi^r = \Gamma \quad \text{with} \quad \mathscr{H} = \frac{\partial}{\partial t} - D\nabla^2 - \mathscr{H}_I \tag{A.0}$$

The discontinuity between spatial structures u_i at r' and u at r is taken into account by considering a discrete nonlocal operator:

$$\mathscr{P}_i : \psi^r \left[r', t - \frac{d(r', r)}{v} \right] \rightarrow \psi^r(r, t) \tag{A.1}$$

which, in the linear case, leads to:

$$(\mathscr{H}_I \psi^r)(r, t) = \sum_{u_i \in D_r} \mathscr{P}_i \psi^r \left[r', t - \frac{d(r', r)}{v} \right] \tag{A.2}$$

where D_r is the set of r'-units connected with the r-unit. This corresponds to the diagram below or (a) in Eq. (A.5)

$$
\begin{array}{ccc}
r'(t') & & r(t) \\
\bullet \text{---} & \bullet \text{---} & \bullet \\
u_i & \mathscr{P}_{i0} & u
\end{array}
\tag{A.3}
$$

where $d(r', r)$ is the distance between r' and r. We have called $\mathscr{P}_i[\psi^s]$ the structural propagator (S-propagator) since the propagation of the functional interaction occurs in the structural organization for the space of units u, including the structural discontinuities at level s with the field variable ψ^s. Now, using the continuous notation for r', the propagation of the field from r' to r occurs, at the lower level, along $d_i(r')$ from r' in u_i to the border of the structural discontinuity denoted as s', then along $d(s)$ inside s, and finally from s to r along $d(r)$ inside the unit u. This propagation corresponds to the mathematical operation per unit time:

$$\mathscr{P}_i[\psi^s] = \mathbf{P}\Psi\mathbf{P}_i \equiv \mathbf{P}\Psi(r)\mathbf{P}(r') \tag{A.4}$$

which is the product of the translevel propagator $\mathbf{P}_i$ in u_i, i.e. $\mathbf{P}(r')$, the in-level propagator Ψ for field variable ψ^s at the level s, which represents the transport through the structural discontinuity, and the translevel propagator $\mathbf{P}$ in u, i.e., $\mathbf{P}(r)$, as shown by the diagrams:

(a) *Field variables*   (b) *Domains*   (c) *Operators*

$$\tag{A.5}$$

where the dotted line shows that s', s belong to the unit at r. Note that:

- The product in Eq. (A.4) must be understood as

$$\mathbf{P}\mathbf{\Psi}(r)\mathbf{P}(r') = [\mathbf{P}(r,s)\mathbf{\Psi}(s,s';r)]\mathbf{P}(r',s'),$$

i.e., an operator $[\mathbf{P}(r,s)\mathbf{\Psi}(s,s';r)]$ that acts on the result of the operation $\mathbf{P}(r')\psi^r$. It is sometimes convenient (however confusing) to note in the same way the operator and the field variable. If there is no discontinuity, then $\mathbf{\Psi}(s,s';r) = \delta(s - s')$ where δ is the Dirac function. Thus, the passage from r' to r through s' gives

$$[\mathbf{P}(r,s')\mathbf{P}(r',s')] \equiv [\mathbf{P}(r)\mathbf{P}(r')].$$

- This relationship includes the density of units and their connectivity (a continuous expression using a density connectivity function π_{rs}, i.e. the product of the density and the probability of connection for the specific units). The pathways in the above diagram represent the action of the operators. Thus, the nonlocal term (A.2) becomes

$$(\mathcal{H}_I \psi^r)(r, t) = \sum_{u_i \in D_r} [\mathbf{P}\mathbf{\Psi}(r)]\mathbf{P}(r')\psi^r \left(r', t - \frac{d(r', r)}{v} \right) \tag{A.6}$$

- With the density of the r'-units denoted as $\rho^r(r')$, this nonlocal term, which describes the action from r' to r, through s' and s, may be written in continuous notation:

$$(\mathcal{H}_I \psi^r)(r, t) = \int_{D_r(r)} \rho^r(r')[\mathbf{P}\mathbf{\Psi}(r)]\mathbf{P}(r')\psi^r \left(r', t - \frac{d(r', r)}{v^r} \right) dr' \tag{A.7}$$

According to this definition, the S-propagator represents the operation of the processes inside the units of the hierarchical structural organization from t' to t, and includes all the processes integrated at the lower level. It gives the global representation of the operation of the processes at each level of the hierarchy. The S-propagator is a nonlocal field operator that transports the field variable ψ^r from point r' in the space of units at time t' to point r at time t. This represents the transport in three sequential steps:

1. a *propagation* of the functional interaction ψ^r inside the source (in this emitting unit, the process is represented by operator $\mathbf{P}(r')$);

2. a *transformation* that is due to the structural discontinuity that provides a propagation at the lower level owing to the functional interaction ψ^s at this lower level (the process is represented by operator $\mathbf{\Psi}$, i.e. the solution of the field equation for ψ^s at this level); and

3. a *propagation* of ψ^r at the higher level in the sink [in this receiving unit, the process is represented by the operator $\mathbf{P}(r)$].

To sum up, it is crucial to note that the S-propagator represents the operation of the processes inside the units of the space of units. In some cases, transport is possible through extra-unit space, inside the physical space. The nonlocal term [Eq. (A.7)] inserted into Eq. (A.0) gives the hierarchical field equation that describes the dynamics at the highest level of structural organization:

In the nonlinear case:

$$\frac{\partial \psi^r}{\partial t}(r,t) = \nabla_r[D^r \nabla_r \psi^r(r,t)] + \int_{D_r(r)} \rho^r(r') \mathbf{P\Psi}(r)\mathbf{P}(r')\psi^r\left[r', t - \frac{d(r',r)}{v^r}\right] dr' + \Gamma_r(r,t)$$

$$(A.8)$$

The non-local term is also a source term because it provides the contribution to the current compartment of a virtual compartment (i.e. from other levels of organization). The "factor" represented by the operator and the integral represents the quantity of ψ brought per unit time into the current compartment. Because operators are generally nonlinear, the operator that is applied to the input function ψ represents the specific local model, i.e., mechanisms that occur during a time interval.

In the linear case, the operator may be replaced by a kernel. The result of each operator, taking into account the interlevel connectivities, is:

$$\mathbf{P}(r')\psi^r(r',t') = \int_{D_r(r)} \pi_{r's'} B(r',s')\psi^r(r',t')\, dr'$$

$$\mathbf{P\Psi}(r)\psi^s(s',t') = \int_{D_s(r',r)} \int_{D_s(r)} \pi_{rs} \mathscr{P}_{s',s}[\psi^c] A(s,r)\psi^s(s',t')\, ds\, ds' \qquad (A.9)$$

where A and B are specific spatiotemporal functions that depend on the local physiological mechanisms. The second equation involves the functional interaction at the lower c-level, through the S-propagator $\mathscr{P}_{s',s}[\psi^c]$. In the same way, the given s is connected to all c, each being connected to all s', and each of these being connected to all r' in the corresponding spaces. Equation (A.8) then becomes:

$$\frac{\partial \psi^r}{\partial t}(r,t) = \nabla_r(D^r \nabla_r \psi^r(r,t)) + \int_{D_r(r)} \int_{D_s(r',r)} \int_{D_s(r)} \rho^r(r') \pi_{rs} \pi_{r's'} \mathscr{P}_{s',s}[\psi^c]$$

$$\times A(s,r) B(r',s')\psi^r\left(r', t - \frac{d(r',r)}{v^r}\right) dr'\, ds\, ds' + \Gamma_r(r,t) \qquad (A.10)$$

where the three levels and their connected units appear through the units at c, s', r'. The local mechanisms associated with the propagators are clearly represented for the s'-unit by the functions $B(r',s')$, and for the s-unit by $A(s,r)$. However, development down to the c-level would require a nonlocal field equation for ψ^s in the same functional organization, i.e., in the same time scale. Most often the field only exists at the highest level.

Appendix B: Functional Organization of the Cerebellar Cortex

Structure	Function	Property
Purkinje cell	Synaptic modifiability between parallel fibers and Purkinje cell, μ_p	Hebbian learning rules
Granule cells	Synaptic modifiability between mossy fibers and granule cells, σ_m	Hebbian learning rules
Purkinje unit: Local Purkinje circuit including the network of granule cells, Golgi cell and basket cells	Learning and memorization of trajectories: *In time*: sampling via the Golgi cell–granule cells circuit *In space*: via the granule cells–Purkinje cell circuits.	Condition for stability (unit k): $$C_1(k) = \left(\sum_{j=1}^{g} \eta_{p,j}^{(k)} \right) \max_{1 \le i \le g} \sigma_{G,i}^{(k)} < 1 \quad \text{(B.1)}$$ where the time lag T_G due to the Golgi cell is involved.
Network of Purkinje units: set of Purkinje units	Learning Learning and memorization of coordinated trajectories (time-space patterns) Dynamic stability Global stability	Functional organization: Time scale $\Rightarrow$ Condition for VLR (see appendix C): $$|dH_0| \gg |dG_0|$$ $$|dH| \gg |dG| \quad \text{(B.2)}$$ where G, H, G_0 and H_0 are defined by $$dX(t) = dG_0(t) + \varepsilon dH_0(t)$$ $$dY(t) = dG(t) + \varepsilon dH(t)$$ derived from $$\mathbf{X} = F_1(\mathbf{U}; \sigma_m) - \underline{\sigma}_G H_0$$ $$Y = F_2(\mathbf{X}; \mu_P) + H \quad \text{(B.3)}$$ Structural organization: Space scale $\Rightarrow$ Condition for stability of the network (condition between units): $$C_2(k) = \left(\sum_{l=1, l \ne k}^{N} \sum_{j=1}^{g} \eta_{e,j}^{(kl)} \right) \max_{1 \le i \le g} \sigma_{G,i}^{(k)} < 1 \quad \text{(B.4)}$$ $$C_1(k) + C_2(k) < 1 \quad \text{(B.5)}$$
Network of Purkinje domains: Purkinje units associated with the cerebellar nuclei	Enhanced learning and memorization of coordinated patterns	Increased learning capacity
Sensorimotor system	Integration of sensorial signals and coordinated patterns	Motor control

Appendix C: The VLRs: An Example of an "Emerging" Property

With H and H_0 being functions representing the external signals that converge from the connected Purkinje units (the "context") to the current Purkinje unit, calculated from the equations for the Purkinje cell subsystem and the granular cell subsystem, the following conditions are always satisfied:

$$|dH_0| \gg |dG_0|, \quad \mathrm{sgn}(dH_0) = \text{constant,}$$

$$H_0 \text{ bound and } \lim_{t \to \infty} dH_0 = 0 \tag{C.1}$$

$$|dH| \gg |dG|, \quad \mathrm{sgn}(dH) = \text{constant,}$$

$$H \text{ bound and } \lim_{t \to \infty} dH = 0 \tag{C.2}$$

Variational learning rules   (applying to the sense of variation of activities as well as synaptic weights):

$$dH_0 > 0 \Rightarrow dX < 0 \quad \text{with } (U_i = 1 \Rightarrow d\sigma_m^i > 0 \text{ and } U_i = 0 \Rightarrow d\sigma_m^i < 0)$$

or $\tag{C.3}$

$$dH_0 < 0 \Rightarrow dX > 0 \quad \text{with } (U_i = 1 \Rightarrow d\sigma_m^i < 0 \text{ and } U_i = 0 \Rightarrow d\sigma_m^i > 0)$$

and

$$dH > 0 \Rightarrow dY > 0 \Rightarrow (dX < 0 \Rightarrow d\mu_p^i > 0 \text{ and } dX > 0 \Rightarrow d\mu_p^i < 0)$$

or $\tag{C.4}$

$$dH < 0 \Rightarrow dY < 0 \Rightarrow (dX < 0 \Rightarrow d\mu_p^i < 0 \text{ and } dX > 0 \Rightarrow d\mu_p^i > 0)$$

for inputs V, X_e represented by the function H_0, and X_e' represented by the function H, and for the presented pattern $\mathbf{U} = (U_1, \ldots, U_i, \ldots, U_g)^T$.

Appendix D: Statistical Equation of Field States

The distribution function of the state variables $f^n(\psi^0, \psi^1, \ldots, \psi^n)$ from the 1-level to the n-level gives the proportion of structural units that are in the state determined by the field. It depends on specific parameters of the system, which describe the influence of the units on the population of these units. This function may be obtained as the solution of the equation that describes the balance of units submitted to numerous and various independent influences, e.g. elementary physiological mechanisms. Two classes of mechanisms are assumed such that:

$$\frac{\partial f^n}{\partial t} = \Delta f_{ext}^n + \Delta f_{\psi^n}^n \tag{D.0}$$

The first class is an external influence on the system, e.g., an excitation from another system in the biological system, or a stimulation, which changes the proportion of units in a given state. Since each unit has an equal probability of passing from one state to another, this process is similar to the change of states in a compartment: the corresponding time variation Δf_{ext}^n of the distribution function is directly related to the number of units at a given time. Let $Q(t)$ be the coefficient that expresses the fraction of units that change their state. Then:

$$\Delta f_{ext}^n = \left[\frac{\partial f^n}{\partial t}\right]_{ext} \Delta t = Q(t) f^n \Delta t \tag{D.1}$$

The second is an internal transformation corresponding to the elementary mechanisms described by the field variable: a state transition $\Delta f_{\psi^n}^n$ occurs as soon as there is a transformation in the biological system, i.e., when a stimulation is applied to the system. The formulation of this term depends on the mechanisms that cause changes in the field variables represented by specific parameters not reducible to individuals, i.e., on the field equations themselves:

$$\Delta f_{\psi^n}^n = \left[\frac{\partial f^n}{\partial \psi^n}\right]_{\psi^n} \Delta t \tag{D.2}$$

The effect of all the state transitions may be assumed to be additive, since each field equation represents a process on a different time scale. Thus, using Eqs. (D.0) to (D.2), the action of the fields on the population of a large number of structural units may be described by a statistical distribution function of the states $f^n(\psi^1, \ldots, \psi^n)$, which is a solution of the equation

$$\frac{\partial f^n}{\partial t} = Q(t) f^n + \sum_{i=1}^{n} \left(\frac{\partial f^n}{\partial t}\right)_{\Delta \psi^i} \tag{D.3}$$

References

Barto, A. G., Fagg, A. H., Sitkoff, N., and Houk, J. C. (1999) A cerebellar model of timing and prediction in the control of reaching. *Neural Comput.* 11(3): 565–594.

Berger, T. W., and Bassett, J. L. (1992) System properties of the hippocampus. In I. Gormezano and E. A. Wasserman, eds., *Learning and Memory: The Biological Substrates*. Hillsdale, N.J.: Lawrence Erlbaum, pp. 275–320.

Bower, J. M., and Beeman, D. (1995) *The Book of Genesis: Exploring Realistic Neural Models with the General Neural Simulation System*. New York: Springer-Verlag/TELOS.

Chauvet, G. A. (1993a) An n-level field theory of biological neural networks. *J. Math. Biol.* 31: 771–795.

Chauvet, G. A. (1993b) Hierarchical functional organization of formal biological systems: A dynamical approach. I. An increase of complexity by self-association increases the domain of stability of a biological system. *Philos. Trans. R. Soc. Lond. Ser. B* 339: 425–444.

Chauvet, G. A. (1993c) Non-locality in biological systems results from hierarchy: Application to the nervous system. *J. Math. Biol.* 31: 475–486.

Chauvet, G. A. (1995) On associative motor learning by the cerebellar cortex: From Purkinje unit to network with variational learning rules. *Math. Biosci.* 126: 41–79.

Chauvet, G. A. (1996a) *Theoretical Systems in Biology: Hierarchical and Functional Integration.* Vol. II. *Tissues and Organs.* Oxford: Pergamon, p. 450.

Chauvet, G. A. (1996b) *Theoretical Systems in Biology: Hierarchical and Functional Integration.* Vol. III. *Organisation and Regulation.* Oxford: Pergamon.

Chauvet, G. A. (1999) S-Propagators: A formalism for the hierarchical organization of physiological systems. Application to the nervous and the respiratory systems. *Int. J. Gen. Syst.* 28(1): 53–96.

Chauvet, G. A. (2002) On the mathematical integration of the nervous tissue based on the S-Propagator formalism. I. Theory, *J. Integrative Neurosci.* 1(1): 31–68.

Chauvet, G. A., and Berger, T. W. (1996) Higher cognitive function of the hippocampus as the integration of a hierarchical model derived from an n-level field theory. In V. Torre and F. Conti, eds., *Neurobiology. Ionic Channels, Neurons, and the Brain.* New York: Plenum, pp. 277–292.

Chauvet, G. A., and Chauvet, P. (1999) The Purkinje local circuits as an example of a functional unit in the nervous system. In M. Baudry, J. L. Davis, and R. F. Thompson, eds., *Advances in Synaptic Plasticity.* Cambridge, Mass.: MIT Press, pp. 277–298.

Chauvet, P. (1993) Sur la stabilité d'un réseau de neurones hiérarchique à propos de la coordination du mouvement. Ph.D. thesis, University of Angers, France.

Chauvet, P., and Chauvet, G. A. (1995) Mathematical conditions for adaptive control in Marr's model of the sensorimotor system. *Neural Networks* 8(5): 693–706.

Chauvet, P., and Chauvet, G. A. (2002) On the mathematical integration of the nervous tissue based on the S-Propagator formalism. II. Numerical simulations for molecular-dependent activity. *J. Integ. Neurosci.* 1(2): 157–194.

Daya, B., and Chauvet, G. A. (1999) On the role of anatomy in learning by the cerebellar cortex. *Math. Biosci.* 155: 111–138.

Hopfield, J. J. (1982). Neural networks and physical systems with emergent collective computational abilities. *Proc. Nat. Acad. Sci. U.S.A.* 79: 2554–2558.

Houk, J. C., Singh, S. P., Fisher, C., and Barto, A. G. (1991) An adaptive sensorimotor network inspired by the anatomy and physiology of the cerebellum. In W. T. Miller, III, R. S. Sutton, and P. J. Werbos, eds., *Neural Networks for Control.* Cambridge, Mass.: MIT Press, pp. 301–347.

Ito, M. (1984) *The Cerebellum and Neural Control.* New York: Raven Press.

Koch, C., and Laurent, G. (1999). Complexity and the nervous system. *Science* 284(5411): 96–98.

Kohonen, T. (1978) *Associative Memory: A System-Theoretical Approach.* Berlin: Springer-Verlag.

Thompson, R. F. (1986) The neurobiology of learning and memory. *Science* 233: 941–947.

Thompson, R. F. (1990) Neural mechanisms of classical conditioning in mammals. *Philos. Trans. R. Soc. Lond. Ser. B* 329: 161–170.

Thompson, R. F. (1994) The cerebellum and memory. In P. Cordo and S. Harnad, eds., *Movement Control.* Cambridge: Cambridge University Press.

Yeckel, M. F., and Berger, T. W. (1998) Spatial distribution of potentiated synapses in hippocampus: Dependence on cellular mechanisms and network properties. *J. Neurosci.* 18(1): 438–450.

8 Real-Time Spatiotemporal Databases to Support Human Motor Skills

Shahram Ghandeharizadeh

The term *multimedia* has a different meaning for different groups. The computer industry uses this term to refer to a system that can display audio- and videoclips. Generally speaking, a multimedia system supports multiple modes of presentation to convey information. Humans have five senses: sight, hearing, touch, smell, and taste. Thus, in theory, a system based on this generalized definition must be able to convey information to all senses. This would be a step toward virtual environments that facilitate total recall of an experience. This chapter explores touch and motor skills as an extension of a multimedia information management system.

Driven by virtual reality applications, the early 1990s witnessed a growing interest in haptic devices. By definition, a haptic interface is a force-reflecting device that enables a user to touch, feel, and manipulate a virtual object. Its application ranges from entertainment to education and patient rehabilitation. In education, for example, the dental curriculum of almost all major universities dedicates a portion of its program to training students on how to perform a procedure, such as a root canal. The objective is to educate students on the dexterity required to perform the procedure at a very fine (millimeter) level. These programs typically require students to observe the instructor and are followed by practice sessions. Haptic devices could complement this curriculum by making it possible for students to experience the dexterity of the instructor (figure 8.1). The instructor could wear a haptic glove and perform the procedure. The haptic glove would be equipped with sensors that monitor the movement of the instructor's joints and the force exerted by each joint. Each sensor would provide a stream of data that is stored in a multimedia database management system. Next, a student would wear the glove. This time, the multimedia database management system would control the movement of the student's hand by streaming recorded data to the glove, enabling the student to experience the instructor's dexterity. The glove could also be used to monitor the student's learning progress and to provide feedback (which is almost identical to an instructor watching and providing feedback). Wearing the glove, the student would perform a procedure while the glove recorded his or her movements. Next, the underlying multimedia

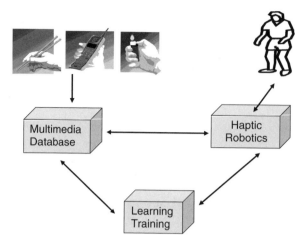

Figure 8.1
Key components of a haptic training system.

database management system would compare this recording with a recording from the instructor to provide the student with detailed feedback. For example, the student might not be moving his or her hand at the right velocity and accuracy at certain corners; the index finger of the student might not be at the right position relative to the other fingers, etc.

Haptic devices can also complement existing physical rehabilitation programs for patients with either a transplant or a prosthetic device that restores a motor skill. As an example, consider Mathew Scott, who was featured in the February 8, 1999 issue of *Newsweek* as the first person in the United States to receive a hand transplant after a 15-hr surgery at the Jewish Hospital of Louisville, Kentucky. He had lost his hand to a fourth of July fireworks accident 15 years earlier. His operation involved a 17-member surgical team that reattached multiple tissues: skin, muscle, tendons, bone, nerves, and blood vessels. Haptic devices would be useful for rehabilitating patients like Mathew. Once again, the idea would be to collect recordings from a haptic glove worn by a trainer who is performing complex activities, such as dialing a telephone, lighting a cigarette lighter, or using chopsticks. Next the patient would be provided with the glove in order to experience the transplant and its stimuli to the nerves. The multimedia database may transform the raw data into knowledge by associating streams of data with different limbs and muscle groups. This would allow patients to ask for activities related to a specific finger (say index) in order to experience and exercise a single limb.

Both examples demonstrate that a haptic device extended with a multimedia database management system (MDBMS) is a valuable tool. (Such a coupling does not exist at the time of this writing.) While both examples illustrate the use of a haptic glove, our research is envisioned to be general and applicable to other haptic devices to support motor skills. However, in order to simplify the discussion, we use the human hand and the haptic glove for the remainder of this chapter.

With a haptic glove, there are three modes of operation:

• *Record:* An instructor (or a physical trainer) performs a complex activity while wearing the glove. Each sensor attached to the glove generates a stream of data that is transmitted to a continuous media server for storage.

• *Play:* A student (or patient) experiences the motor skill required to support a specific activity by wearing the glove and playing back the recorded streams that constitute the activity. During this mode, the MDBMS retrieves the streams to activate the glove.

• *Teach:* The system analyzes the movements of a student (or patient) in a complex activity by providing feedback as to what the user might be doing. If a student informs the system that she (or he) wants to perform a specific procedure (say, a root canal on a mannequin), the glove records the student's actions. When the system detects an error, it identifies which fingers were not in the right position and suggests possible exercises to correct the movement.

At the time of this writing, components of an MDBMS (see e.g., Ghandeharizadeh et al., 1997a) and a haptic glove, for example, the Cyber Grasp, exist independent of one another. Combining these two components raises several questions:

• When the instructor and student's hand have different dimensions, how can the computer process the data to compensate for this difference during the play mode?

• An activity, for example, dialing a telephone, might be performed in a slightly different way every time it is performed by the instructor or trainer during record mode. How can the database management system process the data and extract the sense of the motor-skill movement for the student or patient?

• When a student performs an activity in teach mode, how can the system process the data to evaluate what the student might be doing wrong?

• In teach mode with a given student, how can the system build a profile of the student to use in evaluating when learning is in progress and when it is complete? Assuming that this is successful, how can the system propose other activities that would help the student to move to the next level of dexterity?

Several key technological advances are making it possible to answer these questions. First, computer components are becoming faster and more reliable every year. As predicted by Moore in 1965, central processing units (CPUs) nearly double in speed of operation every 12 to 18 months. While some in the industry predict an end to this trend with compound semiconductors, there are alternatives, such as the superconducting metal niobium that can support 100-GHz processors (Brock et al., 2000; Bunyk et al., 2001). Second, the cost of storing data is dropping by approximately a factor of 2 every 12 to 18 months, with industry offering smaller devices. To illustrate, in 1980, IBM's 3380 offered 1 gigabyte of storage for $40,000. This refrigerator-sized device weighed 550 pounds (250 kg). Twenty-four years later, in 2004, IBM's Micro drive offered the same storage capacity in a 1-inch device that weighed 1 ounce (16 g) for $200. Another trend in the area of storage involves high-density devices. At the time of this writing, 200-gigabyte disk drives are commonplace. With rapid advances in disk head technology that can pack magnetic disks with a large amount of data per square centimeter (Comerford, 2000), magnetic disks that offer terabytes of storage should be available in a few years. Third, rapid advances in both wire-based and wireless communication technology enable devices to exchange data rapidly. One may observe bandwidths on the order of tens of megabits per second from 802.11a/g wireless LAN cards. Fourth, the power consumption of these devices decreases every year, in turn reducing the amount of heat produced. These trends point toward powerful haptic devices with small footprints that can gather a large volume of data from a person's joints and reason about these data in a fraction of a second.

One area that deserves greater scrutiny is the mechanical nature of haptic devices. First, they should be designed to minimize the likelihood of physical injury to their users. Second, they should become more reliable and user friendly in order to be accepted for general use.

The rest of this paper is organized as follows. In the next section we describe techniques to support data retrieval and the spatiotemporal characteristics of data. Then we detail how these data are used for mining and query processing. The last section contains some brief conclusions.

Continous Media and Haptic Devices

The data generated by each sensor of a haptic glove consist of continuous media with a prespecified bit rate requirement. If a system delivers a movement more slowly than its prespecified rate without special precautions, the user might observe logical errors that result in undesirable behavior; for example, with chopsticks, either one or both sticks might fall out of place. A second important characteristic of the haptic glove is the temporal constraints that exist between multiple streams. These temporal constraints are computed during the record mode. Moreover, during the play mode, the system must ensure that the retrieval and rendering of data respect these temporal constraints. Otherwise, once again, the resulting motor activity might fail to perform the required task, for example, causing one or both chopsticks to fall. Both types of logical errors are collectively termed hiccups (Ghandeharizadeh and Ramos, 1993). In the following discussion, we start by describing a scalable server to store the stream generated by a haptic glove and support hiccup-free displays. Next, we focus on how to capture the temporal relationships between the different streams (i.e., sensors) and how to ensure that the retrieval of data respects these constraints. Finally, we explain how we intend to relate the different streams to the different joints and muscle groups in a hand to facilitate query processing.

MITRA: A Scalable Continuous Media Server

From 1993 to 1999, we conducted pioneering research to support a multimedia server that can store and retrieve continuous media. This research focused on multiuser systems that (1) employ off-the-shelf hardware; (2) have a software architecture that can scale as a function of the underlying hardware platform to support thousands of simultaneous streams; (3) utilize hierarchical storage structures to minimize cost; (4) use intelligent data placement techniques, disk scheduling algorithms, and buffering schemes to enhance either the cost-effectiveness of a configuration (competitive cost per stream) or experience by minimizing latency, that is, the amount of delay incurred from the time a user requests a stream to the start of a display. This research result is embodied in MITRA (Ghandeharizadeh et al., 1997a), an experimental prototype developed at the University of Southern California. MITRA's original hardware platform consisted of a cluster of workstations using a UNIX operating system. Currently, MITRA's platform consists of a cluster of personal computers (PCs) using a Microsoft Windows NT operating system. Attached to each PC is an Adaptec small computer system interface (SCSI) card with several magnetic disks. The system can show audio and video data encoded in different formats, for example, Motion Picture Experts Group (MPEG).

Simultaneous with our implementation efforts, other investigators conducted pioneering research on fault-tolerant techniques to support continuous media, for example, Berson et al. (1994) and Brock et al. (2000). MITRA implements a simple mirroring technique to ensure the availability of data when these are disk failures. However, it can be extended to incorporate the more elaborate designs found in the literature.

To minimize the cost of storage with large datasets, MITRA is designed to support a hierarchical storage structure consisting of either one or multiple tertiary storage devices, D disks, and M megabytes of memory (Ghandeharizadeh et al., 1994; Hillyer and Silberschatz, 1996a,b; Sarawagi and Stonebraker, 1996). The database resides permanently on the tertiary storage devices. Streams are materialized on the disk drives on demand (and deleted when the disk storage capacity is exhausted). A small fraction of a stream is staged in memory to support its display (see next paragraph for details). We have analyzed pipelining algorithms that stage portions of a stream intelligently from the tertiary storage onto magnetic storage to minimize the latency incurred when displaying a stream (Ghandeharizadeh et al., 1995; Ghandeharizadeh and Shahabi, 1994).

At the file system level, each stream that constitutes a task is partitioned into a sequence of blocks. When the task is referenced, a block of each stream is staged from disk into memory for display, assuming that they are resident on a disk; otherwise, they must be either staged or pipelined from tertiary; see Ghandeharizadeh et al. (1995) and Ghandeharizadeh and Shahabi (1994). Moreover, resources are scheduled intelligently to prevent data starvation. This ensures the availability of the right block at the right time for rendering (Ghandeharizadeh and Muntz, 1998; Gemmell et al., 1995; Yu et al., 1992, 1993; Martin et al., 1996; Ozden et al., 1995, 1994, 1996b). Moreover, it maximizes the number of simultaneous streams supported by a system configured with a fixed amount of resources. With D disks, the data blocks that constitute a stream are dispersed across all disks to distribute the load imposed by the retrieval of that stream evenly across the D disks (this is an important consideration when scalability is an objective).

There are two ways to partition data blocks across disks (Ghandeharizadeh et al., 1997b; Muntz et al., 1997): (1) deterministic, for example, a round-robin (Berson et al., 1994); and (2) undeterministic, for example, random (Muntz et al., 1997). In addition, there are a variety of ways to schedule resources and perform admission control (Nerjes et al., 1997). In a nutshell, the tradeoff between these choices is one of: (1) saving money versus saving time (Ghandeharizadeh and Muntz, 1998; Ghandeharizadeh et al., 1996b), (2) throughput versus latency (Ghandeharizadeh and Muntz, 1998; Chang and Garcia-Molina, 1996), and (3) guaranteeing continuous display versus the possibility of a slight chance for data starvation and hiccups (Vin et al., 1994; Nerjes et al., 1997). A system designer must understand the requirements of the human motor skill in order to configure the system with the appropriate data placement, scheduling, and admission control strategy.

Assuming that the available bandwidth is scarce, one may assign a different priority to the different streams that constitute an activity (based on the different joints and fingers). Next, each stream is assigned a priority, starting with the least important stream. In essence, a stream with a higher priority is more important. There are a host of scheduling techniques that strive to meet the deadline of as many low-priority requests as possible while meeting the deadline of almost all high-priority requests (Kamel et al., 2000).

Spatiotemporal Multimedia Objects and an Envelope of Limits

We use Allen's temporal constructs (Allen, 1983) to capture the temporal constraints that exist among multiple streams. Using these constructs, we can optimize both the placement of data and scheduling of resources to maximize system performance

(Chaudhuri et al., 1995). In the following paragraphs, we describe each in turn. In passing, it is important to note that storage of streams is not currently supported by the Cyber Glove; here we explain how we intend to capture this information.

During recording of a task, we use Allen's (1983) starts and finishes constructs to mark the beginning and end of those streams that constitute the task. This is accomplished by identifying one stream of 22 as the master and the remaining 21 as slaves. Each of the slaves is synchronized with the master. Moreover, these temporal constructs can be periodically repeated in the recorded streams to prevent drifts during playback.[1] There are alternative ways of capturing this representation (Ghandeharizadeh, 1999). Currently, we plan to use an object-relational database and define a composite object that keeps track of the master and slave streams, along with their temporal constraints (detailed later). Each stream is termed an atomic object.

In Chaudhuri et al. (1995), we analyzed hiccup-free display of composite video and audio streams by scheduling resources intelligently. That study focused on applications that construct composite objects on the fly; for example, CNN's newsroom, where an editor accesses an archive and constructs composite objects to narrate a documentary. It assumed that the placement of data cannot be modified to enhance the utilization of resources to minimize the delay incurred when a user requests the display of a composite object. Based on this assumption, we identified intraobject conflicts where retrievals of multiple streams that constitute the object compete for a single disk of the D disk system, resulting in potential hiccups. Our study proposed a novel framework to identify these conflicts and resolve them by perfecting data. This framework is at the physical file system level and uses the individual blocks that constitute the streams of a composite object. It defines a composite object as a triplet (X, Y, j), indicating that the object consists of streams X and Y. The parameter j is the lag parameter. It indicates that the start time of stream Y (i.e., display of Y_1) is synchronized with the display of block X_j. For example, to designate a complex object where the display of X and Y must start at the same time, we use the notation $(X, Y, 1)$. Similarly, the composite object specification $(X, Y, 3)$ indicates that the display of Y is initiated with the display of the third block of X. This physical definition of a composite object supports the alternative temporal relationships described in Allen (1983). Table 8.1 lists these temporal relationships and their representation using our notation of a composite object.

As detailed in Chaudhuri et al. (1995), our proposed techniques support all temporal constructs because they solve for (1) arbitrary j values, (2) arbitrary sizes for both X and Y, and (3) placement of X and Y starting with an arbitrary disk (assuming a round-robin placement of data).

The environment proposed here is different than that assumed by Chaudhuri et al. (1995) in one fundamental way: Composite objects are static and not created on the fly. With a cyber glove, the composite object may consist of 22 atomic objects

Table 8.1
Representation of temporal relationships

Allen's Construct	Composite Object Representation
X before Y	(X, Y, j) where size $(X) < j$
X equals Y	(X, Y, j) where size $(X) =$ size (Y) and $j = 1$
X meets Y	(X, Y, j) where $j =$ size $(X) + 1$
X overlaps Y	(X, Y, j) where $1 < j \Leftarrow$ size (X)
X during Y	(X, Y, j) where $(j < 1)$ and [size $(X) \Leftarrow$ size $(Y) - j$]
X starts Y	(X, Y, j) where $(j = 1)$ and [size $(X) <$ size (Y)]
X finishes Y	(X, Y, j) where [$j =$ size $(Y) -$ size $(X) + 1$] and [size $(X) <$ size (Y)]

(streams) and be created when the trainer or instructor performs a complex task. During the recording of a composite object, we can control the placement of its data blocks to prevent intraobject conflicts during its retrieval. With a round-robin data placement technique, this is accomplished by starting the storage of each stream with a different disk drive. If there are $D \Leftarrow 22$ disks, then the storage of each stream starts with a unique disk and its blocks are dispersed round-robin across all disks. There will be no intraobject conflicts because this assignment ensures that a unique disk supports the retrieval of each stream. When $D < 22$ disks, we can distribute the load of the composite object evenly across the available resources by uniformly assigning the streams to disks. Of course, the techniques detailed in Chaudhuri et al. (1995) remain applicable whenever intraobject conflicts exhaust the available bandwidth.

In addition to being continuous, these data are both multilevel and spatiotemporal. They are spatiotemporal because each sensor is a spatial point that moves as a function of time. They are multilevel because the points can be combined to form a region that moves in time. For example, a limb, say an index finger, is a region that moves in time. This region consists of the sensors (points) that monitor the joints of this finger. This is applied recursively to support higher representations; for example, a hand is a region that moves in time. An activity performed by a trainer is one multilevel presentation. Moreover, a trainer performing an activity might do it slightly differently each time. This slight variation is important and should be captured as part of an activity's essence. It provides an opportunity to refine the system when it is operating in either the play or teach mode. By capturing the variation, the system might be able to develop a set of boundaries, or "envelope of limits," termed EoL, for the different fingers. An EoL is a continuous stream of data as a function of time. Now, in the play mode, the system can control the movement of the novice's fingers based on the computed EoL. In essence, the EoL captures the statistically significant boundaries across multiple repetitions.

With a novice, the system can enlarge the EoL during playback to prevent stress and injury. In the teach mode, the recorded stream is a measure of the student's training progress. The same EoL is applied to see if the student has gained sufficient dexterity. Once the student satisfies the current EoL, the database can tighten the EoL to train the student to the next level of dexterity. This process is repeated until the EoL is tightened to correspond to that of the instructor. The EoL is similar to a filter superimposed on the streams. Its logical representation and physical storage are challenging topics that require further investigation.

The concept of EoL can also assist the users directly by making the teach mode more interactive. The idea is as follows: Consider a novice who is making a specific mistake consistently from time t_1 to t_2 relative to the start of the display of an activity; term this duration δ_1. The system can detect such errors and bring them to the attention of the user (or trainer). Next, it may switch from the teach to the play mode during δ_1 when the error is encountered. This special mode is termed active-teach. In this mode, if the user does not make an error during δ_1, then the system does not intervene and remains a passive observer. However, if the user starts to make the same mistake, then the system becomes active by switching to the play mode.

In order to detect repetitive errors that are consistent in nature, the system must build an EoL for the student when operating in the teach mode. Next, it can build a profile of errors as a function of time. Next, the system can cross-compare the student's EoL with that of the instructor to compute the spatial difference during δ_1. This spatial difference can be minimized incrementally when the error is encountered during δ_1.

This process builds a profile of a novice and his or her frequent errors. Based on this, the system can analyze its library of activities and their associated EoLs to identify those activities with movements that match the frequent mistake of the students. These can be brought to the students' attention as potential practice activities to help them improve the learning curve.

The concept of EoL as a filter can also compensate for the difference between the trainer's hand and the student's hand. Given the dimensions of two different hands, the system can construct a filter, similar to an EoL, which would be applied to the streams in the play mode. The design of this filter is expected to be simple because it is spatial in nature. (The EoL is a spatiotemporal filter that can be viewed as a stream in its own right.)

Metadata and Data Mining

Storage and retrieval of streams that constitute a composite object is a first step toward information retrieval. It is important to make it possible for a patient or student to divide an activity into its subactivities to simplify the learning experience. For example, with chopsticks, a patient such as Mathew might request the system to display only the movement of the right index finger (with no chopsticks of course). These metadata can also be used to enhance presentation. For example, not all five fingers of a hand are as mobile as one's thumb; in particular, stretching the second finger entails the movement of adjacent fingers. To see this, form a fist with your right hand. Now, while keeping the other fingers in the form of a fist, stretch your thumb out. Put your thumb back to form a complete fist again. Next, proceed to do this with your index finger. Repeat this with other fingers, moving one finger to the right each time. As one approaches the second rightmost (the "ring") finger, it becomes more difficult to maintain a fist with the other four fingers while stretching this finger outward. (It is easy to maintain a fist while stretching the thumb, index, or the rightmost finger.) Such knowledge is useful in designing a haptic glove because it prevents the system from stretching the second finger while keeping the other fingers in an uncomfortable position. This minimizes stress and possible injury. We are investigating data-mining techniques on how to discover and represent this knowledge. These tools analyze the streams and detect patterns of movements in the instructor's hand to compute the dependence between different fingers. They can be made more application specific and powerful with triggers at the metadata level that provide a framework to direct the data-mining tools toward the optimal solution.

As indicated earlier, an activity performed by a trainer is one multilevel representation. We are analyzing tools that can process data at different levels to detect correlations that represent constraints. To illustrate this concept, assume that for each activity, one level of representation corresponds to the movement of different fingers (regions). The MDBMS can scan all such data to build a profile of how the different fingers move relative to each other. If two limbs always move with one another, then it might be feasible to hypothesize that these two limbs are dependent on one another. The objective here is to create a framework that can detect interesting spatio-temporal patterns based on the underlying data. These patterns can serve as a framework when activating the glove to move a single finger. They represent the system's belief about the operation of the human hand. They might be patterns that communicate such simple concepts as "two fingers never occupy the same space" or "all fingers are mobile relative to a single plane." A belief is almost identical to a hypothesis. In Ghandeharizadeh et al. (1992, 1996a), we described how deltas as first-class citizens could facilitate hypothetical query processing. In addition, we introduced novel constructs, such as "merge," "smash," and "when" to facilitate hypothetical query processing, assuming the relational data model. We are now investigating automated techniques that compute deltas.

Query Processing

The database management system should be able to accept spatiotemporal input from the user to retrieve all those spatiotemporal datasets that match the input data. The input data constitute a query against the database. One example would be for a patient to request retrieval of all those activities that involve the folding of the index finger. Another example is an automated system that translates the hand signs performed by a hearing-impaired individual into text to facilitate communication (Murakami and Taguchi, 1991; Fels and Hinton, 1995; Sandberg, 1997; Nam and Wohn, 1996; Lee and Yangsheng, 1996; Wu and Huang, 1999). In this example, the hand signs are represented as spatiotemporal data. Each sign is labeled as either a character or a word. Next, these characters are printed on a screen, conveying what the individual is trying to say.

We have investigated a role for clustering techniques in supporting retrieval of spatial data. Our objectives were to detect a hand sign from a continuous stream of haptic data generated by a glove. For experimental purposes, we used ten subjects performing ten different hand signs (nine corresponding[2] to letters "A" through "I" plus the letter "L"). We used an implementation of K-Means (MacQueen, 1967; Jain and Dubes, 1988; Ng and Yang, 1994) and Adaptive (Martin-Bautista and Vila, 1999; Carrasco et al., 1999) provided by a package called numerical cruncher (Galiano and Talavera, 1999) for experimental purposes. Our study assumed a simplified environment consisting of two steps: training and data lookup. During training, a user issues a fixed number of hand signs and repeats them several times. The system detects the different clusters that represent each class with no prior knowledge of classes. The user then assigns a label to each cluster. During lookup, the user repeats a hand sign, and the system compares it with the available clusters to identify the best match.

The K-Means algorithm requires the user to specify the number of classes K, where each class corresponds to a sign. It forms the cluster by minimizing the sum of squared distances from all patterns in a cluster to the center of the cluster. The pattern samples are constructed using the twenty-two sensors that pertain to the position of different joints that constitute a hand. An assumption of K-Means is that clusters are hyperellipsoidal. Adaptive also determines the number of clusters based on training data. It is more general than K-Means because it does not require a priori knowledge of K. It chooses the first cluster center arbitrarily. It assigns an input training record to a cluster when the distance from the sample to the cluster is below $\theta \times \tau$ where θ is the distance threshold and τ is a fraction between 0 and 1. Adaptive does not create a new cluster when this distance is greater than τ. Moreover, it does not make a decision when the sample record falls in an intermediate region. Once the training ends, it assigns all patterns to the nearest class according to the minimum distance rule, that is, Euclidean distance. It may leave some patterns unclassified if their distances to all cluster centers are greater than τ. With Adaptive, we used $\theta = 0.8$ and $\tau = 4.1$. These values were chosen to guide Adaptive[3] to construct ten clusters. The results obtained demonstrate that both clustering algorithms are dependent on the input training dataset, its size, and the order in which the data are presented to the algorithm. Generally speaking, K-Means is the more sensitive, providing an accuracy that ranges between 55 and 83% (depending on the input data and the order in which they are presented to the algorithm). Adaptive is less sensitive, with its accuracy ranging between 66 and 77%. This is because Adaptive delays the formation of clusters and does not assign a training set to one of them.

As a comparison, we used a classification algorithm, K Nearest Neighbor (termed KNN), to compare with both K-Means and Adaptive clustering. For each data point X, KNN constructs a hypersphere centered on X that is just big enough to include K nearest neighbors (its similarity function is based on Euclidean distance). With $K = 5$, the results demonstrate that KNN provides the best accuracy compared with both K-Means and Adaptive, providing 81 to 88% accuracy. With large training sets, 2000 samples (20 samples per sign per subject), the accuracy of KNN increases to 95%. However, the accuracy of KNN decreases as the value of K is increased from 1 to 15.

We are investigating hybrid techniques that combine clustering, classification, and neural net techniques to query data with a higher accuracy. In particular, we are studying a multilevel approach to data representation, with each abstract layer offering its own context to support query processing. A preliminary design of this system is detailed in Eisenstein et al. (2003). This system employs multiple neural nets to detect a vector of different hand postures that are present in a hand sign. This vector is compared with prestored vectors of hand signs to detect a specific sign.

Conclusion and Direction of Future Research

This chapter has described research issues, some solutions, and some challenges of real-time spatiotemporal databases to support human motor skills. It focused on wearable haptic devices that produce spatiotemporal data for a motor skill, and analyzed techniques to facilitate data storage and retrieval. These spatiotemporal data streams are almost always multidimensional, continuous, large in size, and noisy. As indicated, we are investigating a multilayer framework that represents these data at different levels of abstraction. The key characteristics of this framework are as follows: First, in addition to raw data streaming bottom-up from sensors to layers of higher abstraction, the framework streams context (whenever available) from the higher layers down toward the sensors. The context is used to compensate for noise and improve accuracy. Second, intermediate representations produced by each layer are maintained in temporary buffers to support delayed decision making. This enables a layer to delay detection of an uncertain pattern until further data are available from either sensors or context. Third, with those layers that can be incrementally trained, the buffers can be used to detect mistakes and retrain the layer. This produces an adaptable framework that learns from its past mistakes and refines itself over time. The metrics used to evaluate our framework are its accuracy in detecting spatiotemporal features, robustness to noise, time and space complexity, extensibility, and adaptation to other devices. This in-progress activity is shaping our immediate research.

Acknowledgments

This research is supported in part by National Science Foundation grants IIS–0091843 and IIS–0307908.

Notes

1. With multiple streams being rendered simultaneously, it is important for the software to resynchronize them periodically. Otherwise, over the course of a long display, the streams might drift apart. This phenomenon was first observed with synchronized audio- and videoclips, where over a period of time the lips of speakers were no longer synchronized with their spoken works.

2. The letter "J" was omitted because it is spatiotemporal. In Eisenstein et al. (2003) we focused only on spatial data.

3. This is based on trial and error by manipulating θ and τ multiple times. It took us four trials to realize ten clusters.

References

Allen, J. F. (1983) Maintaining knowledge about temporal intervals. *Comm. ACM* 26(11): 832–843.

Berson, S., Ghandeharizadeh, S., Muntz, R., and Ju, X. (1994) Staggered striping in multimedia information systems. In *Proceedings of the ACM SIGMOD International Conference on Management of Data*. New York: ACM Press. Available from http://perspolis.usc.edu/User/shkim/dblab_papers.html.

Berson, S., Golubchik, L., and Muntz, R. R. (1995) A fault-tolerant design of a multimedia server. In *Proceedings of the ACM SIGMOD International Conference on Management of Data*. New York: ACM Press, pp. 364–375.

Brock, S., Track, E., and Powell, J. (2000) Superconductor ICs: The 100-GHz second generation. *IEEE Spectrum* 37(12): 40–46.

Bunyk, P., Likharev, K., Zinoviev, D., and Brock, D. (2001) RFSQ technology: Physics, devices, circuits, and systems. *Int. J. High-Speed Electron. Systems* 11: 257–362.

Carrasco, R., Galindo, J., Medina, J. M., and Vila, M. A. (1999) Clustering and classification in a financial data mining environment. In *Proceedings of the Third International ICSC Symposium on Soft Computing*. Millet, Alberta, Canada: ICSC, pp. 713–772.

Chang, E., and Garcia-Molina, H. (1996) Reducing initial latency in a multimedia storage system. In *Third International Workshop on Multimedia Database Systems*.

Chaudhuri, S., Ghandeharizadeh, S., and Shahabi, C. (1995) Avoiding retrieval contention for composite multimedia objects. In *Proceeding of the VLDB Conference*. Available from http://perspolis.usc.edu/User/shkim/dblab_papers.html.

Comerford, R. (2000) Magnetic storage: The medium that would not die. *IEEE Spectrum* 37(12): 36–39.

Eisenstein, J., Ghandeharizadeh, S., Golubchik, L., Shahabi, C., Yan, D., and Zimmermann, R. (2003) Device independence and extensibility in gesture recognition. In *IEEE Virtual Reality Conference (VR)*. New York: Institute of Electrical and Electronics Engineers, pp. 207–216.

Fels, S., and Hinton, G. (1995) Glove-talk: An adaptive gesture-to-format interface. In *Proceedings of SIGCHI 95 Human Factors in Computing Systems*. New York: ACM Press, pp. 456–463.

Galiano, F. B., and Talavera, J. C. C. (1999) Data mining software. In *Front DB Research*.

Gemmell, D. J., Vin, H. M., Kandlur, D. D., Rangan, P. V., and Rowe, L. A. (1995) Multimedia storage servers: A tutorial. *IEEE Comp.* 28(5). Los Alamitos, CA: IEEE Computer Society Press, pp. 40–49.

Ghandeharizadeh, S. (1999) Multimedia servers. In F. Borko, ed., *Handbook of Multimedia Computing*. Boca Raton, Fla.: CRC Press.

Ghandeharizadeh, S., and Muntz, R. (1998) Design and implementation of scalable continuous media servers. *Parallel Computing* 24(1): 91–122. Available from: http://perspolis.usc.edu/User/shkim/dblab_papers.html.

Ghandeharizadeh, S., and Ramos, L. (1993) Continuous retrieval of multimedia data using parallelism. *IEEE Trans. on Knowl. Data Eng.* 5(4): 658–669.

Ghandeharizadeh, S., and Shahabi, C. (1994) On multimedia repositories, personal computers, and hierarchical storage systems. In *ACM Multimedia Conference*. New York: ACM Press, pp. 407–416.

Ghandeharizadeh, S., Hull, R., and Jacobs, D. (1992) Design, implementation of delayed updates in Heraclitus. In *Proceedings of the 1992 Extending Data Base Technology Conference*. New York: Springer, pp. 261–276.

Ghandeharizadeh, S., Dashti, A., and Shahabi, C. (1994) A pipelining mechanism to minimize the latency time in hierarchical multimedia storage managers. Technical report. Los Angeles: University of Southern California.

Ghandeharizadeh, S., Dashti, A., and Shahabi, C. (1995) A pipelining mechanism to minimize the latency time in hierarchical multimedia storage managers. *Comp. Comm.* 18(3): 170–184. Available from http://perspolis.usc.edu/User/shkim/dblab_papers.html.

Ghandeharizadeh, S., Hull, R., and Jacobs, D. (1996a) Design, implementation, and application of Heraclitus[Alg,C]. *ACM Trans. Database Syst.* 21(3): 370–426.

Ghandeharizadeh, S., Kim, S., Shahabi, C., Zimmermann, R. (1996b) Placement of continuous media in multi-zone disks. In Soon M. Chung, ed., *Multimedia Information Storage and Management*, chap. 2. Boston: Kluwer Academic Publishers.

Ghandeharizadeh, S., Zimmermann, R., Shi, W., Rejaie, R., Ierardi, D., and Li, T. W. (1997a) Mitra: A scalable continuous media server. In *Kluwer Multimedia Tools and Applications*. 5(1): 79–108. Available from http://perspolis.usc.edu/User/shkim/dblab_papers.html.

Ghandeharizadeh, S., Kim, S., Shi, W., and Zimmermann, R. (1997b) On minimizing startup latency in scalable continuous media servers. In *Multimedia Computing and Networking Conference*. Available from http://perspolis.usc.edu/User/shkim/dblab_papers.html.

Hillyer, B., and Silberschatz, A. (1996a) On the modeling and performance characteristics of a serpentine tape drive. *ACM Sigmetrics*. New York: ACM Press, pp. 170–179.

Hillyer, B., and Silberschatz, A. (1996b) Random I/O scheduling in online tertiary storage systems. *ACM Sigmetrics*. New York: ACM Press, pp. 195–204.

Jain, A. K., and Dubes, R. C. (1988) *Algorithms for Clustering Data*. Englewood Cliffs, NJ: Prentice Hall.

Kamel, I., Niranjan, T., and Ghandeharizadeh, S. (2000) Novel deadline driven disk scheduling algorithm for multi-priority multimedia objects. In *IEEE Data Engineering Conference*. New York: Institute of Electrical and Electronics Engineers, pp. 349–358.

Laubach, M., Wessber, J., and Nicolelis, M. (2000) Cortical ensemble activity increasingly predicts behavior outcomes during learning of a motor task. *Nature* 405(6786): 567–571.

Lee, C., and Yangsheng, X. (1996) Online interactive learning of gestures for human/robot interfaces. In *Proceedings of IEEE International Conference on Robotics and Automation.* New York: Institute of Electrical and Electronics Engineers, pp. 2982–2987.

MacQueen, J. B. (1967) Some methods for classification and analysis of multivariate observations. In *Proceedings of the Fifth Berkeley Symposium on Mathematical Statistics and Probability.* University of California Press, Berkeley, CA, pp. 281–297.

Martin, C., Narayan, P. S., Ozden, B., Rastogi, R., and Silberschatz, A. (1996) The Fellini multimedia storage server. In Soon M. Chung, ed., *Multimedia Information Storage and Management*, chap. 5. Boston: Kluwer Academic Publishers.

Martin-Bautista, M. J., and Vila, M. A. (1999) A survey of genetic selection in mining issues. In *IEEE Conference on Evolutionary Computation.* New York: Institute of Electrical and Electronics Engineers, pp. 1314–1321.

Muntz, R., Santos, J., and Berson, S. (1997) RIO: A real-time multimedia object server. *ACM Sigmetrics Perform. Eval. Rev.* 25(2): 29–35.

Murakami, K., and Taguchi, H. (1991) Gesture recognition using recurrent neural networks. In *Proceedings of CHI91 Human Factors in Computing Systems.* New York: ACM Press, pp. 237–242.

Nam, Y., and Wohn, K. (1996) Recognition of space-time hand-gestures using hidden Markov model. In *Proceeding of ACM Symposium on Virtual Reality Software and Technology.* New York: ACM Press, pp. 51–58.

Nerjes, G., Muth, P., and Weikum, G. (1997) Stochastic service guarantees for continuous data on multizone disks. In *Sixteenth Symposium on Principles of Database Systems* (PODS'97). New York: ACM Press, pp. 154–160.

Ng, R., and Yang, J. (1994) Maximizing buffer and disk utilization for news on-demand. In *Proceedings of the 20th International Conference on Very Large Databases.* San Francisco: Morgan Kaufman, pp. 451–462.

Ozden, B., Rastogi, R., Shenoy, P., and Silberschatz, A. (1994) A low-cost storage server for movie On-demand databases. In *Proceedings of the 20th International Conference on Very Large Data Bases.* San Francisco: Morgan Kaufman, pp. 594–605.

Ozden, B., Biliris, A., Rastogi, R., and Silberschatz, A. (1995) A disk-based storage architecture for movie on demand servers. *Inform. Syst. Journal* 20(6): 465–482.

Ozden, B., Rastogi, R., and Silberschatz, A. (1996a) Buffer replacement algorithms for multimedia databases. In *IEEE International Conference on Multimedia Computing and Systems.* New York: Institute of Electrical and Electronics Engineers.

Ozden, B., Rastogi, R., Shenoy, P., and Silberschatz, A. (1996b) Fault-tolerant architectures for continuous media servers. *ACM Sigmod.* 79–90.

Sandberg, A. (1997) Gesture recognition using neural networks. Master's Thesis TRITA-NA-E9727 Dept. Numerical Analysis and Computing Science, Stockholm University.

Sarawagi, S., and Stonebraker, M. (1996a) Reordering query execution in tertiary memory databases. In *Proceedings of the 22nd International Conference on Very Large Databases.* San Francisco: Morgan Kaufman, pp. 156–157.

Vin, H. M., Goyal, P., and Goyal, A. (1994) A statistical admission control algorithm for multimedia severs. In *Proceedings of the ACM Intl. Conf. on Multimedia.* New York: ACM Press, pp. 33–40.

Wu, Y., and Huang, T. (1999) Vision-based gesture recognition: A review. In *Proceedings of the International Gesture Recognition Workshop.* Hildelberg: Springer-Verlag, pp. 103–115.

Yu, P. S., Chen, M. S., and Kandlur, D. D. (1992) Design and analysis of a grouped sweeping scheme for multimedia storage management. In *Proceedings of the Third International Workshop on Networks and Operating System Support for Digital Audio and Video.* London: Springer-Verlag, pp. 44–55.

Yu, P. S., Chen, M. S., and Kandlur, D. D. (1993) Grouped sweeping scheduling for DASD-based multimedia storage management. *Multimedia Systems* 1(1): 99–109.

III NEURON/SILICON INTERFACES

9 Long-Term Functional Contact between Nerve Cell Networks and Microelectrode Arrays

Guenter W. Gross, Emese Dian, Edward G. Keefer, Alexandra Gramowski, and Simone Stuewe

The interface between biological tissue and nonbiological materials such as structural implants or microelectrodes has shown itself to be a challenging scientific and engineering problem. The concept of biocompatibility has grown beyond studies of toxicity to include long-term cell–surface interactions, with emphasis on maintenance of normal cellular functions. These studies are difficult to perform exclusively in vivo because it is not possible to monitor the cellular dynamics at implants as a function of time under controlled chemical and physiological conditions. However, such conditions can be obtained in vitro, where developing tissue responses can be monitored with time-lapse photography, fluorescence, intracellular microelectrodes, and extracellular multichannel recording, and where the physical and chemical environments can be maintained and manipulated with great precision.

In the past two decades, methods have been developed that allow the growth of primary cultures, derived from a variety of dissociated central nervous system (CNS) tissues, on surfaces decorated with substrate-integrated microelectrodes. These cultures form spontaneously active neuronal networks that allow the simultaneous monitoring of neuronal spike activity at sixty-four or more sites and provide a concomitant optical monitoring of major features of network morphology over relatively long periods of time. Such cultures have been maintained in an electrophysiologically active and pharmacologically responsive state for a maximum of 312 days in vitro. It is the purpose of this chapter to acquaint the reader with some of the characteristics of culture networks, describe the stability of the cell electrode coupling, and summarize the remaining challenges in this research domain.

Generation of Networks on Microelectrode Arrays

In order to achieve strong and stable adhesion, long culture life, and reproducibility (as measured with responses to pharmacological substances), we consider it desirable to generate mixed cultures that contain both neurons and glia in somewhat predictable ratios. Therefore glia are considered an important component of these cultures. Although the resulting flat arrangement of cells is often called a monolayer, the culture is actually a three-dimensional structure of cells. Neuronal somata are always situated on top of the glia layer (carpet); however, axonal processes can be found both on top and underneath the carpet. The initial stages of organization seem to be determined by a competition between cell-cell and cell-substrate adhesion. A poorly prepared surface will favor cell-cell adhesion, resulting in cell aggregates on the surface and floating cell clumps in the medium.

General Cell Culture Methods

Primary cultures are prepared according to the basic method established by Ransom et al. (1977) from embryonic murine CNS tissues (BALB-c/ICR). Because of different developmental rates of CNS regions, spinal cord and brain tissues are harvested from embryonic mice at gestation days 14–15 and 16–18, respectively. The tissues are dissociated enzymatically and mechanically, seeded at a density of 0.2–0.5×10^6 cells/cm^2 onto microelectrode array (MEA) surfaces confined by a $2 \times$ 3-cm^2 silicone gasket (figure 9.1; Gross and Kowalski, 1991; Gross, 1994). Cultures are incubated at $37°C$ in a 10% CO_2 atmosphere until ready for use, generally 3 weeks to 3 months after seeding. The culture medium is replenished twice a week with minimum essential medium (MEM, Gibco, Carlsbad, Calif.) containing 10% horse serum. Spontaneous activity starts at approximately 1 week in the form of random spiking and stabilizes in terms of coordinated spike and burst patterns by 15 days in vitro. Such networks can remain spontaneously active and pharmacologically responsive for more than 6 months (Gross, 1994). Although the general experimental approaches are quite similar, different parent tissues may require slightly different treatments or maintenance. For example, spinal cultures that contain both glycine and γ-aminobutyricacid (GABA) inhibitory circuits are maintained in MEM that is devoid of glycine. Cortical cultures that do not have active glycine inhibition are maintained in DMEM (Dulbecco's minimum essential medium), which contains 3 mM glycine.

Using the methods described, cell cultures have been found to survive and remain electrophysiologically active and pharmacologically responsive for many months (table 9.1). Since the data in this table were not obtained from designed longevity experiments, but resulted from routine procedures and culture usage, it is likely that with special care, such primary cultures can survive for up to a year or longer. Present feeding methods subject cultures to substantial osmotic shocks and metabolite and pH fluctuations. If these stressors could be avoided, culture survival should exceed 6 months in vitro (Potter and DeMarse, 2001).

Surface Preparation and Cell-Surface Adhesion

The dynamics involved in the generation of stable adhesion may be described in terms of three major events (Doherty and Walsh, 1992): (1) initial apposition (in

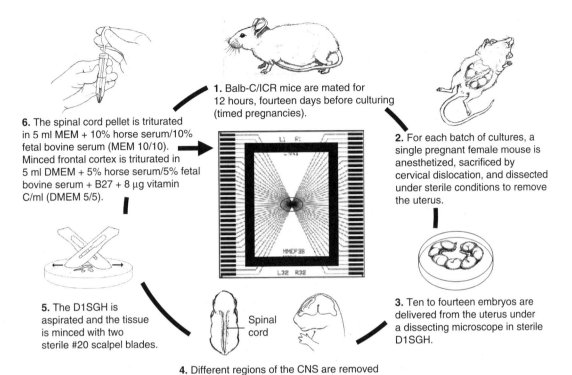

6. The spinal cord pellet is triturated in 5 ml MEM + 10% horse serum/10% fetal bovine serum (MEM 10/10). Minced frontal cortex is triturated in 5 ml DMEM + 5% horse serum/5% fetal bovine serum + B27 + 8 µg vitamin C/ml (DMEM 5/5).

1. Balb-C/ICR mice are mated for 12 hours, fourteen days before culturing (timed pregnancies).

2. For each batch of cultures, a single pregnant female mouse is anesthetized, sacrificed by cervical dislocation, and dissected under sterile conditions to remove the uterus.

5. The D1SGH is aspirated and the tissue is minced with two sterile #20 scalpel blades.

Spinal cord

3. Ten to fourteen embryos are delivered from the uterus under a dissecting microscope in sterile D1SGH.

4. Different regions of the CNS are removed (spinalcord, frontal cortex, auditory cortex, brain stem) and placed in D1SGH at room temperature.

Figure 9.1
Summary of major steps required to obtain primary cultures growing on microelectrode arrays (MEA). The dissociated cells are seeded onto an adhesion island prepared in the center of the MEA. After 24 hr, the entire area within the gasket (heavy black rectangle) is filled with medium. Thereafter, cultures are maintained with biweekly feeding for up to 6 months in incubators under 10% CO_2 to maintain pH. For ease of handling and to minimize contamination, the MEAs are contained in covered petri dishes.

Table 9.1
Cell culture survival

Tissue Experiments	No. of Experiments	Max. Active Culture Age (days)	Mean Age for Experiments (days)
Spinal cord	720	312	47
Cortex (whole)	58	137	57
Cortex (frontal)	117	94	48
Cortex (auditory)	209	189	58
Olfactory bulb	62	172	54

which nonspecific adhesion plays a role), (2) diffusional recruitment [assembly of cell adhesion molecules (CAMs) in a transient cluster], and (3) stable adhesion (critical mass of CAMs and coupling to cytoskeleton). In the nervous system, certain components may alternate between stable and transient adhesion in order to achieve morphological remodeling, which is an important component of plasticity. It has been observed in *Aplysia* that cell adhesion molecules can be internalized via coated pits, a process that is thought to induce instability in the synaptic structure and could be a prerequisite for circuit restructuring (Mayford et al., 1992; Bailey et al., 1992). The majority of the specific adhesion molecules found to date belong to one of four large families: the immunoglobin superfamily, the cadherins, the integrins, and the selectins (Pigott and Power, 1993). However, except for adhesion to laminin, glia-to-substrate adhesion in a culture is largely nonspecific and appears dominated by ionic and hydrogen bonding.

The primary materials we have used for insulation of the microelectrode arrays are polysiloxane resins (dimethylpolysiloxane, Dow Corning DC 648) and a methylsilicone resin (PS233, Glasclad RC, United Chemical Technologies, Bristol, Pa.). Both surfaces are decorated with methyl groups that render the surface hydrophobic and unsuitable for cell adhesion. Surface activation can be achieved by a short (1-s) exposure to a hot flame (butane) that oxidizes the methyl groups to hydroxyl moieties and other radicals (Lucas et al., 1986; Harsch et al., 2000).

Using our methods, the chemical nature of the adhesion surface is quite complex (figure 9.2). The dominant covalently attached surface adhesion molecule is covered by poly-D-lysine (PDL, mol. wt. 70–120 kD, Boehringer, Mannheim, Germany). After allowing the PDL to settle overnight, the solution is aspirated, dried, and the surface covered with laminin on the day of seeding. When the suspension of dissociated cells is added, a large variety of dissolved soluble molecules (DSM) are also added and settle onto the laminin and PDL adhesion structure. Since we always

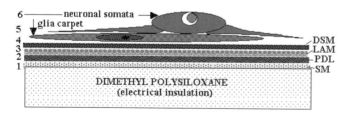

Figure 9.2
Realistic view of neuronal adhesion to a substrate. The dominant surface moiety (SM) of the polysiloxane is covered sequentially by poly-D-lysine (PDL) and laminin (LAM). Upon adding the suspension of dissociated cells, dissolved soluble molecules (DSM) are added to the laminin and PDL adhesion layer. Dissociated spherical glia and neurons form weak adhesion with this complex surface within 15–30 min, flatten, and extend short processes by 1–2 hr. The system then stratifies, with neuronal somata situated on top of the glial layer.

culture in a serum-containing medium, serum albumin is most likely the dominant soluble molecule. However, even if serum is avoided, it is impossible to dissociate tissue without causing extensive cell death, resulting in cell debris and soluble molecules that modify the surface. Spherical glia and neurons form weak adhesion with this complex surface within 15–30 min and flatten and extend short processes by 1–2 hr. The system then stratifies, with neurons situated on top of the glial layer.

Although the sequential addition of polylysine and laminin provides a good surface for subsequent cell attachment, neurons prefer glia and are rarely seen outside the glial domain. When glia retract locally, neuronal processes generally fasciculate, lift off the surface, and become bundles. If the glial carpet is not confluent during culture development, neurites usually follow glial structures. Somata are always found on segments of the glial carpet (figure 9.3).

Strength of Adhesion

For a particular contact area, the greater the cell mass adhering to that area, the more unstable the adhesion. Cell clumps and fascicles of neurites have relatively large vertical dimensions and are therefore subject to greater lateral hydrodynamic forces associated with even slight movement of culture dishes (Goslin et al., 1998). This is often encountered during attempts to create ordered networks. Narrow adhesion patterns limit the contact area and encourage process fasciculation. Fascicles develop tension and often pull away from the substrate. The same is true of cell aggregates that arise under most culture conditions but are again favored by

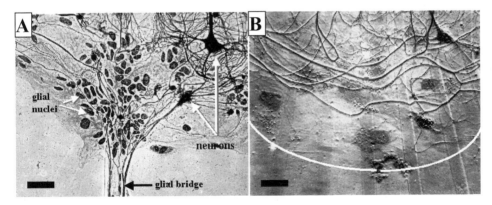

Figure 9.3
Phase-contrast (*A*), Bodian-stained and (*B*) interference-contrast microscopy of peripheral areas of adhesion islands produced by flame activation of polysiloxane and surface decoration with polylysine and laminin. Despite the presence of these two adhesion proteins, neuronal somata and their neurites prefer adhesion to the glia carpet and are rarely found on glia-free surfaces. A glial bridge in *A* demonstrates the strong preference of neurites for a glial carpet. The white curve in *B* represents the edge of the adhesion island. Bar: 25 μm.

adhesion patterns that limit the overall adhesion area. To establish strong, stable adhesion with present methods, there is little choice but to grow shallow, highly dispersed monolayers that maximize cell contact with the substrate.

The strength of adhesion varies greatly with procedure, tissue, and technique. It is also difficult to measure quantitatively. However, a study of rapid acceleration injury in dispersed monolayer cultures by Lucas and Wolf (1991) allows some estimation of how strongly glia and neurons adhere to their respective substrates. Using a novel application of a ballistic pendulum, culture flasks with most of the medium removed were subjected to 220 g impacts every 3–5 s tangential to the adhesion surface. Cumulative impact forces of 440 g were required to reach a threshold for neuronal death, and forces of 1100 g were required to achieve 50% neuronal death. Glia were not affected at these impact levels.

Neuronal death thresholds were also moved higher by the addition of 100 µM ketamine to the medium 1 day prior to the impact experiments. Lucas and Wolf suggested that Ca^{2+} entry through N-methyl-D-aspartate (NMDA) channels weakened the cytoskeleton, allowing an increasing degree of nuclear displacement during impacts and leading to subsequent catastrophic membrane damage and necrotic cell death. Of interest to the topic of this chapter are the observations that neurons did not lose adhesion to glia, and that glia did not lose their adhesion to the substrate as long as the glial carpet was confluent, the neurons were highly dispersed, and fasciculation was at a minimum. These interesting results indicate that under appropriate conditions, neuronal and glial adhesion in primary cultures is remarkably stable unless compromised by pH fluctuations, low calcium, or rapid changes in osmolarity of the medium. In addition, adhesion islands that do not have adequate coverage with PDL or laminin at their periphery often show partial glial carpet retraction in areas where glia ventured beyond the PDL regions onto the flamed areas. Elastic forces generated within the glial carpet then overcome the weak adhesion to the flamed surface. Retraction usually stablilizes over the optimum PDL-laminin surfaces.

Cellular Constituents of the Cultures

Despite substantial progress in immunocytochemistry, a quantitative cell identification in mixed neuronal-glial cultures is still extremely difficult. Neuronal counts per microscope field are greatly dependent on seeding densities and early adhesion conditions that are difficult to determine accurately. An estimate of neurons in culture as percentage of total cells depends as much on neuronal survival as on glial survival and proliferation. Antibody staining depends on culture age, tissue source, and level of differentiation of cells. For these reasons we consider the Bodian stain (Bodian, 1936) or Loots-modified Bodian (Loots et al., 1979) the most convenient method for neuron identification.

Table 9.2
Percentage of neurons in spinal cultures at 2 and 4 weeks

Seeding Density	Culture Date	% neurons at 14–15 days in vitro	N	n	% neurons at 29–30 days in vitro	N	n
5×10^5 cells/ml	2-3-00	27.2	2	2	18.5 (7.1)	2	10
5×10^5 cells/ml	8-3-00	28.2 (8.4)	2	8	18.1 (3.7)	1	4
2.5×10^5 cells/ml	7-20-00	17.8 (8.2)	2	10	9.6 (9.8)	1	3

Notes: N, number of different cultures used; n, total number of fields counted. Neurons were stained with neurofilament monoclonal antibodies (Sigma; catalog no. N-5139). Glia counts were determined from counting nuclei under phase contrast. Percent values represent number of neurons over total nuclei counted. Standard deviations are given in parentheses.

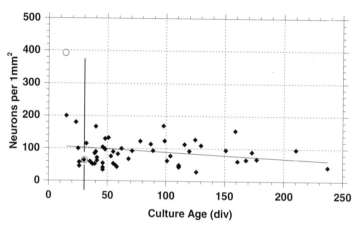

Figure 9.4
Neuronal cell counts over recording matrix (1-mm² area) from 54 Bodian-stained cultures, and from 9 and 14 cultures stained with neurofilament antibody at 15 and 30 days, respectively (o). Despite density fluctuations, a stabilization of neuronal counts past 30 days (vertical line) is apparent. After 30 days, neuronal loss is approximately 10% in 100 days or 3% per month. All Bodian-stained cultures were treated with 50 μM FdU. Cultures used for neurofilament staining were treated with 7.5 μM ara-C.

Table 9.2 summarizes neuronal percentages based on neurofilament staining and counts of all nuclei per microscope field for young cultures at 15 and 30 days in vitro. All cultures were treated with 7.5 μM cytosine arabinoside (ara-C) at days 4–5 after seeding. Although the percentage is influenced by variable glial proliferation, primarily before treatment, the table clearly shows a substantial neuronal cell death (approximately 35%) between 15 and 30 days in vitro. It is difficult to estimate the neuronal cell death during the first 2 weeks after seeding because molecular markers are not expressed reliably (Whithers and Banker, 1998). However, Segal et al. (1998) has estimated that 50% of the neurons obtained from postnatal rat brain survive the

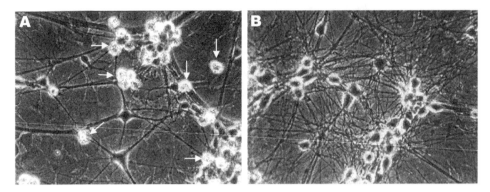

Figure 9.5
Comparison of electrophysiological parameters for untreated cultures and cultures treated with ara-C and FdU. (*A*) The percent of channels with activity greater than 2:1 (active channels) is the same for ara-C and FdU, but is significantly lower for the untreated cultures. (*B*) Signal-to-noise ratios (S/N, both maximum and mean) were not significantly different. (*C*) and (*D*) Global means of spike and burst rates (per minute) also show a significant difference ($p < 0.05$) in the native (normal medium) state among untreated and treated cultures. The numbers on the columns in *A* and *B* indicate the number of different cultures in each dataset. The numbers in *C* also represent the number of cultures and are the same for each set of columns in *C* and *D*.

first 30 days in vitro. Thereafter, the rate of neuronal cell death is greatly reduced. Figure 9.4 shows data from 54 Bodian-stained cultures where all neurons situated in a 1-mm^2 area centered on the recording matrix were counted. The cell seeding concentration was 500k cells/ml. A linear regression for the scatter plot shows a neuron loss of approximately 3% per month. The large open circles represent the neurofilament data (table 9.2) normalized to 1-mm^2 areas for 15 and 30 days in vitro and show the cell death that occurs within the second 2-weeks in culture. These results are in general accord with the more qualitative observations found in the literature.

Control of Glia in Culture
In the adult CNS, there can be found at least ten times as many glia cells as neurons (Streit, 1995). Microglia represent 5–20% of the entire central nervous system glial cell population, and there are at least as many microglia as there are neurons (Kreutzberg, 1987; Perry and Gordon, 1988). Although these ratios are not the same at the time embryonic tissue is isolated for culturing, glia represent a major constituent of the dissociated tissue and continue to develop after seeding. Cultures overgrown with glia provide poor optical data and were at one time thought to lose more neurons than cultures treated with antimitotics. We have recorded from cultures that were allowed to grow unrestrained (untreated) and cultures treated with either cytosine arabinoside (Ara-C, 7.5 μM) or fluorodeoxyuridine (FdU, 50 μM) (figure 9.5). The results show a difference in electrode yield (number of electrodes

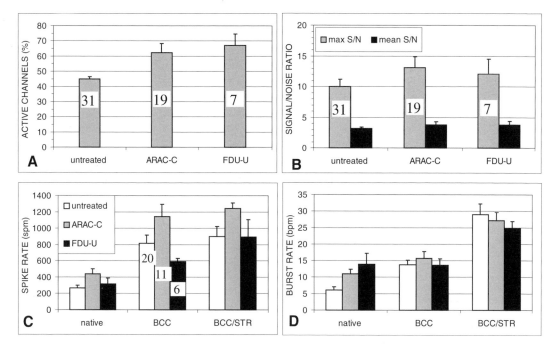

Figure 9.6
Comparison of spinal cord culture for (*A*) untreated and (*B*) ara-C-treated conditions at 7 days in vitro. Untreated cultures have more microglia and reaveal a thicker glial carpet with a typical cobblestone effect. Treated cultures at 7 days have fewer microglia, reveal more processes, and have a thinner glial carpet. At 4 weeks in vitro, cultures such as the one shown in *A* will have most neurites covered by glia and reveal only the tops of neurons as phase-bright bodies.

with measurable activity expressed as percent of all functional electrodes) and burst and spike rates (figure 9.6). The percent of channels with activity greater than 2:1 is the same for ara-C and FdU, but is significantly lower for the untreated cultures. Whether this relates to a reduced number of neurons, reduced axonal growth, or increased glial insulation of recording craters is not known at this time. Signal-to-noise ratios (SNRs, both maximum and mean) were not significantly different; global means of spike and burst rates (per minute) also show a significant difference ($p < 0.05$, Student-t) in the native state (normal medium) among untreated and treated cultures.

FdU inhibits thymidylate synthase, the enzyme that produces thymidine, thus preventing DNA replication (Liu et al., 1999). In AraC, the arabinose ring is phosphorylated on the side opposite the phosphorylation site of the ribose ring. This results in inhibition of DNA synthase. The characteristics of untreated and treated cultures are compared in table 9.3.

Table 9.3
Characteristics of treated and untreated cultures

	Untreated Cultures	Treated Cultures (FdU or ara-C)
General architecture	Multiple layers of glia intermixed with neurons	Monolayer glial carpet with axons above and below the carpet and neuronal somata always on top of the carpet
Recording	Good	Good
Adhesion strength	Good, retraction at periphery due to internal tension	Optimal
Cell-electrode coupling	Good	Good
Resistance to medium movement and flow	Excellent, very robust	Sensitive to high to medium flow rates
Microscopy	Fair to poor, neurites and cell bodies covered by glia	Excellent; well-defined cell bodies and many neurites unobscured by glia
Neuronal survival	Good	Good
Microglia	Many	Few

Microelectrode Arrays and Cell-Electrode Coupling

The techniques used to fabricate and prepare microelectrode arrays have been described elsewhere (Gross, 1979; Gross et al., 1985; Gross and Kowalski, 1991). Two MEAs with different electrode patterns are now in routine use (figure 9.7). Cell-electrode coupling is complex and depends on random crater crossing (or near crossing) of axons (figure 9.8). Although signals are also obtained from somata, more than 80% of the signals show a sharp negative-going wave of approximately 300 µs duration and are considered to be of axonal origin. The presence of glia and their greatly differing morphological arrangement relative to the recording sites makes a determination of maximum recording distances as a function of process size very difficult. So far we have not seen signal pickup by nearest-neighbor electrodes (40 µm distant). However, axons will occasionally cross two different recording sites, resulting in the pickup of the same temporal spike pattern on two electrodes. Spike wave shapes still will differ because of different cell-electrode coupling at each recording crater. The highest signal-to noise ratios are obtained when axons are trapped in recording craters by glia cells (cf. figure 9.9).

Seeding of mammalian cell suspensions onto planar arrays has been done in our laboratory since 1980 (Gross and Lucas, 1982). Two adhesion areas are formed on the array by flaming through masks: a centrally located island (usually 3–4 mm in diameter) and a separate 1 × 2-cm region used for medium conditioning. Polylysine and laminin are then added as described earlier. The adhesion areas receive, respectively, 50-µl and 450-µl volumes from a cell suspension at a concentration of

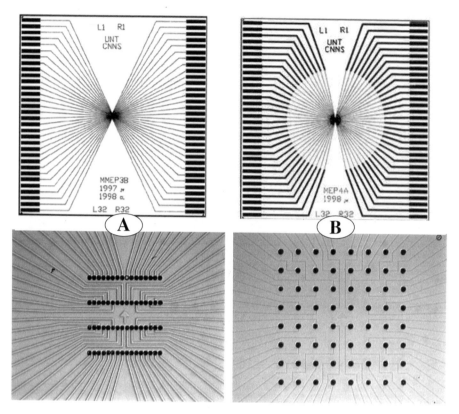

Figure 9.7
MEAs in use. CNNS MMEP3 (*A*) and 4 (*B*) showing electrode arrangement in the recording area. The bottom panels represent phase-contrast micrographs of the recording matrices of either MMEP version after fabrication and gold electroplating of recording craters. Under bright-field microscopy, the conductors are invisible. MMEP3 has four rows separated by 200 μm, with 16 electrodes per row spaced 40 μm apart. MMEP4 has an 8 × 8 matrix of electrodes spaced at 150-μm intervals. Impedances: 3 MΩ and 1 MΩ (at 1 kHz) for each version, respectively.

approximately 500k cells/ml. After 1 hr, 450 μl of medium are added between the two regions so that the fluid volumes merge. After 24 hr, 1 ml of medium is added, increasing the total volume confined by the gasket to 2 ml. This volume is maintained for the duration of the cultures life span in the incubator. It is essential to monitor the osmolarity of the solutions and minimize osmotic shocks. Although neurons osmoregulate, rapid osmolarity changes are detrimental. At present we use Dulbecco's minimum essential medium (Sigma Chemical Co., St. Louis, Mo.) with 5% fetal bovine and 5% horse serum for the cortical tissues, and MEM with 10% fetal bovine and 10% horse serum for the spinal cord cultures.

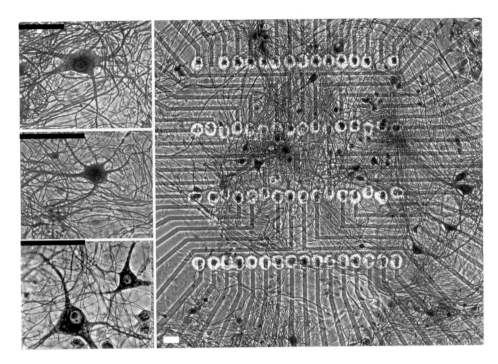

Figure 9.8
Neuronal network on a microelectrode array. Medium-density spinal culture on MEA, 98 days after seeding. Conductors in the recording matrix are 10 μm wide; lateral spacing between electrodes (center to center) is 40 μm.

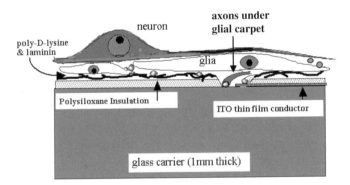

Figure 9.9
Trapping of neurites in recording craters under glia provides optimal recording conditions. In treated cultures, glia do not overgrow neuronal somata, but do grow over neurites in the first few days of network
development on MEAs. ITO, indium tin oxide.

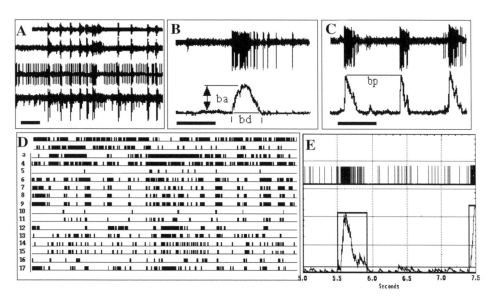

Figure 9.10
Examples of data formats. (*A*) Complex 4-channel, multiunit activity as seen on oscilloscopes. (*B*) and (*C*) Whole-channel integration showing the derivation of the activity variables' burst duration (bd), burst period (bp), and integrated burst amplitude (ba). (*D*) Spike raster display showing multiple simultaneous spike and burst patterns. (*E*) Digital simulation of Resistor-capacitor filter (RC) integration.

Extracellular Recording: Procedures and Data Analysis

MEAs are placed into either sterililized (via autoclaving) constant-bath recording chambers or closed perfusion chambers (Gross and Schwalm, 1994; Gross, 1994) and maintained at 37°C on a microscope stage. For the open-chamber configuration, the pH is maintained at 7.4 with a continuous stream of filtered, humidified, 10% CO_2 in air. Neuronal activity is recorded with a two-stage, 64-channel amplifier system (Plexon Inc., Dallas, Texas), and digitized simultaneously via a Dell 410 workstation (spike analysis) and a Masscomp 5700 computer (burst analysis). Total system gain is normally 10 to 12K. Spike identification and separation is accomplished with a template-matching algorithm (Plexon, Inc.) in real time to provide single-unit spike rate data. In addition, whole-channel (multiple units/channel) data are analyzed offline using custom programs for burst recognition and analysis. Burst patterns derived from spike integration ($\tau = 200$ ms) provide a high signal-to-noise feature extraction that reveals the major modes of neuronal network behavior (Gross, 1994). Using this approach, burst rate, duration, and interburst interval can be quantified from individual recording sites (figure 9.10). Action potentials are stored as time stamps, using the threshold crossing of the negative-going wave. Time stamp data are usually processed in 60-s bins, a convenient measure that allows the plotting of activity variables to show the evolution of network activity patterns over periods of many hours.

Figure 9.11 shows nineteen action potential (AP) wave shapes recorded in a closed flow chamber on day 1 and day 7 after chamber assembly. The flow rate of the medium was 20 µl/min and the culture was not subjected to any pharmacological manipulation. The medium was recirculated into a 15-ml medium supply flask (a totally closed system). It can be seen that the AP shapes are not constant, but undergo slow changes. We assume that this stems from fluctuations in cell-electrode coupling, which is influenced by movement or swelling and shrinking of glial components.

Figure 9.12 demonstrates the stability of basic recording parameters, electrode yield, and signal-to-noise ratios as a function of age. The results are from a recent (1994–2000) database and confirm earlier assertions (Gross, 1994) that there is no major deterioration in these characteristics over 5 months (probably up to 9 months). The scatter of the data, however, is substantial and reflects culture problems, minor experimentation with seeding densities, and mistakes during chamber assembly that lead to cell stress. Most important, sudden osmotic stresses through rapid additions of medium at different osmolarities are common mistakes made by beginning experimenters in this field. The electrophysiological consequences of sudden osmotic shocks should not be underestimated. Optimization of recording conditions (in terms of number of electrodes showing activity) is also reached by the fourth week and stabilizes thereafter (figure 9.13).

Data are observed in both analog and digital formats (figure 9.14). Two to four oscilloscopes are usually employed to monitor the most interesting or most representative channels. In parallel, up to thirty-two channels can be digitized via a Plexon Multiple-Neuron Acquisition Processor system. A real-time spike separation feature allows 4 units to be discriminated and separated (when SNRs are large) so that a maximum of 128 units can be processed simultaneously. A data flow summary is provided in figure 9.14.

The main data display format available at present is shown in figure 9.15. This massive amount of information can be presented in real time and provides an overview of major pattern changes or loss of channels during the course of the experiment. In addition, gross changes in burst durations, phase delays for burst onsets, and some fine structure for spiking within bursts can be observed. However, a simple display of all channels obviously is not the answer to the data-processing problems. It is necessary to select key activity variables and process them quantitatively.

As a first step, a dual graph of spike and burst rates per minute should be available (preferably in real time) to follow the evolution of activity with time during all

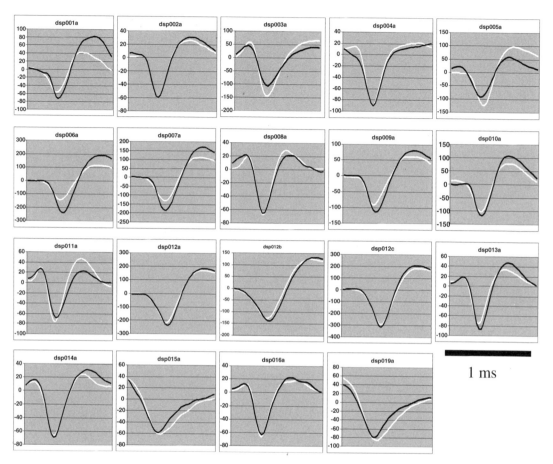

Figure 9.11
Spike signals at individual electrodes over a 7-day period. Each trace represents the mean of forty action potentials recorded on day 1 (white trace) and day 7 (black). Although changes in spike shape occur, they are slow and attributed to gradual rearrangements of glia and/or active neuronal components near the recording site. Both increases and decreases in spike amplitudes occur as a result of this restructuring. Age of culture: 33 days in vitro.

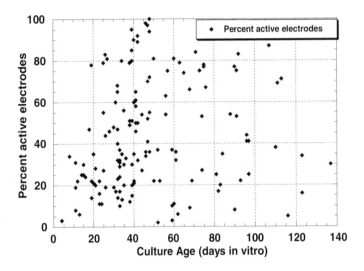

(a)

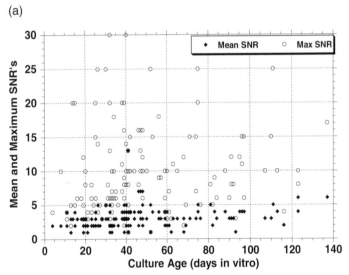

(b)

Figure 9.12
Basic activity parameters as a function of age. (*A*) Percent of functional electrodes with measurable signals
(1.5:1 or greater). (*B*) Signal-to noise ratios (SNRs) as a function of culture age. Neither the electrode yield
nor the maximum mean SNRs show a trend of decreasing with age. The mean SNRs include values of
1.5:1.

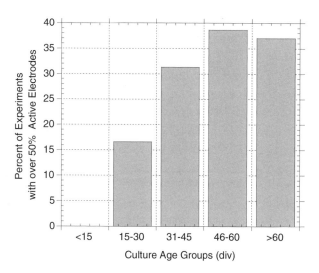

Figure 9.13
Age distribution of results from experiments when more than 50% of the electrodes showed activity. Electrode yield appears to optimize by 4 weeks and become stable over time.

experimental manipulations. We have found bins of 1 min to be a good compromise between plotting too much detail and losing real-time contact with the network. Minute means from all channels with standard deviations allow a minute-to-minute evaluation of network activity and channel variability and an immediate comparison with past network activity. In these bins, activity variables such as spike and burst production remain numbers, whereas other variables such as burst duration, period, and integrated amplitude are averaged and form "minute means."

More quantitative steps can be taken by extracting coefficients of variation (CV) from the minute values for each activity variable. Two types of CVs have been used (Keefer et al., 2001): one that describes the degree of synchronization among channels (termed $CV_{network}$), and one that represents the degree of temporal fluctuation of the burst pattern (termed CV_{time}). The values for $CV_{network}$ are obtained by averaging the binned values (60 s) across all channels, followed by calculations of a new average across time for a particular experimental episode. These for CV_{time} are obtained from activity variables per minute that are averaged for each channel across time (i.e., often the stationary activity domain of an experimental episode), followed by an averaging of the individual channel CVs obtained across all channels (figure 9.16). Hence, if a population is synchronized but the activity varies with time, a low $CV_{network}$ and high CV_{time} are obtained. Conversely, a nonsynchronized network with several simultaneous regular (periodic) patterns yields a high $CV_{network}$ with a

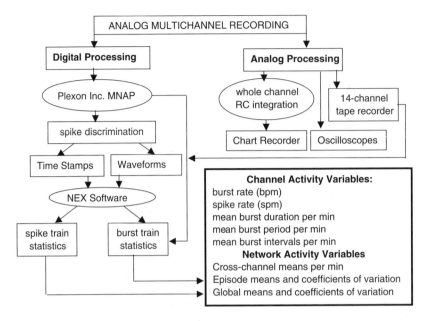

Figure 9.14
Flow chart of digital and analog signal-processing steps. The 64-channel (maximum) analog data are processed digitally via the Plexon Inc. MNAP/NEX software, which allows a multitude of conventional data manipulations. Spike profiles on single channels are usually discriminated, but can also be lumped as whole-channel responses for displays of total spike production and major burst patterns. Parallel analog processing involved display on an 8- or 12-channel chart recorder after RC integration (integration constant approximately 700 ms). Storage on tape is used occasionally to back up the digital processing.

low CV_{time}. In the latter case, each channel could be periodic, but with different periods and patterns on each channel or subsets of channels.

Although the calculation of CVs is an effective tool for quantifying the states of oscillatory networks and burst coordination, which are always seen as steady states during disinhibition (i.e., the blocking of inhibitory synapses), this approach is less effective for describing transient network states. In fact, the recognition and quantification of transient spatiotemporal patterns that are continually generated by networks in vitro present a formidable challenge. Here, extensive application of nonlinear dynamics and sophisticated schemes of pattern recognition will be necessary before substantial progress can be made in dealing with subtle pattern changes in nonlinear and nonstationary systems. However, changes induced by toxins and other neuroactive compounds are generally robust and relatively large in magnitude and therefore quantifiable. Such compounds can be detected rapidly and produce reliable responses. Thus, pharmacological investigations and applications are realistic with present techniques and methods.

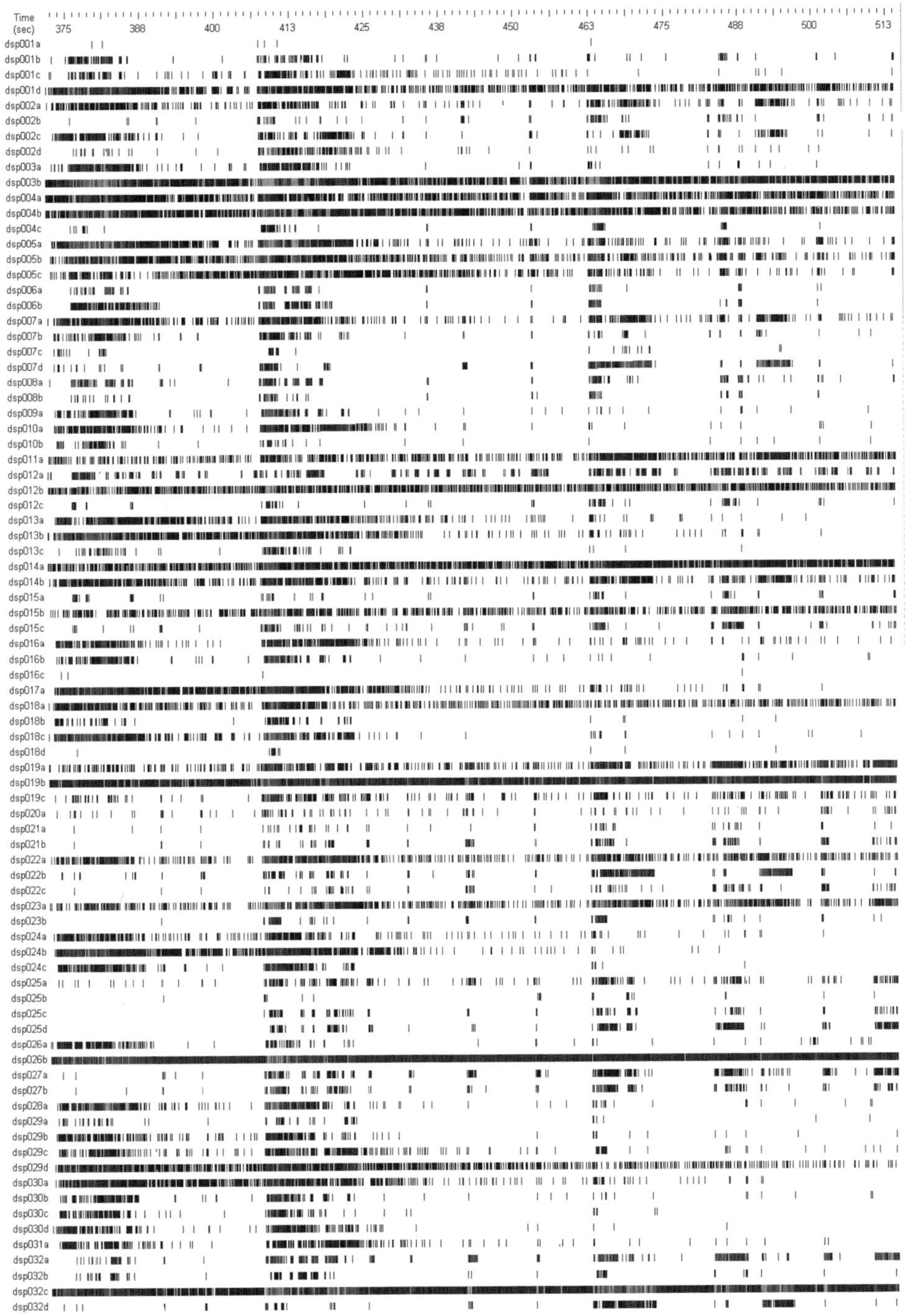

Figure 9.15
Raster display of all spikes from 83 discriminated active units generated by 32 digital signal processors. The width of the panel represents 30 s. Note the coordinated burst patterns on most of the channels and variable phase delays for burst onsets. Spinal cord culture, 48 days in vitro, native activity.

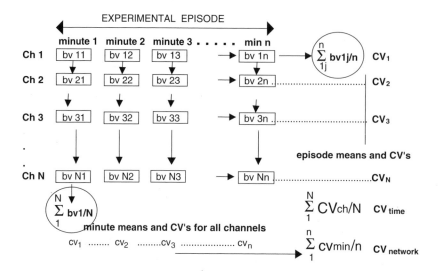

Figure 9.16
Determination of temporal regularity and network synchronization using coefficients of variation (CV). All
calculations are based on 1-min bins where a specific burst variable (bv) is either logged as a number for
burst rate or averaged for burst duration and interburst interval. These values are used to obtain episode
means with CVs for experimental episodes (left/right), or minute means for each minute of the experimental episode (top to bottom). The episode CVs for each channel represent a measure of temporal pattern
fluctuation for that channel. Averaged across the network, these CVs reflect pattern regularity even if several patterns exist and even if they are not synchronized. Conversely, the minute CVs represent channel
coordination. Averaged across the experimental episode, they reflect the degree of synchronization even if
the pattern fluctuates in time. For simplicity, they have been designated CV_{time} and $CV_{network}$, respectively
(from Keefer et al., 2001a).

Applications: Toxicology, Drug Development, and Biosensors

Neuronal cell cultures in vitro are isolated systems for which the culture medium
becomes the extracellular space. Consequently, their chemical or pharmacological
environment can be controlled precisely and kept constant for long periods of time.
Results achieved so far indicate that the networks formed by primary cultures are
pharmacologically histiotypic, that is, they mimic the pharmacological responses of
the parent tissue (Gross, 1994; Gramowski et al., 2000; Morefield et al., 2000). This
behavior of cell cultures allows the development of unique platforms for systematic
investigations of many neurobiological and pharmacological mechanisms. In light
of the now-demonstrated longevity of neurons in culture (6–9 months, Gross, 1994;
Kamioka et al., 1996), such test systems also will allow chronic studies and investigations of developmental influences. Extensive preliminary data suggest this concept is
viable and that responses will be obtained from all substances able to stop or alter
nervous system activity, as well as from general metabolic toxins.

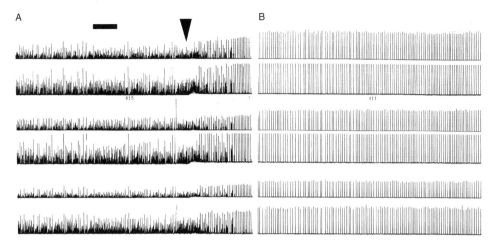

Figure 9.17
Burst pattern changes in response to 100 μM trimethylolpropane phosphate (TMPP) shown with integrated spike data as displayed on a chart recorder. (*A*) Native activity consists of bursts of short and long durations, with irregular burst amplitudes. Within 2 min after application of TMPP to the culture (arrow), the activity transitions to a much more regular and synchronized burst pattern. (*B*) 20 min after TMPP application, the network has reached a quasi-periodic oscillatory state. The bar represents 1 min. The amplitude of the traces is proportional to spike frequencies within bursts.

Figure 9.17 shows a network response to the convulsant trimethylolpropane phosphate (TMPP). Such pattern regularization is typical for compounds that generate epilepsy in mammals and represents a classic disinhibitory response. The blocking of inhibitory synapses such as GABA synapses in frontal cortex tissue or GABA and/or glycine synapses in spinal cord tissue always results in pattern regularization and highly coordinated bursting. Although an increase in spike production is frequently associated with such a response, this is not the salient feature. Excitatory compounds such as glutamate or NMDA increase spike production but never generate such regular burst patterns. Hence any unknown compound that generates the response shown in figure 9.17 can be classified with high reliability as a potential convulsant.

In contrast to the excitation and pattern regularization shown in figure 9.17, many compounds terminate activity reversibly or irreversibly. The manner in which activity terminates is substance specific (Gross et al., 1997a,b) and may be used to identify or at least classify a substance. An example of activity termination is shown in figure 9.18. While testing a set of novel acetylcholinesterase (AChE) blockers (Keefer et al., 2001b) that were expected to increase activity in cultures derived from frontal cortex tissue, two of seven substances inhibited activity irreversibly. Such unexpected responses reflect secondary binding that is difficult to predict biochemically.

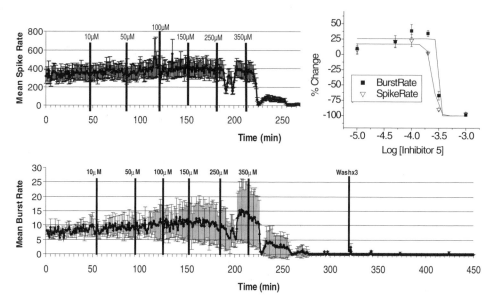

Figure 9.18
Irreversible inhibition of network activity in response to acctylcholinesterase blocker (inhibitor 5). (*A*) Mean ± SD of 28 discriminated units. Titration to 200 μM produces very little effect on spike rates; raising the concentration to 350 μM causes a rapid reduction in spiking. All spike activity is abolished within approximately 30 min. (*B*) The effect on spike rates is paralleled by inhibition of burst rate (mean ± SD of 12 channels). However, the standard deviation of the burst rates begins to increase at 50 μM, indicating a lessened cross-channel coordination. The inhibition was not reversible by three complete changes of medium at 320 min (from Keefer et al., 2001b).

Spontaneously active networks, as pharmacologically functional systems that contain the synaptic mechanisms present in the parent tissue, reveal the effects of all binding sites targeted by the new compound and are therefore predictors of physiological responses.

Figure 9.18 displays the mean spike rates ± SD from twenty-eight discriminated units (A) and mean burst rates from a subset of twelve channels (B) as a function of time, and shows the termination of activity after application of 350 μM of a choline compound with a six-carbon hexylene spacer (Keefer et al., 2000). Three complete changes of medium at 320–325 min did not reactivate the network. After 2 hr of observation, the loss of spontaneous activity was considered "irreversible." The insert shows the dose-response curves for the inhibition of spiking and bursting activity, with median effective concentration (EC_{50}) values of 260 and 340 μM, respectively. It is also interesting to note that the standard deviations remain constant for spike production, but increase substantially for network bursting activity. This reflects a loss of coordination among channels that starts right after the application of 10 μM at 55 min.

Network responses are highly specific and not all compounds produce alterations in the spontaneous activity. This is illustrated in figure 9.19, which summarizes responses to nerve gas hydrolysis products. Isopropyl methylphosphonate (IMP) and methylphosphonate (MP) are metabolites of sarin; pinacolyl methylphosphonate (PMP) is a breakdown product of soman. Panel A shows that IMP decreased spike production by an average of 37% ($n = 3$ cultures) at 5 mM, without significantly altering burst rates. A 72-hr chronic exposure to 6 mM IMP (arrow) produced no visible cytotoxicity or significant loss of network activity. Test responses to the NMDA receptor antagonist APV and to 20 μM bicuculline (BIC) were normal. However, a lack of recovery of higher spike rates after a medium change at 0 is unexplained. Panel B reveals that increasing concentrations of MP up to 5 mM did not change bursting or spiking during acute exposures. In contrast, PMP (panel C) inhibited both bursting and spiking at concentrations above 2 mM. The loss of activity was not associated with observable cytotoxicity, and was reversible by washing.

Such results, together with the monitoring of cells through the light microscope, imply that none of these nerve gas metabolites are toxic, but some are neuroactive at high concentrations. These results were already deduced from animal experiments (Brown and Brix, 1998; Munro et al., 1999), and the compounds discussed here are listed as irritants in chemical catalogs. We have used them to illustrate the reliability of the physiological predictions; networks neither exaggerate nor dismiss the effects of toxic or neuroactive chemicals. They respond to concentrations at which animals also show effects. It is interesting to speculate if better methods of pattern recognition would provide early warning at lower concentrations. This is entirely possible, but has not yet been demonstrated.

Research in the past 3 years has also demonstrated that with the proper life support, it is feasible to use networks as tissue-based biosensors. In this role, the networks are not artificial "olfactory systems," but rather "function deficit detectors" that respond reliably to all compounds capable of interfering with the normal neuronal function of an organism. Such interference can occur on several levels: metabolic, synaptic and nonsynaptic channels, and cytotoxic. The network mirrors the physiological changes that occur in intact nervous systems. Although a termination of activity is the easiest change to detect, epileptiform states (as demonstrated in figure 9.17) and even responses to mind-altering drugs, such as the cannabinoid mimetics anandamide and methanandamide (Morefield at al., 2000), can be detected and classified. Networks are not supersensitive; responses occur at concentrations similar to those that cause effects in animals (Gramowski et al., 2000; Morefield et al., 2000; Keefer et al., 2001a). As a consequence, they do not generate false positives because of high sensitivities, but report the presence of compounds at concentrations that will affect the nervous systems of mammals.

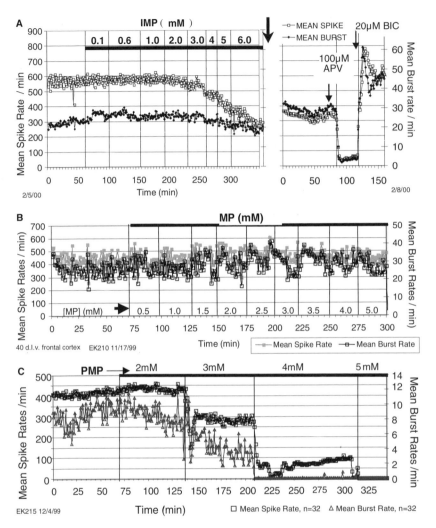

Figure 9.19
Differential effects of nerve gas hydrolysis products. IMP (isopropyl methylphosphonate) and MP (methyl-phosphonate) are metabolites of sarin; PMP (pinacolyl methylphosphonate) is a breakdown product of soman. (*A*) IMP decreased spike production by an average of 37% (*n* = 3) at 5 mM, without significantly altering burst rates. A 72-hr constant exposure to 6 mM IMP (arrow) produced no visible cytotoxicity or significant loss of network activity. The culture still responded normally to test applications of D-2-amino-5-phosphonovaleric acid (APV, stopped the activity) and bicuculline (BIC, return to a bursting state.) (*B*) 5-mM MP did not change either bursting or spiking during acute exposures. (*C*) PMP inhibited both bursting and spiking at concentrations above 2 mM. The loss of activity was not associated with observable cytotoxicity and was reversible by washing.

Summary

Spontaneously active networks growing on microelectrode arrays are effective "test-beds" for a large number of investigations. Cell-surface adhesion and cell-electrode coupling, tissue survival, and the dynamics of cellular interactions with nonbiological materials and even with special geometries can all be studied quantitatively in vitro. Local stimulation through recording electrodes is possible, with responses often exciting the entire network (Gross et al., 1993; Gross, 1994). Although the three-dimensional environment of tissue in vivo is more difficult to mimic in culture, it is important to note that even optically observable "monolayers" are shallow three-dimensional constructs. Also, all implants, regardless of their structural complexity, will have surfaces to which tissue must adhere. Finally, three-dimensional growth of tissue in culture is being investigated (O'Connor et al., 2000) with confocal microscopy so that cellular dynamics in thick tissue layers can also be studied.

At present, it appears that data processing and display in a multichannel environment may be the most complex and most challenging of all remaining problems in implanted prostheses. Although substantial progress has already been achieved with implanted electrodes in behaving animals (Sasaki et al., 1989; Wilson and Mc-Naughton, 1993; Nicolelis et al., 1998; Chapin, 1998; Hampson and Deadwyler, 1998), cultured networks generally provide a larger number of channels over a longer period of time. Also, they are well suited for investigating the internal dynamics of small networks because of the high electrode density that can be achieved without causing tissue disruption. This allows investigation of structure and function relationships, pattern generation and processing, fault tolerance, and even storage mechanisms. Networks in culture provide experimentally simple and highly economical test-beds for exploring the frontiers of multichannel data processing.

As isolated systems, networks in culture allow quantitative, repeated pharmacological manipulations over long periods of time. In this domain, response repeatability is remarkable because the networks react to molecules introduced into the medium, which simultaneously affects all target receptors or other binding sites. Indications of tissue specificity (Morefield et al., 2000) complicate applications, but also reflect a welcome retention of parent tissue characteristics in culture. These network properties immediately suggest the development of massively parallel systems for systematic screening and evaluation of compounds for toxicity and neuroactive and pharmacological potential. Finally, as a consequence of their pharmacological sensitivity and reliable neurophysiological responses, networks can be used to provide early warning of the presence of chemical toxicants. The networks represent broadband sensors that react to known and unknown compounds that have the capability of altering the performance of nervous system functions.

References

Bailey, C. H., Chen, M., Keller, F., and Kandel, E. R. (1992) Serotonin-mediated endocytosis of apCAM: An early step of learning-related synaptic growth in *Aplysia*. *Science* 256: 645–649.

Bodian, D. (1936) A new method for staining nerve fibers and nerve endings in mounted paraffin sections. *Anat. Rec.* 65: 89–97.

Brown, M. A., and Brix, K. A. (1998) Review of health consequences from high-, intermediate and low-level exposure to organophosphorus nerve agents. *J. Appl. Toxicol.* 18: 393–408.

Chapin, J. K. (1998) Population-level analysis of multi-single neuron recording data: Multivariate statistical methods. In M. A. L. Nicolelis, ed., *Methods for Neural Ensemble Recordings*. Boca Raton, Fla.: CRC Press, pp. 193–228.

Doherty, P., and Walsh, F. S. (1992) Cell adhesion molecules, second messengers and axonal growth. *Curr. Opin. Neurobiol.* 2: 595–601.

Goslin, K., Asmussen, H., and Banker, G. (1998) Rat hippocampal neurons in low-density culture. In G. Banker and K. Goslin, eds., *Culturing Nerve Cells*. Cambridge, Mass.: MIT Press, pp. 339–370.

Gramowski, A., Schiffmann, D., and Gross, G. W. (2000) Quantification of acute neurotoxic effects of trimethyltin using neuronal networks cultured on microelectrode arrays. *Neurotoxicology* 21: 331–342.

Gross, G. W. (1979) Simultaneous single unit recording in vitro with a photoetched laser deinsulated gold multi-microelectrode surface. *IEEEE Trans. Biomed. Eng.* BME-26: 73–279.

Gross, G. W. (1994) Internal dynamics of randomized mammalian neuronal networks in culture. In D. A. Stenger and T. M. McKenna, eds., *Enabling Technologies for Cultured Neural Networks*. New York: Academic Press, pp. 277–317.

Gross, G. W., and Kowalski, J. M. (1991) Experimental and theoretical analysis of random nerve cell network dynamics. In P. Antogenetti and V. Milutinovic, eds., *Neural Networks: Concepts, Applications, and Implementations*, vol. 4. Englewood Cliffs, N.J.: Prentice-Hall, pp. 47–110.

Gross, G. W., and Lucas, J. H. (1982) Long-term monitoring of spontaneous single unit activity from neuronal monolayer networks cultured on photoetched multielectrode surfaces. *J. Electrophys. Tech.* 9: 55–69.

Gross, G. W., and Schwalm, F. U. (1994) A closed chamber for long-term electrophysiological and microscopical monitoring of monolayer neuronal networks. *J. Neurosci. Meth.* 52: 73–85.

Gross, G. W., Wen, W., and Lin, J. (1985) Transparent indium-tin oxide patterns for extracellular, multisite recording in neuronal cultures. *J. Neurosci. Meth.* 15: 243–252.

Gross, G. W., Rhoades, B. K., Reust, D. L., and Schwalm, F. U. (1993) Stimulation of monolayer networks in culture through thin-film indium-tin oxide recording electrodes. *J. Neurosci. Meth.* 50: 131–143.

Gross, G. W., Harsch, A., Rhoades, B. K., and Göpel, W. (1997a) Odor, drug, and toxin analysis with neuronal networks in vitro: Extracellular array recording of network responses. *Bisosensors Bioelectron.* 12: 373–393.

Gross, G. W., Norton, S., Gopal, K., Schiffmann, D., and Gramowski, A. (1997b) Nerve cell network in vitro: Applications to neurotoxicology, drug development, and biosensors. In *The Neuro-Electronic Interface. Cellular Engineering* 2: 138–147.

Hampson, R. E., and Deadwyler, S. A. (1998) Pitfalls and problems in the analysis of neuronal ensemble recordings during behavioral tasks. In M. A. L. Nicolelis, ed., *Methods for Neural Ensemble Recordings*. Boca Raton, Fla.: CRC Press, pp. 229–248.

Harsch, A., Calderon, J., Timmons, R. B., and Gross, G. W. (2000) Pulsed plasma deposition of allylamine on polysiloxane: A stable surface for neuronal cell adhesion. *J. Neurosci. Meth.* 98: 135–144.

Kamioka, H., Maeda, E., Jimbo, Y., Robinson, H. P., and Kawana, A. (1996) Spontaneous periodic synchronized bursting during formation of mature patterns of connections in cortical cultures. *Neurosci. Lett.* 15: 109–112.

Keefer, E. W., Gramowski, A., and Gross, G. W. (2001a) NMDA receptor dependent periodic oscillations in cultured spinal cord networks. *J. Neurophysiol.* 86: 3030–3042.

Keefer, E. W., Norton, S. J., Boyle, N. A. J., Talesa, V., and Gross, G. W. (2001b) Acute toxicity screening of novel AChE inhibitors using neuronal networks on microelectrode arrays. *Neurotoxicology* 22: 3–12.

Kreutzberg, G. W. (1987) Microglia. In *Encyclopedia of Neuroscience*, G. Adelman, ed., Cambridge, Mass.: Birkhauser, pp. 661–662.

Liu, J., Skradis, A., Kolar, C., Kilath, J., Anderson, J., Lawson, T., Talmadge, J., and Gmeiner, H. (1999) Increased cytotoxicity and decreased in vivo toxicity of FdUMP[10] relative to 5-FDU. *Nucleosides Nucleotides* 18: 1789–1802.

Loots, G. P., Loots, J. M., Brown, J. M. M., and Schoeman, J. L. (1979) A rapid silver impregnation method for nervous tissue: A modified protargol-peroxide technique. *Stain Technol.* 54: 97–101.

Lucas, J. H., Czisny, L. E., and Gross, G. W. (1986) Adhesion of cultured mammalian CNS neurons to flame-modified hydrophobic surfaces. *In Vitro Cell Dev. Biol.* 22: 37–43.

Lucas, J. L., and Wolf, A. (1991) In vitro studies of multiple impact injury to mammalian CNS neurons: Prevention of perikaryal damage and death by ketamine. *Brain Res.* 543: 181–193.

Mayford, M., Barzilai, A., Keller, F., Schacher, S., and Kandel, E. R. (1992) Protein, nucleotide modulation of an NCAM-related adhesion molecule with long-term synaptic plasticity in *Aplysia. Science* 256: 638–644.

Morefield, S. I., Keefer, E. W., Chapman, K. D., and Gross, G. W. (2000) Drug evaluations using neuronal networks cultured on microelectrode arrays. *Biosensors Bioelectron.* 15: 383–396.

Munro, N. B., Talmage, S. S., Griffin, G. D., Waters, L. C., Watson, A. P., King, J. F., and Hauschild, V. (1999) The sources, fate, and toxicity of chemical warfare agent degradation products. *Environ. Health Perspect.* 107: 933–874.

Nicolelis, M. A., Ghazanfar, A. A., Stambaugh, C. R., Oliveira, L. M., Laubach, M., Chapin, J. K., Nelson, R. J., and Kaas, J. H. (1998) Simultaneous encoding of tactile information by three primate cortical areas. *Nature Neurosci.* 1: 621–630.

O'Connor, S. M., Andreadis, J. D., Shaffer, K. M., Pancrazio, J. J., and Stenger, D. A. (2000) *Biosensors Bioelectron.* 14: 871–881.

Perry, V. H., and Gordon, S. (1988) Macrophages and microglia in the nervous system. *Trends Neurosci.* 11: 273–277.

Pigott, R., and Power, C. (1993) *The Adhesion Molecule Facts Book*. New York: Academic Press.

Potter S. M., and DeMarse, T. B. (2001) A new approach to neuronal cell culture for long-term studies. *J. Neurosci. Math.* 110: 17–24.

Ransom, B. R., Neile, E., Henkart, M., Bullock, P. N., and Nelson, P. G. (1977) Mouse spinal cord in cell culture. *J. Neurophysiol.* 40: 1132–1150.

Sasaki, K., Bower, J. M., and Llinas, R. (1989) Multiple Purkinje cell recording in rodent cerebellar cortex. *European J. Neurosci.* 1: 572–581.

Segal, M. M., Baughman, R. W., Jones, K. A., and Huettner, J. E. (1998) Mass cultures and microislands of neurons from postnatal rat brain. In G. Banker and K. Goslin, eds., *Culturing Nerve Cells*. Cambridge, Mass.: MIT Press, pp. 309–338.

Streit, W. J. (1995) Microglial cells. In H. Kettenmann and B. R. Ransom, eds., *Neuroglia*. New York: Oxford University Press, pp. 85–96.

Wilson, M. A., and McNaughton, B. L. (1993) Dynamics of the hippocampal ensemble code for space. *Science* 261: 1055–1058.

Whithers, G. S., and Banker, G. (1998) Characterizing and studying neuronal cultures. In G. Banker and K. Goslin, eds., *Culturing Nerve Cells*. Cambridge, Mass.: MIT Press, pp. 113–152.

10 Building Minimalistic Hybrid Neuroelectric Devices

James J. Hickman

The objective of our research efforts is to learn how to handle and prepare cells to serve as components for microdevices and engineered tissues, and then to demonstrate the practicality of this approach by manipulating them to build hybrid systems and engineer functional tissues. We are developing test-beds based on the signals generated between two neurons that can react to changes in the neuronal circuit's environment. Since it will be necessary to predict the outputs of the neuronal circuits in the test-beds, which will depend on geometry, synapse placement, and cell phenotype(s), we have modeled various circuit configurations as well. The ability to control the surface composition of an in vitro system, as well as other variables, such as growth media and cell preparation, plays an important role in creating a defined system for fabricating a hybrid device and in vitro evaluation of surface modifications and their effect on cellular materials.

We have reproducibly created patterned neuronal circuits and shown that we can successfully measure the signals from these circuits in our defined in vitro culture system (Das et al., 2003; Ravenscroft et al., 1998). We have also modeled modes of cell-cell communication that could be monitored and investigated the electrical properties of the neuronal circuits in contact with the designed biological interfaces in these systems (Peterson, 2001; Jung et al., 1998; Ravenscroft et al., 1998). One application of this concept is for drug development or new biomedical diagnostics. These function-based test-beds could also detect drug efficacy or toxicity through effects ranging from the obvious (cell death) to those that are more subtle (impairment of function). This wide range of responses can be measured because cells and the networks they form are exceedingly sensitive to certain changes in their environment.

We have developed surface chemistry that can be used to create templates that enable the patterning of discrete cells and networks of cells in culture (Stenger et al., 1998; Ravenscroft et al., 1998); the networks can then be aligned with transducers. This advance allows the construction of a test-bed that measures changes in the potential of cells and/or their processes. Thus, any changes in the electrical signals upon exposure to a compound could be detected. Other types of sensors currently in use or under development include ion-sensitive electrodes (Solsky, 1990; Uhlig et al., 1997) sensors based on antibody binding (Aizawa, 1991; Bernard and Bosshard, 1995), living cells (Parce et al., 1989; Leech and Rechnitz, 1993), and other types (Hughes et al., Edelman and Wang, 1991). Most assays rely on the fact that the agonist is known and are targeted for a specific compound. Preliminary work has been reported on measuring signals from neurons using solid-state devices (Regher et al., 1989; Fromherz et al., 1991; Jung et al., 1998; Offenhausser and Knoll, 2001; Gross et al., 1997). However, sensors that can determine a compound's efficacy or toxicity that affects motor function, cognitive function, or other higher-order processes are primitive or do not exist. At present, the only available "test-beds" based on cognitive or motor function are living creatures. It would be beneficial to develop sensors to function as precursors to these epidemiological studies.

In vitro cell cultures of embryonic rat tissue have been used to study rudimentary cellular organization and communication. Neurons in culture are generally disorganized in the sense that the connections between the cells are not controllable. Historically, this has made it difficult to relate specific signals to specific functions, as well as to make the system reproducible. If one could control the connections between living neurons, new paradigms in in vitro cellular networks could be realized. A major benefit would come from sorting out all of these complex connections and arrangements and making them reproducible. We are using a reductionist approach to in vitro cellular networks by using the minimum number of neurons to construct simple reproducible circuits and connecting them to silicon devices. These new hybrid neuroelectric devices can then be connected in a multitude of configurations, much like the components and devices that comprise computational devices.

The most difficult tasks in developing the fabrication protocol are controlling the placement of neurons, the processes, and the number and placement of synapses. Building a network composed of neurons into the preferred synaptic configuration requires high-resolution surface patterns that guide the geometry and outgrowth of the elements of the circuit. The use of hippocampal neurons is of particular interest for studies of cell-cell communication because the hippocampus is thought to play a central role in learning and memory function. It is known that the ability of neuronal processes to extend to their targets is dependent on adhesion to underlying substrata, which in vivo appears to be spatially and temporally patterned. The ability to culture mammalian neurons on patterned substrata would allow the investigation, and possible control, of the factors involved in the formation of basic neuronal circuits.

The use of surface modification techniques allows the interface between biological and nonbiological materials to be tailored independently of the bulk composition of the nonbiological material. We are using SAMs to control the intrinsic and geometric properties of surfaces in contact with biological systems. A self-assembled monolayer (SAM) is a modifying layer composed of organic molecules, one molecule thick, that can spontaneously form strong interactions or covalent bonds with reactive groups on an exposed surface. The utilization of SAMs for modifying surfaces has been demonstrated on silicon dioxide (Stenger et al., 1992), biodegradable polymers (Hickman et al., 1993), and other polymers such as Teflon (Vargo et al., 1992). A large variety of functional groups or a combination of functional groups can be located on the terminal opposite the attachment point of a SAM, and the chemical composition can be manipulated to systematically vary the surface free energy (Stenger et al., 1992). We have used the geometric control of the surface composition afforded by SAMs to create in vitro circuits of mammalian neurons (Stenger et al., 1998).

Patterning of surfaces to control the growth of neurons and other cells in culture has been achieved by numerous investigators (Stenger et al., 1992; Vargo et al., 1992; Cooper et al., 1976; Hammarback et al., 1985; Kleinfeld et al., 1988; Corey et al., 1991; Singhvi et al., 1994; St. John et al., 1997; Stenger et al., 1998; Ravenscroft et al., 1998) and most important, several photolithographic methods utilizing SAMs have emerged that allow high-resolution patterning for biological applications (Stenger et al., 1992; Kleinfeld et al., 1988; Corey et al., 1991; Singhvi et al., 1994; St. John et al., 1997; Stenger et al., 1998; Ravenscroft et al., 1998). We have demonstrated functional control of these systems by recording the electrophysiological signals produced by neurons on the patterned SAMs in response to stimuli, successfully modeled the neuronal networks, and demonstrated geometric control of synaptic development (Ravenscroft et al., 1998). In addition, geometric only cues have been used to define axonal-dendrite polarity in developing hippocampal neurons, which is a key step in creating engineered neuronal networks (Stenger et al., 1998). The surfaces have been characterized by X-ray photoelectron spectroscopy (XPS), imaging XPS, and contact-angle measurements.

A key requirement for fabricating a test-bed from rudimentary circuits is that the neuronal cultures be located in a defined environment. By this we mean that in order to reproducibly determine how factors and modifications affect a system, it is important to have as many conditions defined as possible. It is also necessary to be able to assay the effect of unknown samples that may contain toxic compounds. The use of serum-free media in combination with the SAM surface modifications allows systematic investigation of optimal growth conditions for different neurons or combinations of neurons. In previous work, we studied the effect of maintaining hippocampal neurons in medium containing serum and in serum-free medium, while varying the nature of the culture plate surface, dissociation methods, and other factors. The results reported in Schaffner et al. (1995) established a good in vitro model for hippocampal culture.

We have found that by analyzing the surface through all phases of modification, it is possible to establish a cell culture system in which the surface composition and geometry, growth medium, and cell preparation method are reproducible and defined. The ability to define these characteristics enables the fabrication and study of neuronal circuits in a controlled environment. In conjunction with our continuing patterning work, we have determined some of the possible modes of communication between cells and constructed models of simple logic circuits to test our hypothesis that sensors can be based on cell-cell communication.

Patterning Neuronal Circuits

The complete experimental details for the neuronal patterning and electrophysiology can be found in Ravenscroft et al. (1998). The metal microelectrode recording details can be found in Jung et al. (1998). The modeling parameters are described here for clarity.

An analysis of the surface both before and after culture, as well as X-ray photo-electron spectroscopy imaging of the patterns as the laser conditions were varied, was crucial to understanding the effect of different combinations of fabrication variables. Optimized high-resolution circuit patterns successfully guided the neuronal adhesion and neurite outgrowth of E18–19 hippocampal neurons in a defined serum-free medium as shown in figure 10.1A (Ravenscroft et al., 1998).

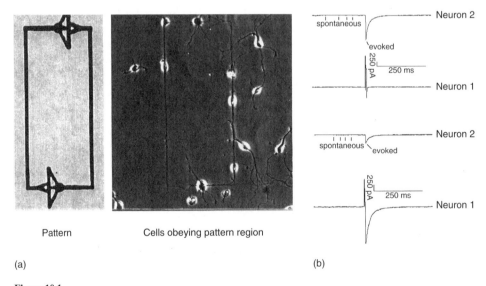

Pattern   Cells obeying pattern region

(a)   (b)

Figure 10.1
(*a*) Micrograph of circuit-patterned day 2 in vitro hippocampal neurons plated onto DETA/15F modified glass coverslips. (*b*) Electrophysiology of day 12 in vitro hippocampal neurons displaying both spontaneous and evoked activity on a DETA/15F line-space patterned surface. The top two traces are the control, and the bottom two are from the circuit pattern. Neuron 1, stimulated presynaptic neuron. Neuron 2, postsynaptic neuron.

We have successfully recorded from the patterned neurons using dual patch-clamp electrophysiology (figure 10.1B). With the dual patch-clamp technique, we monitored the emergence of spontaneous (single-cell) and evoked (two-cell) synaptic activity for both the patterned and unpatterned (control) neuronal cultures. The electrophysiology trace from neuron 2 represents the postsynaptic neuron, and neuron 1 the electrophysiology trace for the stimulated presynaptic neuron. No evoked electrophysiology data were obtained for day 8 hippocampal neurons on a circuit-patterned surface.

These results suggest that synapses form on the pattern at different rates than in random undissociated cultures, which suggests a geometry-mediated development of synaptic events. This indicates that we may be able to control synaptic development by controlling the cell growth parameters and surface geometry. This makes sense when you consider data that show most neurons remain "plastic" or are capable of synaptic change during their lifetime.

Another important issue is how to orient the neurons once they are placed in the correct position. Much like an electronic transistor, not only the construction but the orientation of the device is critical for function. Banker and Cowan (1977) showed that the longest neurite from a developing embryonic neuron would become the axon. Our hypothesis was that if we gave the neurites many paths, but put "speed bumps" on all but one path, this would be sufficient to make the unimpeded neurite the axon. Figure 10.2 (left to right) shows the mask pattern used; a micrograph of a neuron plated on this pattern using DETA as the permissive surface and 13F as the repulsive surface; immunocytochemical labeling with anti-MAP-5 primary

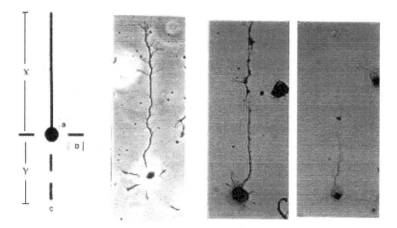

Figure 10.2
Directional axonal outgrowth by geometric manipulation of a surface as well as immunocytochemical identification of the axon and dendrites.

antibody for axonal identification; and labeling with anti-MAP-2 for dendrites and the cell body. This experiment indicates that polarity can also be achieved by geometric means alone (Stenger et al., 1998).

The accurate spatial placement of a neuronal cell network allows a wide spectrum of circuit and fabrication technology to be applied to the detection of signals transmitted within the network. Preliminary work by Fromherz et al. (1991) demonstrated that field-effect transistors (FETs) can detect changes in membrane potential from cell bodies. We have also developed an electronic interface to a microelectrode chip and have successfully tested it by recording electrical activity from single unpatterned hippocampal neurons using metal microelectrodes (Jung et al., 1998). The neurons were grown on a silicon nitride (Si_3N_4)-coated microelectrode, and the signals were recorded from gold microelectrodes in serum-free media. This demonstrates that we can culture the cells in a defined media on the Si_3N_4 surface and record the signals, and that the electronic interface can process and display the electrophysiological signals. The results demonstrate that the signals produced by the mammalian cells are strong enough to be picked up by the electrodes, and the signal-to-noise ratio can approach that achieved with patch-clamp electrophysiology. We have also shown that the cells' activity can be attenuated by the introduction of a toxin to the in vitro environment, which is experimental proof of concept for the sensor (data not shown). This result demonstrates the feasibility of using the sensor to evaluate drug candidates if we can establish the modes of cell-cell communication that could be monitored as an indicator of cell function.

Modeling Cell-Cell Communication

We believe that there will be different modes of operation of the system based on the number and location of synapses, which will permit the fabrication of neuroelectric devices with distinct input-output relationships. To address this question, preliminary simulations of simple two-neuron circuits were made using the neural modeling program GENESIS (Wilson et al., 1989; Bower and Beeman, 1998; Peterson, 2001). In these models, the interaction between an excitatory and an inhibitory neuron was simulated. For the sake of simplicity, both current injection and voltage measurements were performed at the soma of each neuron, as represented by the microelectrodes in figure 10.3. We typically ran the modeling experiments using current injection on both neurons. The full details of these simulations can be found in Peterson (2001). Characterization of the neuronal model example includes (1) examination of the time response of each circuit branch, (2) verification of the reproducibility of the model network's synaptic connections, and (3) verification of circuit behavior and properties over time in culture.

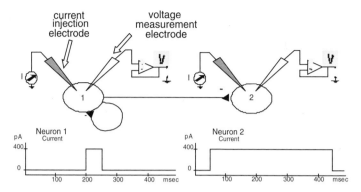

Figure 10.3
Basic setup for dual patch-clamp electrophysiological recordings from simple neuronal circuits.

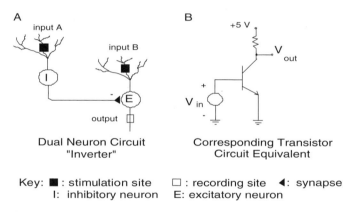

Figure 10.4
(*A*) First circuit model and (*B*) a corresponding transistor logic circuit.

Circuit 1

The circuit model (figure 10.4A) consists of an inhibitory neuron forming a single synaptic connection on the cell body of an excitatory neuron. With appropriately chosen stimuli, this simple circuit can produce distinctive behavior, as demonstrated by the simulation efforts in figure 10.5. For example, a constant stimulation train applied at input B would be gated based on the state of input A. Stimulation of input A would inhibit the transmission of excitation, whereas the lack of stimulation of input A would permit the propagation of excitability. The behavior of this circuit model is similar to that of a simple transistor-logic circuit where the state of the transistor gate influences circuit output (figure 10.4B). Furthermore, this circuit model is the core element of a circuit to explain directional selectivity in the mammalian retina

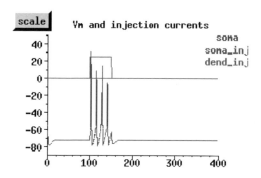

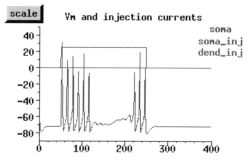

Figure 10.5
Voltage traces for neurons L1 (*top*) and R1 (*bottom*). The synaptic connection from L1 to R1 is inhibitory and is set at a weight of 600. For 100 ms, cell R1 received no somatic current input and then a constant pulse soma input of 0.00025 μA was applied for 50 ms and then turned off. Cell L1 received a similar pulse, which started later and lasted for 200 ms.

(Barlow and Levick, 1965) and thalamocortical processing of visual information (Douglas et al., 1991; Douglas and Martin, 1991). With a stimulus moving in the nonpreferred direction (A to B), the inhibition decreases the excitability of the post-synaptic excitatory neuron, whereas in the preferred direction, excitation passes freely (Anton et al., 1992). As a result, the action potential's amplitude may carry information on stimulus strength, providing the basis for a principle in the mamma-lian nervous system for multilevel logic.

In the experiment we employed two neurons (the top is L1 and the bottom is R1) with standard sodium (Na) and potassium (K) channels and linked the two cells with an inhibitory connection from the cell L1 to the cell R1. The simulation was done in GENESIS using simple Hodgkins dynamics with the following results:

· Cell L1 turns on 50 ms after R1 and, after a delay, inhibits the output of cell R1.
· Once cell L1 turns off, after a delay, the output of cell R1 resumes.

We have simulated this circuit, and as seen in figure 10.5, the inhibition from neuron L1 inactivates the neuron R1 output as expected. While this simulation dem-

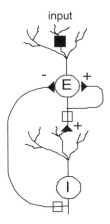

Figure 10.6
Circuit modeling illustrating excitatory train suppression.

onstrates the behavior of a binary device, neuronal circuits such as these are capable of much more complex processing, including temporal integration of asynchronous inputs. We speculate that two aspects of complexity may emerge upon examination of patterned neuronal circuits. First, synaptic connections may undergo long-term potentiation (LTP) or long-term depression (LTD), which require substantial and persistent postsynaptic activity (Juusola et al., 1996). Thus, LTP or LTD would create use-dependent alterations in synaptic strength to affect information processing. Second, there is evidence of the use of graded, rather than "all-or-nothing," action potentials to transmit information in many neurons, including cultured rat hippocampus (Johansson and Arhem, 1990). These could then form the basis for signals that could be modeled and used in determining drug efficacy and toxicity.

Circuit 2

The second circuit model (figure 10.6), in response to a stimulus, produces an excitatory output train, which is then suppressed by the downstream inhibitory neuron. The length of the excitation train would depend on the propagation delay of the inhibitory feedback loop. This particular neuronal model is the key component of a winner-take-all (WTA) circuit that has been characterized in the layer II olfactory cortex (Van Hoesen and Pandya, 1975) and in cutaneous mechanoreception in skin (Van Hoesen and Pandya, 1975), and may have an important role in perceptual decision making in primates (Gardner and Palmer, 1989). In addition, this circuit bears a strong resemblance to the Renshaw cell-spinal motor neuron circuit, where activation of the motor neuron excites the inhibitory Renshaw cell, which then slows or stops the discharge rate of the motor neuron (Van Keulen, 1979). The ion channel settings for the neurons were the same as those in the earlier examples.

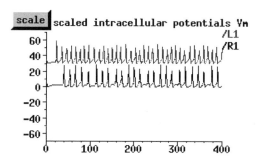

Figure 10.7
Triggered cell output for cells L1 (*top*) and R1 (*bottom*).

We started with the following synaptic connections: a self-excitatory connection on L1 of weight 40 plus a small excitatory connection to R1 of weight 40. R1 does not connect back to L1 at this time. We now allow cell L1 to excite cell R1:

• For 20 ms, cell L1 receives no somatic current input, and then a constant pulse soma input of 0.00025 μA is applied for 380 ms. Cell L1 is strongly connected to cell R1 with excitatory connections, so in the absence of any inhibitory feedback from cell R1, we expected the output from cell L1 to trigger a corresponding output in cell R1.

• Cell R1 received no somatic current and had no synaptic connections with cell L1.

We expected cell R1 to turn on and pulse with a frequency similar to that of cell L1. This was indeed what we observed. The L1 voltage and input current trace can be seen in figure 10.5 (we used the same L1 settings for the rest of the simulation experiments in this section, so the graph is not repeated). The L1 and R1 membrane voltage traces are shown in figure 10.7. It was seen clearly that the output from L1 triggers R1's output.

Now we added the desired inhibition from cell R1 of weight 4000 and ran the simulation as follows:

• For 20 ms, cell L1 receives no somatic current input and then a constant pulse soma input of 0.00025 μA is applied for 380 ms. Cell L1 is strongly connected to cell R1 with excitatory connections, so in the absence of any inhibitory feedback from cell R1, we expected the output from cell L1 to trigger a corresponding output in cell R1.

• Cell R1 received no somatic current and had a large inhibitory synaptic connection with cell L1.

We expected cell R1 to turn on and pulse with a frequency similar to that of cell L1, but the inhibition from R1 shut down L1. The traces of the cell L1 and cell R1

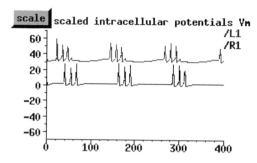

Figure 10.8
Output shutdown caused by inhibition.

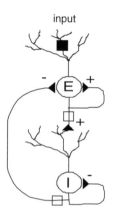

Figure 10.9
Circuit modeling illustrating reactivation via self-inhibition.

voltages are seen in figure 10.8. It is clear that the inhibition from R1 to L1 shuts down the output from L1.

Circuit 3

The third neuronal circuit (figure 10.9) extended the fourth model by including an autoinhibitory synapse to terminate the inhibitory feedback. We expected to be able to shut down cell L1 and then reactivate it using the self-inhibition from R1 to cancel R1's inhibitory signal to L1. The experiment was as follows:

• For 20 ms, cell L1 receives no somatic current input and then a constant pulse soma input of 0.00025 μA is applied for 380 ms. Cell L1 is strongly connected to cell R1 with excitatory connections, so in the absence of any inhibitory feedback from cell R1, the output from cell L1 then triggers a corresponding output in cell R1.

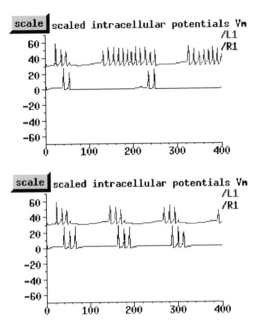

Figure 10.10
Cell firing reinitiates.

• Cell R1 received no somatic current but now has a large inhibitory synaptic connection with cell L1, as well as a large self-inhibitory connection.

We expected cell R1 to turn on and pulse with a frequency similar to that of cell L1 but the inhibition from R1, which was used to seriously affect the frequency of the L1 trace, was now cancelled by the self-inhibition. Hence L1 began to turn on again. The inhibitory R1 to L1 synaptic connection was set to be 4000 as in the previous experiment, and the new self-inhibition on R1 was set to be 400,000. The traces of the cell L1 and R1 voltages are shown in figure 10.10. Note that L1 does indeed begin firing again.

Conclusions

We have developed the tools for creating hybrid neuronal-silicon devices and have successfully modeled basic designs of neuronal circuits. The next step will be to combine these tools to create an integrated device. Our approach to developing this hybrid device in many ways parallels the development of the early transistor. The first transistor involved using two dissimilar systems—p-type and n-type germanium—and taking advantage of the combination's characteristics that resulted from their interaction at the interface. In a similar fashion, we are proposing to take two dissimilar systems composed of a neuron and an FET or metal microelectrode on a silicon chip and tailor the interface to take advantage of the resultant device's characteristics. We believe that using living neurons as indicators of a compound's efficacy is a promising future technology. These neurons can elicit a modified action potential (digital signal) when they are acted upon by different compounds. For example, some compounds operate by inhibition of the sodium channels, some act on the potassium channels, while still others activate intracellular cascades, leading to calcium mobilization and activation of a specific gene. We have achieved neuronal survival on patterned self-assembled monolayers in serum-free media for over a month. In addition, we seek to design the solid-state portion of the toxin detector for our neuronal systems and devices. Work is underway in a number of groups to develop the circuitry to analyze the signals, and progress is rapid. Finally, our modeling experiments indicate numerous candidate circuits for sensor fabrication.

In future work, to determine the response range of the neuronal circuits, we will test their response to drugs or toxins that are known to affect synaptic transmission. For example, anticholinesterase agents (e.g., pesticides, carbamate insecticides) are a class of agents known to potentiate cholinergic transmission by inhibiting acetylcholinesterase, which causes a depolarization block of transmission at cholinergic synapses. Another class of antagonists, which also includes pesticides (e.g., chlorinated cyclodienes, bicuculline picrotoxin), is called GABA antagonists. These antagonists function by blocking the chloride channels in nerve cells at GABA receptors, causing uncontrolled excitation of postsynaptic central neurons. GABA is known to be the chief inhibitory transmitter in the hippocampus. Glycine antagonists, which are often called rodenticides (e.g., strychnine), function by blocking the inhibitory neurotransmitter glycine in the spinal cord, causing convulsions. Glutamate receptor-modulating agents comprise a large class of substances [e.g., zinc, phencyclidine (angel dust), polyamines, redox reagents] that function by disrupting glutamate neurotransmission. This wide range of compounds should give a clear picture of the sensitivity and flexibility of the circuit combinations we have developed.

There is an important caveat to our results to date. From a practical standpoint, implementation of these circuit models requires the ability to distinguish excitatory from inhibitory neurons in a mixed population during dissociation and culture of hippocampal tissue. There is evidence that inhibitory (γ-aminobutyricacid, GABA-ergic) hippocampal neurons exhibit morphological features distinct from excitatory (non-GABA-ergic) hippocampal neurons. For example, most GABA-ergic neurons have more polygonal-shaped cell bodies, nonspiny and less tapering dendrites, and fewer dendrites than excitatory hippocampal neurons (Benson et al., 1994). Still, we cannot be certain that such morphological differences will be apparent under our culture conditions after attachment to SAM or SAM-modified surfaces.

To address this concern, using our standard patterning techniques, we generate a large number of two-neuron patterns on a single surface. We can then expect some significant fraction of the neuronal circuits to exhibit the desired excitatory or inhibitory orientation. Individual circuits we chose for their morphologic characteristics will be examined electrophysiologically and correlated with immunocytochemistry to verify the phenotype of the neurons within each patterned circuit.

This is one of the first attempts to combine all of the required parts to create a useful system for understanding neuronal circuits and for beginning to create multicellular systems using cells as *components*. These biological/nonbiological hybrid devices would be a major demonstration of the ability to combine surface chemistry and microsystems to create systems and to provide a novel, biologically founded solution to many neurological conditions. We believe that the demonstration of this concept and its availability as a new model system will further the aims of the biomedical community and that the idea of bioengineering cells to build natural but also unnatural constructs also has major implications. As biology becomes increasingly integrated with other disciplines, easily *reproducible* recipes for manipulating cells as materials will be necessary. Much like molecular biology used to be a "black art" practiced by a few experts, now a variety of sophisticated analysis tools including PCR, capillary electrophoresis, and Western and Northern blots are routine experiments or "kits" available to all. Cellular manipulation needs to rise to this level of accessibility where the metric of success is not that "they didn't die" but, instead, that the cells can be spatially placed, integrated with other structures, and their reaction to controlled changes in their environment determined, in a defined system, where the results are easily interpretable. The assembly of the cells in homogenous or heterogeneous systems will then become a straightforward process.

Acknowledgment

We wish to acknowledge the U.S. Department of Energy's Office of Science, Basic Engineering Science, for their support of our research under grant DE-FG02-00ER-45856. It should be noted that portions of the work were previously published in the *Proceedings of the Twentieth Symposium on Energy Engineering Sciences*, Argonne National Laboratory, Argonne, Illinois, 2002.

References

Aizawa, M. (1991) Immunosensors. In L. J. Blum, and P. R. Coulet, eds., *Biosensor Principles and Applications*, New York: Marcel Dekker, pp. 249–266.

Anton, P. S., Granger, R., and Lynch, G. (1992) Temporal information processing in synapses, cells, and circuits. In T. McKenna, J. Davis, and S. F. Zornetzger, eds., *Single Neuron Computation*. San Diego: Academic Press, pp. 291–314.

Banker, G. A., and Cowan, W. M. (1977) Rat hippocampal neurons dispersed in cell culture. *Brain Res.* 126: 397–425.

Barlow, H. B., and Levick, W. R. (1965) The mechanism of directionally selective units in the rabbit's retina. *J. Physiol. (London)* 178: 477–504.

Benson, D. L., Watkins, F. H., Steward, O., and Banker, G. (1994) Characterization of GABAergic neurons in hippocampal cell cultures. *J. Neurocytol.* 23: 279–295.

Bernard, A., and Bosshard, H. R. (1995) Real-time monitoring of antigen-antibody recognition on a metal oxide surface by an optical grating coupler sensor. *Eur. J. Biochem.* 230: 416–423.

Bower, J., and Beeman, D. (1998) *The Book of Genesis: Exploring Realistic Neural Models with the General Neural Simulation System*, 2nd ed. New York: Springer/TELOS.

Cooper, A., Munden, H. R., and Brown, G. I. (1976) The growth of mouse neuroblastoma cells in controlled orientations on thin films of silicon monoxide. *Exp. Cell Res.* 103: 435–439.

Corey, J. M., Wheeler, B. C., and Brewer, G. J. (1991) Compliance of hippocampal neurons to patterned substrate networks. *J. Neurosci. Res.* 30: 300–307.

Das, M., Molnar, P., Devaraj, H., Poeta, M., Hickman, J. J. (2003) Electrophysiological and morphological characterization of rat embryonic motorneurons in a defined system. *Biotechnol. Prog.* 19: 1756–1761.

Douglas, R. J., and Martin, K. A. C. (1991) A functional microcircuit for cat visual cortex. *J. Physiol. (London)* 440: 735–769.

Douglas, R. J., Martin, K. A. C., and Whitteridge, D. (1991) An intracellular analysis of the visual responses of neurons in cat visual cortex. *J. Physiol. (London)* 440: 735–769.

Edelman, P. G., and Wang, J. (1991) *Biosensors and Chemical Sensors*. ACS Symposium Series 487. Washington, D.C.: American Chemical Society.

Fromherz, P., Offenhausser, A., Vetter, T., and Weis, J. (1991) A neuron-silicon junction: A Retzius cell of the leech on an insulated-gate field-effect transistor. *Science* 252: 1290–1293.

Gardner, E. P., and Palmer, C. I. (1989) Simulation of motion on the skin II. Cutaneous mechanoreceptor coding of the width and texture of bar patterns displaced across the OPTACON. *J. Neurophysiol.* 62: 1437–1460.

Gross, G. W., Harsch, A., et al. (1997). Odor, drug and toxin analysis with neuronal networks in vitro: Extracellular array recording of network responses. *Biosens. Bioelectron.* 12(5): 373–393.

Hammarback, J. A., Palm, S. A., Furcht, L. T., and Letourneau, P. C. (1985) Guidance of neurite outgrowth by pathways of substratum-adsorbed laminin. *J. Neurosci. Res.* 13: 213–220.

Hickman, J. J., Testoff, M. A., Stenger, D. A., Spargo, B. J., Rudolph, A. S., and Chu, C. C. (1993) *Surface Characterization of Bioadsorbable Polymers Modified with Self-Assembled Monolayers*, ACS Monograph. Washington, D.C.: American Chemical Society.

Hughes, R. C., Ricco, A. J., Butler, M. A., and Martin, S. J. (1991) Chemical microsensors. *Science* 254: 74–80.

Johansson, S., and Arhem, P. (1990) Graded action potentials in small cultured rat hippocampal neurons. *Neurosci. Lett.* 118: 155–158.

Jung, D. R., Cuttino, D. S., Pancrazio, J. J., Manos, P., Custer, T., Sathanoori, R. S., Aloi, L. E., Coulombe, M. G., Czarnaski, M. A., Borkholder, D. A., Kovacs, G. T. A., Stenger, D. A., and Hickman, J. J. (1998) Cell-based sensor microelectrode array characterized by imaging x-ray photoelectron spectroscopy, scanning electron microscopy, impedance measurements, and extracellular recordings. *J. Vac. Sci. Technol. A* 16: 1183–1188.

Juusola, M., French, A. S., Uusitalo, R. O., and Weckstrom, M. (1996) Information processing by graded-potential transmission through tonically active synapses. *Trends Neurosci.* 19: 292–297.

Kleinfeld, D., Kahler, K. H., and Hockberger, P. E. (1988) Controlled outgrowth of dissociated neurons on patterned substrates. *J. Neurosci.* 8: 4098–4120.

Leech, D., and Rechnitz, G. A. (1993) Biomagnetic neurosensors. *Anal. Chem.* 65: 3262–3266.

Offenhausser, A., and Knoll, W. (2001). Cell-transistor hybrid systems and their potential applications. *Trends Biotechnol.* 19(2): 62–66.

Parce, J. W., Owicki, J. C., Kercso, K. M., Sigal, G. B., Wada, H. G., Muir, V. C., Bousse, L. J., Ross, K. L., Sikic, B. I., and McConnell, H. M. (1989) Detection of cell-affecting agents with a silicon biosensor. *Science* 246: 243–247.

Peterson, J. Neuronal models. (2001) Available at http://www.ces.clemson.edu/~petersj/NeuronalModels.

Ravenscroft, M. S., Bateman, K. E., Shaffer, K. M., Schessler, H. M., Jung, D. R., Schneider, T. W., Montgomery, C. B., Custer, T. L., Schaffner, A. E., Liu, Q. Y., Li, Y. X., Barker, J. L., and Hickman, J. J. (1998) Developmental neurobiology implications from fabrication and analysis of hippocampal neuronal networks on patterned silane-modified surfaces. *J. Am. Chem. Soc.* 120: 12169–12177.

Regher, W. G., Pine, J., Cohan, C. S., Mischke, M. D., and Tank, D. W. (1989) Sealing cultured invertebrate neurons to embedded dish electrodes facilitates long-term stimulation and recording. *J. Neurosci. Meth.* 30: 91–106.

Schaffner, A., Barker, J. L., Stenger, D. A., and Hickman, J. (1995) Investigation of the factors necessary for growth of hippocampal neurons in a defined system. *J. Neurosci. Meth.* 62: 111–119.

Singhvi, R., Kumar, A., Lopez, G. P., Stephanopoulos, G. N., Wand, D. I. C., Whitesides, G. M., and Ingber, D. E. (1994) Engineering cell shape and function. *Science* 264: 696–698.

Solsky, R. L. (1990) Ion-selective electrodes. *Anal. Chem.* 62: 21R–33R.

St. John, P. M., Kam, L., Turner, S. W., Craighead, H. G., Issacon, M., Turner, J. N., and Shain, W. (1997) Preferential glial cell attachment to microcontact printed surfaces. *J. Neurosci. Meth.* 75: 171–177.

Stenger, D. A., Georger, J. H., Dulcey, C. S., Hickman, J. J., Rudolph, A. S., Nielsen, T. B., McCort, S. M., and Calvert, J. M. (1992) Coplanar molecular assemblies of amino- and perfluorinated alkylsilanes: Characterization and geometric definition of mammalian cell adhesion and growth. *J. Am. Chem. Soc.* 114: 8435–8442.

Stenger, D. A., Hickman, J. J., Bateman, K. E., Ravenscroft, M. S., Ma, W., Pancrazio, J. J., Shaffer, K. M., Schaffner, A. E., Cribbs, D. H., and Cotman, C. W. (1998) Microlithographic determination of axonal/dentritic polarity in cultured hippocampal neurons. *J. Neurosci. Meth.* 82: 167–173.

Uhlig, A., Lindner, E., Teutloff, C., Schnakenberg, U., and Hintsche, R. (1997) Miniaturized ion-selective chip electrode for sensor application. *Anal. Chem.* 69: 4032–4038.

Van Hoesen, G., and Pandya, D. (1975) Some connections of the entorhinal (area 28) and perirhinal (area 35) cortices of the rhesus monkey: I. Temporal lobe afferents. *Brain Res.* 95: 1–24.

Van Keulen, L. (1979) Axon projections of Renshaw cells in the lumbar spinal cord of the cat, as reconstructed after intracellular staining with horseradish peroxidase. *Brain Res.* 167: 157–162.

Vargo, T. G., Thompson, P. M., Gerenser, L. J., Valentini, R. F., Aebischer, P., Cook D. J., and Gardella, J. A., Jr. (1992) Monolayer chemical lithography and characterization of fluoropolymer films. *Langmuir* 8: 130–134.

Wilson, M. A., Bhalla, U., Uhley, J. D., and Bower, J. M. (1989) GENESIS: A system for simulating neural networks. In D. Touretzky, ed., *Advances in Neural Information Processing Systems*. San Mateo, Calif.: Morgan Kaufman, pp. 485–492.

11 The Biotic/Abiotic Interface: Achievements and Foreseeable Challenges

Roberta Diaz Brinton, Walid Sousou, Michel Baudry, Mark Thompson, and
Theodore W. Berger

Implantable microelectronic systems—first as cardiac pacemakers, then as cochlear implants, and most recently as deep brain stimulators to treat the motor symptoms of Parkinson's disease—have transformed the lives of many and will benefit many more in the future (Loeb, 1990; Humayun et al., 1996). A biomimetic neural prosthetic device, while having stimulation as a component of its function, is envisioned to assume the actual function of neurons, replacing those lost from damage or disease (Berger et al., 2001). Implanted replacement silicon neurons would have functional properties matching those of the damaged neurons, and would both receive and send electrical information to regions of the brain with which the damaged region previously communicated. The design of a biomimetic neural prosthetic device is described in Berger et al. (2001); see also chapter 12 in this volume.

Considered here is the challenge to develop a seamless interface between the electronics and the complex cellular topography of the brain. This chapter summarizes our collective progress to date in developing the underlying science and technology that will make possible an effective long-term interface between specific brain regions and multichip modules consisting of novel, hybrid analog-digital microchips.

Essential Requirements for an Implantable Neural Prosthesis

Integration of a neuroprosthetic implant into the nervous system is a multifactorial challenge that will require developments in (1) the long-term viability of intimate contact between cells of the brain and the neuroprosthetic implant, (2) methods to sustain neuronal survival, and (3) regulation of the glial immune response to promote favorable regeneration conditions while repressing responses that can lead to glial scarring and encapsulation of the implant (see figure 11.1). Surmounting each of these challenges will require strategies that capitalize on existing knowledge and forging new hybrid strategies that provide novel solutions to previously intractable problems. This chapter reviews recent progress and thinking on each of these issues.

Neuron / electrode interface

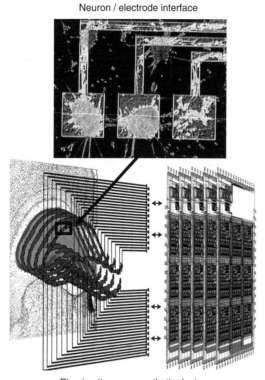

Biomimetic neuroprosthetic device

Figure 11.1
Challenges for the biotic/abiotic interface: (1) Sustaining long-term neuron-electrode compatibility and adhesion; (2) preventing or minimizing an inflammatory response over the lifetime of the prothesis. Representation of a biomimetic neural prosthesis for the hippocampus and the interface between the signal detection component, the electrodes, and neurons (by T. W. Berger).

The Neuron/Silicon Interface

Neuron survival and reorganization is paramount to long-term functional connectivity with a microelectronic neural prosthetic implant. The foreseeable challenges to the seamless integration of such a device center on the longevity of adhesion and survival strategies. To date, all tested strategies have been short-term trials. For a neural prosthetic implant to be effective, its surface must be engineered to promote intimate contact with neural tissue while simultaneously avoiding activation of an inflammatory response.

An integral part of achieving this is the development of surface coatings for the packaging materials, electrodes, and platforms. Ideally, the surface coatings will be tuned to the properties of each surface to match their function within the implant. One can anticipate that platform materials will include both rigid substrates, such as

Table 11.1
Analysis of biocompatibility of hippocampal neurons cultured on silicon-based substrates

Silicon Surface	Neuronal Growth	Characterization
Silicon	Excellent	Excellent neuronal adhesion and process outgrowth
Silicon dioxide	Excellent	Excellent adhesion and outgrowth
Silicon nitride (insulation material used in multisite electrode arrays)	Nonexistent	No neuronal adhesion. Requires coating with organic adhesion molecule (poly-D-lysine, laminin, etc.) for neuronal attachment to occur
Si coated with $\sim$1200 Å MgO_2	Poor	Little to no neuronal adhesion

ceramics, glass, and silicon, as well as flexible polymer materials, such as poly di methyl siloxane (PDMS), parylene, and polyimide. Electrode materials will include simple metals, such as platinum or gold, as well as metal oxides and nitrides, such as iridium oxide (IrO_2), indium tin oxide (ITO), and TiN. The packaging materials will include some of the same materials, that is, ceramics and glass, as well as other environmentally stable materials, such as titanium and stainless steel. The surface treatment chemistries being developed for controlling cell attachment and specific cell recognition must be effacious for each of these surfaces and be adaptable to new materials that we have not yet envisioned.

Neuron/silicon interfaces will have to be tailored to the material requirements of the device. Hence, we have embarked upon a strategy of developing a "toolbox" of materials that can be used to selectively coat abiotic surfaces with a stable, tailorable, biocompatible material so that a device's surface will have a chemical and molecular composition comparable to that of the cellular region of the nervous system being replaced and hence will perform like natural tissue in vivo. The development of such a coating "toolbox" will require analysis of the stability of coating chemistries (Abdelrazzaq et al., 2002; Vijayamohanan and Aslam, 2001; Fendler, 2001; Ulman, 1991) under biologically relevant conditions in vitro and in vivo. Next, these processes can be used to anchor groups chosen to carry out specific operative functions, including selective cell binding, cell repulsion, and controlled release of a substance (Mohajeri et al., 1996; Hailer et al., 1997; Kiss, 1998; Lee and Benveniste, 1999; Esch et al., 2000).

Our previous work, as well as that of others in the field, indicates that selected silicon surfaces (table 11.1), electrode metals (table 11.2), and a variety of bioamine substrates (figure 11.2 and table 11.3) are effective in promoting neuronal adhesion on electrodes and silicon-based surfaces whereas others are ineffective (Gross et al., 1982; James et al., 1998, 2000; Branch et al., 2000; Sorribas et al., 2001; Soussou, 2002). Different substrates result in different neuron topographies (see table 11.4).

Table 11.2
Analysis of biocompatibility of hippocampal neurons cultured on metal ion-based electrodes

Electrode Metal	Neuronal Growth	Characterization
Aluminum	Excellent	Neurons attach, remain adhered for several weeks; permits neuronal process outgrowth. Potential problem with oxidation that would limit signal detection.
Gold	Excellent	Neurons attach, adhere for an extended time; permits neuronal process outgrowth. Easily amenable to cross-linking. High impedance and low charge-transfer capacity. Cheap and easy deposition.
Indium tin oxide (ITO)	No neuronal adhesion	Thin-film transparent microelectrodes that permit visualization of cells on top of microelectrodes. Requires coating with organic substrate for neuronal adhesion. High impedance, resulting in greater noise. Low charge-transfer capacity.
Platinum black	No neuronal adhesion	Requires coating with organic substrate for neuronal adhesion. Low impedance. High charge transfer. Falls off with stimulation. Mechanically unstable.
Titanium nitride	No neuronal adhesion	Requires coating with organic substrate for neuronal adhesion. Microcolumnal shape results in low impedance ($80–250$ kΩ) and high charge-transfer capacity, which enables greater stimulation intensities. More mechanically stable, allows electrodes to be used multiple times.

For example, the density of positive charges and polymer size dramatically affects neuronal cluster development (see figure 11.1 and table 11.4). Dissociated single neurons seeded onto 30,000–70,000 molecular weight polymers of poly-D-lysine and poly-D-ornithine substrates migrate to form small clusters, whereas neurons seeded onto polyethylenimine, which is more highly positively charged, do not migrate to form clusters and suffer a higher degree of cell death. Inclusion of basement membrane, a complex extract of extracellular matrix from a mouse tumor cell line, with any of these substrates greatly increases the capacity of neurons to migrate into clusters (see figure 11.2 and table 11.4).

Poly-D-lysine and laminin are known to be particularly effective in promoting adhesion of dissociated neuron cultures onto inorganic materials, and we investigated their efficacy with regard to our hippocampal conformal multisite electrode arrays (Soussou et al., 2000, 2002). Poly-D-lysine and laminin were applied to the surface of the conformal arrays, with application limited to linear tracks aligned with the long axis of each column of electrode sites in the rectangular array (figure 11.3). When dissociated hippocampal neurons were prepared on the surface of the array, the adhesion of cells and the extension of their processes were restricted to the treated regions. Neural networks that formed were predominantly in parallel, linear tracks over the columns of electrodes.

Poly-D-Lysine Substrate

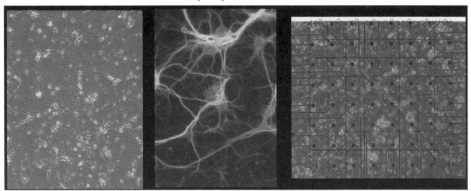

Poly-D-Lysine with Basement Membrane Matrix

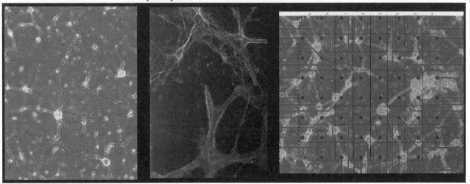

Figure 11.2
Morphological development of hippocampal neurons on polyamine-coated surface in the absence or presence of basement membrane matrix on glass and multisite electrode arrays. The panels on the far left show hippocampal neurons grown on glass coated with poly-D-lysine in the absence (top) and in combination with basement membrane matrix (bottom). Note that in the presence of basement membrane, neuronal clusters appear more frequently and a modest degree of process fasciculation occurs. The middle panels show phenotypic development of neuronal processes on these two substrates. Dendritic processes are labeled with the dendrite selective marker MAP2 shown, while axons are labeled with the axon-selective marker, GAP43. In the third panel are dissociated hippocampal neurons cultured onto multisite electrode arrays. Note that in the presence of basement membrane, a much greater degree of clustering of neurons and fasciculation of their processes occurs. Bar: 50 μm.

Table 11.3
Organic adhesion substrates and their properties

Organic Substrate	Structure	Properties
Poly-D-lysine (PDL)	**PDL** $$\left(\underset{\displaystyle \overset{H_2NCH_2CH_2CH_2CH_2}{\diagdown}}{\underset{\displaystyle NH-\overset{\displaystyle H}{C}-\overset{\displaystyle \overset{O}{\|}}{C}-}{}} \right)_n$$	Most commonly used substrate. Branched cationic polymer, with peptide bonds. D-conformation prevents proteolytic degradation.
Polyornithine (PO)	**PO** $$\left(-NH-CH_2CH_2CH_2\overset{\displaystyle \overset{H_2N}{\diagdown}}{C}-\overset{\displaystyle \overset{O}{\|}}{C}- \right)_n$$	Structurally very similar to PDL, but unbranched cationic polymer, with peptide bonds.
Polyethyleneimine (PEI)	**PEI** $$\left(-NH\,CH_2\,CH_2- \right)_x \left(\overset{\displaystyle CH_2CH_2NH_2}{\underset{\displaystyle N-CH_2\,CH_2-}{\|}} \right)_y$$	Branched cationic polymer with no carboxylic group, thus more positively charged. Lack of peptide bond prevents proteolytic degradation. Reported to enhance cell maturation compared with PDL (Lelong et al., 1992).
Basement membrane (BM)	Contains: Laminin 56% Collagen IV 31% Entactin 8% Heparan sulfate proteoglycan Matrix metalloproteinases Growth factors: EGF, bFGF, NGF, PDGF, IGF-1, TFG-β	Extracellular matrix extracted from EHS mouse tumor. Similar in structure, composition, physical property, and functional characteristics to in vivo BM.

Table 11.4
Analysis of morphological features of hippocampal neurons cultured on various organic substrates

Organic Substrate	Individual Cells	Clusters	Thin Branches	Fasciculated Branches
PDL	Intermediate	Intermediate	High	Below average
PEI	Most	None	Above average	None
PO	Intermediate	Above average	High	Below average
BM	Below average	Above average (highly variable)	Intermediate	Above average (highly variable)

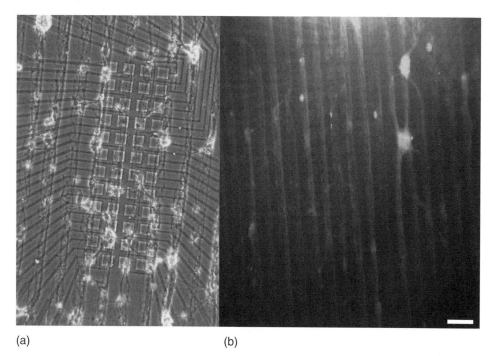

(a)   (b)

Figure 11.3
A designed morphology of a conformal multisite electrode array. (*A*) Dissociated hippocampal neurons grown on a conformal multisite electrode array coated with poly-D-lysine in a linear pattern aligned on top of the electrodes. Both nerve cell bodies and their processes were predominantly attached to the linear tracts of poly-D-lysine, with minimal crossing of processes across the 50-mm gap between electrode pads and leads. (*B*) Axons attached to linear tracts of poly-D-lysine labeled with a fluorescent marker for the axon-selective marker, GAP43. Bar: 50 μm.

Impact of Surface Composition on Electrophysiological Signaling of Neurons

Our most recent work has addressed the impact of surface composition on the electrophysiological properties of neurons, with the long-term intent of manipulating the excitability of neurons that would interface with the electrodes of a neural prosthesis. Our initial data indicate that the morphologies induced by different substrates are associated with different electrophysiological phenotypes (see figure 11.4) (Soussou et al., 2000). It is important to note that the differences in electrophysiological phenotype are not due to changes in neuronal viability because neurons cultured on titanium nitride-silicon nitride multisite electrode arrays coated with poly-D-lysine exhibit markers of viability comparable to that of neurons cultured onto similarly coated glass coverslips (see figure 11.5).

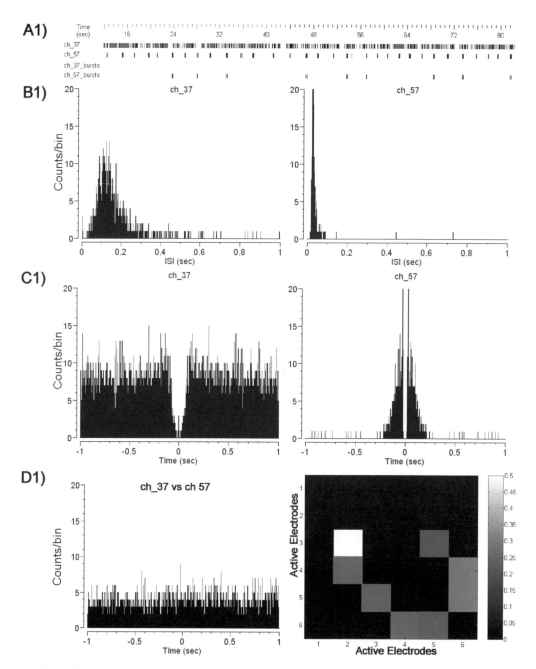

Figure 11.4

Analysis of spontaneous activity of cultured hippocampal neurons on multisite electrode arrays. Electro-physiological recordings are derived from the same dissociated hippocampal neuron culture on a polyethy-leneimine (PEI)-coated multisite electrode array at days 15 (1) and 18 (2). (*A1*) and (*A2*) Rastergrams of two channels and limits of detected bursts. (*A1*) One channel fires almost continuously, whereas the other has short bursts (some too short to be detected as bursts by this algorithm and the set parameters). (*A2*) Both channels fire long and short bursts sporadically but synchronously. (*B1*) and (*B2*) Interstimulus inter-val (ISI) histograms of the two channels in *A*. The continuously firing cell has a wider and delayed histo-gram, while the histograms of the bursting cells get narrower with shorter burst durations. (*C1*) and (*C2*) The autocorrelograms of the activity in the four cells show the refractory period as a drop in the center (the

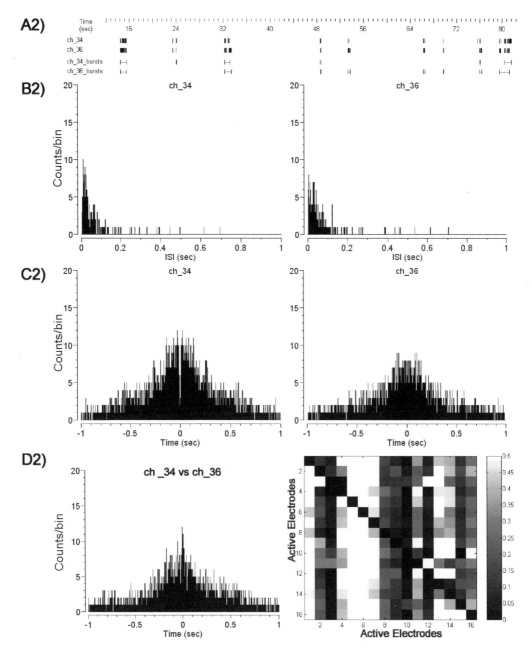

second cell in *C2* has some noise included that occurred during the refractory period and occludes the drop). The flat histogram reflects uncorrelated continuous firing, while the broad peaks in *C2* reflect longer bursts than *C1*'s bursting cell. (*D1*) and (*D2*) Cross-correlograms of the two channels. (*D1*) Flat correlogram indicates nonsynchronous firing between the two cells, while *D2* indicates that the two cells are well synchronized in time. The gray-scale correlation matrices plot the cross-correlation indices of all the active electrodes in that particular multisite electrode array, so that each pair of electrodes has two small squares coding their indices (one above the midline and one below). The indices are calculated as the area between ±0.02 s that is above the average baseline divided by the number of spikes in the reference channel (this normalization generates an unsymmetrical matrix). A higher (white) index indicates highly correlated channels. The autocorrelation indices are set to zero.

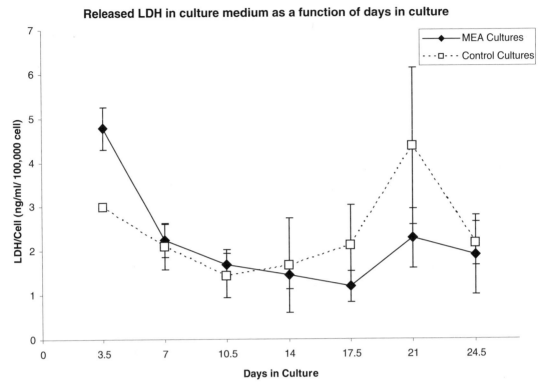

Figure 11.5
Neuronal viability on multisite electrode arrays compared with control hippocampal cells cultured on glass coverslips. The culture medium was collected following specified days from hippocampal neuron cultures plated onto glass or multisite electrode arrays and analyzed for lactate dehydrogenase (LDH) content in the culture medium. LDH is a stable cytoplasmic enzyme expressed in all cells, including neurons. It is rapidly released into the cell culture supernatant upon damage to the plasma membrane. The spectophotometric results are translated to nanograms per milliliter by interpolation on a standard reference curve and normalized to the cell plating density. Both multisite electrode array cultures and control cultures show similar aging patterns: initially high LDH release into the medium as a result of the initial damage at seeding, followed by low level of LDH release for 10 days, and aging followed by a modest rise in LDH release likely due to related oxidative damage to the plasma membrane after 20 days in culture, which occurs in the absence of antioxidants.

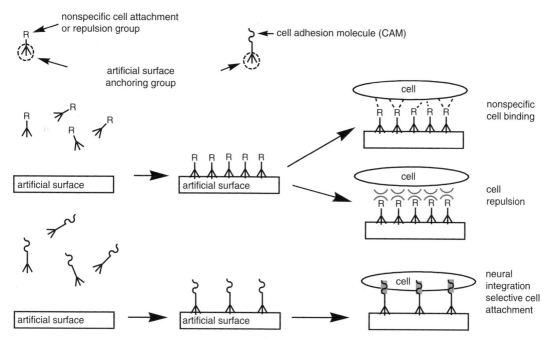

Figure 11.6
Schematic representation of the preparation of surface coatings to promote cell-selective attachment. Surface chemistries can be designed to promote selective cell attachment, prohibit nonspecific cell binding, and prevent inflammation through cell repulsion chemistry to thwart activation of the inflammatory response in glial cells. Integration of the neural component with the artificial surface of the neuroprosthesis could be achieved by specific recognition between either an nCAM sequence or receptors selectively expressed on specific neuron populations (shown as bars).

Although much of the electrophysiological testing of interfaces to date has been completed using hippocampal slices (which remain physiologically viable for 12–18 hr), we also have begun using hippocampal slice cultures to test the long-term viability of the neuron/silicon interface. The latter preparations involve placing slices of hippocampus on a semipermeable membrane in contact with tissue culture media and maintaining them long term in a culture incubator (Gholmieh et al., 2003). Slice cultures can be prepared directly on multisite electrode arrays, which then can be tested periodically to examine the robustness of the electrophysiological interaction with the hippocampal tissue. Preliminary findings have revealed that bidirectional communication remains viable for at least several weeks, although we have yet to systematically test long-term functionality.

For effective signal detection and transmission, intimate contact between neurons and electrode components of a neural prosthesis is necessary. To review, dendrites are the "input" regions of neurons; cell bodies and axons are their "output" regions. A neural prosthesis will inevitably be sandwiched between two surfaces so that it will

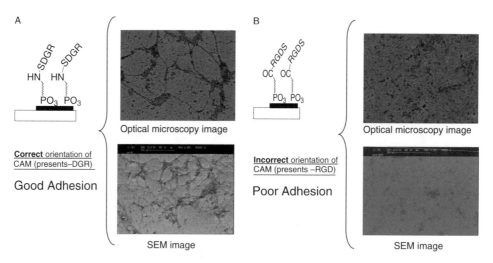

Figure 11.7
Cell adhesion molecule (CAM) sequences to promote neuron adhesion to a neural implant surface. TiN substrates (shown as black bars) were coated with (*A*) aminoalkyl-phosphonic and (*B*) carboxyl-phosphonic acids. The RGDS peptide (arginine-glycine-aspartate-serine) was then coupled to each surface as shown. The substrates were then cultured with dissociated neurons. Both optical (*top*) and scanning electrical micrographs (*bottom*) show string cell adhesion and growth on the amino-treated surface and no adhesion on the carboxyl surface. The four images are of areas that are roughly 500 μm wide.

have to function as neurons do—as a receptive postsynaptic element to receive information, a processing element to transform the incoming signal, and as a transmission presynaptic element to communicate the processed signal. Implanted in the brain, a neural prosthesis would reconnect two disconnected regions of the brain and would have to interface between four surfaces in three-dimensions. Axons from the surviving neural tissue will have to provide input to the device, with the device functioning as the postsynaptic element, whereas dendrites will have to be functionally connected to its output, with the device functioning as the presynaptic element and the dendrite as the postsynaptic element.

Achieving such selective portioning of neuronal elements will require the use of adhesion and attraction strategies that will promote, at the very least, the attachment of neural elements to the reception and transmission electrodes of the prosthesis. In parallel, repulsion of glial cells from the signal detection and transmission electrodes, must be achieved. However, the repulsion of glial cells will have to be very limited in order to keep glial cells in close enough proximity to promote long-term neuron survival. One potential strategy to achieve selective adhesion is to use cell adhesion molecules (CAMs) to generate adhesion or antiadhesion surfaces (see figure 11.6) that promote the selective adhesion of neurons and astrocytes to specific compartments of the interface with the device (see figure 11.7). Our approach will be to develop specific surface modifications using a combination of cell-specific adhesion

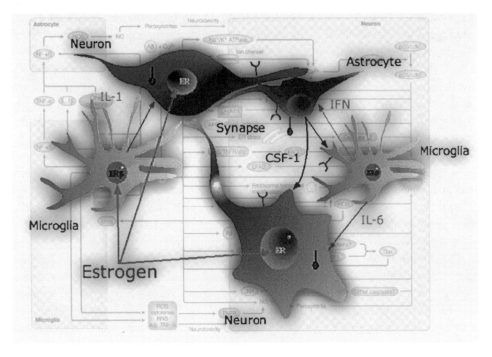

Figure 11.8
Schematic of neuroinflammatory response cascade and cell types involved in neuroinflammation. The background illustrates the complexity of neuroimmune signaling in the brain, whereas the foreground illustrates the types of cells involved in the inflammatory response. Of particular importance are the microglia and resistive astrocytes that are the principal inflammatory cells of the brain. Also shown are factors that can regulate the inflammatory response, including endogenous factors such as estrogen and exogenous anti-inflammatory drugs such as rapamycin, which is both an anti-inflammatory and an antiproliferative agent.

molecules that will promote selective couplings between interface input pads and cell bodies and axons, and between interface output pads and dendrites.

Biocompatibility and Long-Term Viability

Long-term viability of the implant requires the maintenance of effective functional interactions between the microchip and brain tissue on a time scale of years, as periodic replacement of a neural prosthetic implant is not a realistic option. While not all of the biocompatibility and long-term viability challenges can be fully appreciated until the working prototypes of implant devices have been developed, preventing or suppressing the inflammatory response to foreign objects is likely to be a problem for all implantable neural prosthetics and will be chief among the factors that will impede the long-term viability of a neural implant (see figure 11.8).

Regulating the Glial Immune Response: Managing the Inflammatory Response
Managing the multicellular, multifaceted glial response is crucial to the success of
the neuron/neuroprosthetic interface (Cui et al., 2001; Sorribas et al., 2001). In laboratories conducting chronic electrophysiological recordings, it has been well known
for decades that the quality of electrophysiological signals generated by many standard recording methods designed for long-term use in behaving animals gradually
degrades over the course of weeks. However, not all electrophysiological recording
methods are always subject to such degradation in signal quality over time. For example, multimicrowire recording methods using a small number of wires can record
in a stable manner for many months (approaching a year). While it is widely
accepted that the "window" for stable, high-quality electrophysiological recordings
is on the order of days to weeks, only relatively recently (i.e., within the past 5 years)
have detailed histological descriptions of the encapsulation of the electrodes begun to
appear (A. M. Turner et al., 2000; Szarowski et al., 2003).

The inflammatory response begins immediately upon insertion of electrodes into
the brain, reaches steady state within several weeks, and is correlated with a gradual
decrease in the quality of electrophysiological signals recorded from target neurons
(A. M. Turner et al., 2000; Szarowski et al., 2003). To be considered viable, any
strategy for a long-term, implantable, cortical prosthetic system must overcome the
inflammatory encapsulation response. For images of the encapsulation process and
the contribution of astrocytes and microglia, the reader is referred to the web site of
the Craighead laboratory at http://www.hgc.cornell.edu/neupostr/lrie.htm.

The challenge of the glial inflammatory response is complicated. Astrocyte function is crucial to neuron viability because astrocytes are the repository of growth factors vital to neuron survival (Anderson and Swanson, 2000; Aschner, 2000; Dong
and Benveniste, 2001; Gates and Dunnett, 2001; Gimenez y Ribotta et al., 2001).
However, astrocyte proliferation is well known to be a principal culprit in blocking
regeneration of central nervous system neurons and encapsulation of implanted devices (Eclancher et al., 1996; Davies et al., 1997; DiProspero et al., 1997; Yang
et al., 1997; Fawcett and Asher, 1999; Fitch et al., 1999; Logan et al., 1999; J. N.
Turner et al., 1999; Asher et al., 2000, 2001; A. M. Turner et al., 2000; Yang et al.,
2000; Menet et al., 2001). The production of the glial-derived cytokines that lead to
inflammation is highly complex but, in general, activation of actrocytes and especially microglia leads to the inflammatory response and ultimately to encapsulation
of the device and degeneration of neurons (see figure 11.8) (Anderson and Swanson,
2000; Aschner, 2000; Dong and Benveniste, 2001; Gates and Dunnett, 2001; Gimenez y Ribotta et al., 2001; Eclancher et al., 1996; Davies et al., 1997; DiProspero
et al., 1997; Yang et al., 1997, 2000; Fawcett and Asher, 1999; Fitch et al., 1999;
Logan et al., 1999; J. N. Turner et al., 1999; Asher et al., 2000, 2001; A. M. Turner

et al., 2000; Menet et al., 2001). In contrast, radial glia can function as progenitor cells for neurogenesis (Yang et al., 1997; Gotz et al., 2002).

Despite their role in the inflammatory response, astrocytes also serve as sources of growth factors and nutrients and function to remove toxins from the extracellular compartment. The close proximity of astrocytes to neurons is essential to neuronal long-term survival. One strategy to achieve the benefits of astrocytes while potentially obviating their deleterious effects is to develop a method for selective attachment of neurons and glia to specific compartments of a neural prosthesis. Our initial approach will involve differential surface coatings of specific cell adhesion molecules, such as decapeptide (KHIFSDDSSE) or L1, to bind glial cells and repulsion molecules, such as the integrin-ligand peptide RGDS (arginine-glycine-aspartate-serine) or the amino acids serine or polyethylene glycol (Mohajeri et al., 1996; Hailer et al., 1997; Kiss, 1998; Lee and Benveniste, 1999) (see figure 11.7).

An alternative approach could use inhibitors of glial proliferation (cycloheximide) at the time of implantation to permit neuronal contact and adhesion with the neuroprosthetic electrodes to occur and then allow normal glial proliferation to proceed. The risk of this approach is that while antiproliferative agents would inhibit the proliferative response of activated and hence inflammatory glial cells, they would also inhibit proliferation of neural progenitor and stem cells, thereby potentially eliminating a crucial source of neurons necessary for successful interfacing between the biomimetic device and the brain tissue surrounding the device. A third approach could be to couple surface coatings of CAMs and repulsion molecules with hydrogels for release of chondroitinase to inhibit the chondroitin sulfate proteoglycans required for glial scarring and/or inflammatory response inhibitors such as vasopressin or anti-interleukin 1 (figure 11.9) (Zhao and Brinton, 2004; Sanderson et al., 1999).

The aforementioned strategies of creating biomimetic surfaces with membrane proteins found on the extracellular side of the membrane, such as cell adhesion molecules, coupled with anti-inflammatory strategies that capitalize on the advances in neuroimmunology, may prove to be sufficient to sustain the viability of a neural prosthesis over the lifetime of the user.

Conclusions

The goal of this chapter was to bring into focus several of the major challenges for the development of implantable neural prostheses that can coexist and bidirectionally communicate with living brain tissue. Although these problems are formidable, advances in the field of microelectronics, surface chemistry, materials science, neuroimmunology, neuroscience, and therapeutic formulation provide the scientific and engineering scaffolding necessary to generate solutions to the challenges at the biotic/abiotic interface.

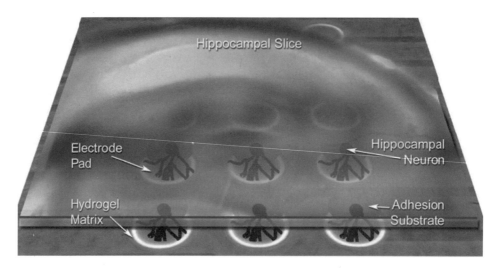

Figure 11.9
In vitro model system for demonstrating proof of principle for biotic/abiotic interface strategies. It shows a diagrammatic representation of a multifunctional system to achieve long-term neuron survival and a neuronal interface with an electrode (pads or penetrating) while simultaneously suppressing glial proliferation, activation, invasion, and the ensuing inflammatory response. Conformal multisite electrode arrays can be coated with specific adhesion substrates, followed by microstamping of hydrogel matrices that contain neuronal survival and glial suppression factors around the electrode. Hippocampal slices can be cultured on top of the electrode-adhesion substrate-hydrogel matrix to test for optimal in vitro conditions prior to in vivo analyses.

Acknowledgments

This work was supported by Office of Naval Research grants to T.W.B., M.T., M.B.; grants from the Defense Advances Research Projects Agency to T.W.B.; and National Institutes of Heath grants to R.D.B.

References

Abdelrazzaq, F. B., Kwong, R. C., and Thompson, M. E. (2002) Photocurrent generation in multilayer organic-inorganic thin films with cascade energy architectures. *J. Am. Chem. Soc.* 124: 4796–4803.

Anderson, C. M., and Swanson, R. A. (2000) Astrocyte glutamate transport: Review of properties, regulation, and physiological functions. *Glia* 32: 1–14.

Aschner, M. (2000) Neuron–astrocyte interactions: Implications for cellular energetics and antioxidant levels. *Neurotoxicology* 21: 1101–1107.

Asher, R. A., Morgenstern, D. A., Fidler, P. S., Adcock, K. H., Oohira, A., Braistead, J. E., Levine, J. M., Margolis, R. U., Rogers, J. H., and Fawcett, J. W. (2000) Neurocan is upregulated in injured brain and in cytokine-treated astrocytes. *J. Neurosci.* 20: 2427–2438.

Asher, R. A., Morgenstern, D. A., Moon, L. D., and Fawcett, J. W. (2001) Chondroitin sulphate proteoglycans: Inhibitory components of the glial scar. *Prog. Brain Res.* 132: 611–619.

Berger, T. W., Baudry, M., Brinton, R. D., Liaw, J. S., Marmarelis, V. Z., Park, A. Y., Sheu, B. J., and Tanquay, A. R. (2001) Brain-implantable biomimetic electronics as the next era in neural prosthetics. *Proc. IEEE* 89: 993–1012.

Branch, D. W., Wheeler, B. C., Brewer, G. J., and Leckband, D. E. (2000) Long-term maintenance of patterns of hippocampal pyramidal cells on substrates of polyethylene glycol and microstamped polylysine. *IEEE Trans. Biomed. Eng.* 47: 290–300.

Cui, X., Lee, V. A., Raphael, Y., Wiler, J. A., Hetke, J. F., Anderson, D. J., and Martin, D. C. (2001) Surface modification of neural recording electrodes with conducting polymer/biomolecule blends. *J. Biomed. Mat. Res.* 56: 261–272.

Davies, S. J., Fitch, M. T., Memberg, S. P., Hall, A. K., Raisman, G., and Silver, J. (1997) Regeneration of adult axons in white matter tracts of the central nervous system. *Nature* 390: 680–683.

DiProspero, N. A., Meiners, S., and Geller, H. M. (1997) Inflammatory cytokines interact to modulate extracellular matrix and astrocytic support of neurite outgrowth. *Exp. Neurol.* 148: 628–639.

Dong, Y., and Benveniste, E. N. (2001) Immune function of astrocytes. *Glia* 36: 180–190.

Eclancher, F., Kehrli, P., Labourdette, G., and Sensenbrenner, M. (1996) Basic fibroblast growth factor (bFGF) injection activates the glial reaction in the injured adult rat brain. *Brain Res.* 737: 201–214.

Esch, T., Lemmon, V., and Banker, G. (2000) Differential effects of NgCAM and N-cadherin on the development of axons and dendrites by cultured hippocampal neurons. *J. Neurocytol.* 29: 215–223.

Fawcett, J. W., and Asher, R. A. (1999) The glial scar and central nervous system repair. *Brain Res. Bull.* 49: 377–391.

Fendler, J. H. (2001) Chemical self-assembly for electronic applications. *Chem. Materials* 13: 3196–3210.

Fitch, M. T., Doller, C., Combs, C. K., Landreth, G. E., and Silver, J. (1999) Cellular and molecular mechanisms of glial scarring and progressive cavitation: In vivo and in vitro analysis of inflammation-induced secondary injury after CNS trauma. *J. Neurosci.* 19: 8182–8198.

Gates, M. A., and Dunnett, S. B. (2001) The influence of astrocytes on the development, regeneration and reconstruction of the nigrostriatal dopamine system. *Restorative Neurol. Neurosci.* 19: 67–83.

Gholmieh, G., Courellis, S., Fakheri, S., Cheung, E., Marmarelis, V., Baudry, M., and Berger, T. (2003) Detection and classification of neurotoxins using a novel short-term plasticity quantification method. *Biosensors Bioelectron.* 18: 1467–1478.

Gimenez y Ribotta, M., Menet, V., and Privat, A. (2001) The role of astrocytes in axonal regeneration in the mammalian CNS. *Prog. Brain Res.* 132: 587–610.

Gotz, M., Hartfuss, E., and Malatesta, P. (2002) Radial glial cells as neuronal precursors: A new perspective on the correlation of morphology and lineage restriction in the developing cerebral cortex of mice. *Brain Res. Bull.* 57: 777–788.

Gross, G. W., William, A. N., and Lucas, J. H. (1982) Recording of spontaneous activity with photo-etched microelectrode surfaces from mouse spinal neurons in culture. *J. Neurosci. Meth.* 5: 13–22.

Hailer, N. P., Bechmann, I., Heizmann, S., and Nitsch, R. (1997) Adhesion molecule expression on phagocytic microglial cells following anterograde degeneration of perforant path axons. *Hippocampus* 7: 341–349.

Humayun, M. S., de Juan, E., Jr., Dagnelie, G., Greenberg, R. J., Propst, R. H., and Phillips, D. H. (1996) Visual perception elicited by electrical stimulation of retina in blind humans. *Arch. Ophthalmol.* 114: 40–46.

James, C. D., Davis, R. C., Kam, L., Craighead, H. G., Isaacson, M., Turner, J. N., and Shain, W. (1998) Patterned protein layers on solid Substrates by thin stamp microcontact printing. *Langmuir* 14: 741–744.

James, C. D., Davis, R., Meyer, M., Turner, A., Turner, S., Withers, G., Kam, L., Banker, G., Craighead, H., Isaacson, M., Turner, J., and Shain, W. (2000) Aligned microcontact printing of micrometer-scale poly-L-lysine structures for controlled growth of cultured neurons on planar microelectrode arrays. *IEEE Trans. Biomed. Eng.* 47: 17–21.

Kiss, J. Z. (1998) A role of adhesion molecules in neuroglial plasticity. *Molec. Cell. Endocrinol.* 140: 89–94.

Lee, S. J., and Benveniste, E. N. (1999) Adhesion molecule expression and regulation on cells of the central nervous system. *J. Neuroimmunol.* 98: 77–88.

Loeb, G. E. (1990) Cochlear prosthetics. *Ann. Rev. Neurosci.* 13: 357–371.

Logan, A., Green, J., Hunter, A., Jackson, R., and Berry, M. (1999) Inhibition of glial scarring in the injured rat brain by a recombinant human monoclonal antibody to transforming growth factor-beta2. *Eur. J. Neurosci.* 11: 2367–2374.

Menet, V., Gimenez y Ribotta, M., Chauvet, N., Drian, M. J., Lannoy, J., Colucci-Guyon, E., and Privat, A. (2001) Inactivation of the glial fibrillary acidic protein gene, but not that of vimentin, improves neuronal survival and neurite growth by modifying adhesion molecule expression. *J. Neurosci.* 21: 6147–6158.

Mohajeri, M. H., Bartsch, U., van der Putten, H., Sansig, G., Mucke, L., and Schachner, M. (1996) Neurite outgrowth on non-permissive substrates in vitro is enhanced by ectopic expression of the neural adhesion molecule L1 by mouse astrocytes. *Eur. J. Neurosci.* 8: 1085–1097.

Sanderson, K. L., Raghupathi, R., Saatman, K. E., Martin, D., Miller, G., and McIntosh, T. K. (1999) Interleukin-1 receptor antagonist attenuates regional neuronal cell death and cognitive dysfunction after experimental brain injury. *J. Cerebral Blood Flow Metabol.* 19: 1118–1125.

Shimono, K., Baudry, M., Panchenko, V., and Taketani, M. (2002) Chronic multichannel recordings from organotypic hippocampal slice cultures: Protection from excitotoxic effects of NMDA by non-competitive NMDA antagonists. *J. Neurosci. Meth.* 120: 193–202.

Sorribas, H., Braun, D., Leder, L., Sonderegger, P., and Tiefenauer, L. (2001) Adhesion proteins for a tight neuron-electrode contact. *J. Neurosci. Meth.* 104: 133–141.

Soussou, W., Yoon, G., Gholmieh, G., Brinton, R., and Berger, T. W. (2000) Network responses of dissociated hippocampal neurons cultured onto multi-electrode arrays. Paper presented at Society for Neuroscience Annual Meeting.

Soussou, W. B. R. D., and Berger, T. W. (2002) The effects of surface biomolecules on neuronal network morphology and electrophysiology. Paper presented at BioDevice Interface Science and Technology Workshop.

Szarowski, D. H., Andersen, M. D., Retterer, S., Spence, A. J., Isaacson, M., Craighead, H. G., Turner, J. N., and Shain, W. (2003) Brain responses to micro-machined silicon devices. *Brain Res.* 983: 23–35.

Turner, A. M., Dowell, N., Turner, S. W., Kam, L., Isaacson, M., Turner, J. N., Craighead, H. G., and Shain, W. (2000) Attachment of astroglial cells to microfabricated pillar arrays of different geometries. *J. Biomed. Mat. Res.* 51: 430–441.

Turner, J. N., Shain, W., Szarowski, D. H., Andersen, M., Martins, S., Isaacson, M., and Craighead, H. (1999) Cerebral astrocyte response to micromachined silicon implants. *Exp. Neurol.* 156: 33–49.

Ulman, A. (1991) *Introduction to Ultrathin Organic Films: From Langmiur-Blodgett to Self-assembly.* Boston: Academic Press.

Vijayamohanan, K., and Aslam, M. (2001) Applications of self-assembled monolayers for biomolecular electronics. *Appl. Biochem. Biotechnol.* 96: 25–39.

Yang, H. Y., Lieska, N., Kriho, V., Wu, C. M., and Pappas, G. D. (1997) A subpopulation of reactive astrocytes at the immediate site of cerebral cortical injury. *Exper. Neurol.* 146: 199–205.

Yang, T., Wu, S. L., Liang, J. C., Rao, Z. R., and Ju, G. (2000) Time-dependent astroglial changes after gamma knife radiosurgery in the rat forebrain. *Neurosurgery* 47: 407–415; discussion 415–416.

Zhao, L., and Brinton, R. D. (2003) Vasopressin-induced cytoplasmic and nuclear calcium signaling in cortical astrocytes: Dynamics of calcium and calcium-dependent kinases translocation. *J. Neurosci.* 23: 4228–4239.

IV HARDWARE IMPLEMENTATIONS

12 Brain-Implantable Biomimetic Electronics as a Neural Prosthesis for Hippocampal Memory Function

Theodore W. Berger, Roberta Diaz Brinton, Vasilis Z. Marmarelis, Bing J. Sheu, and Armand R. Tanguay, Jr.

One of the true frontiers in the biomedical sciences is repair of the human brain: developing prostheses for the central nervous system to replace higher thought processes that have been lost through damage or disease. The type of neural prosthesis that performs or assists a cognitive function is qualitatively different than the cochlear implant or artificial retina, which transduce physical energy from the environment into electrical stimulation of nerve fibers (Loeb, 1990; Humayun et al., in press), and qualitatively different than functional electrical stimulation (FES), in which preprogrammed electrical stimulation protocols are used to activate muscular movement (Mauritz and Peckham, 1987). Instead, we consider here a neural prosthesis designed to replace damaged neurons in central regions of the brain with silicon neurons that are permanently implanted into the damaged region. The replacement neurons would have the same functional properties as the damaged neurons, and would receive electrical activity as inputs and send it as outputs to regions of the brain with which the damaged region previously communicated. Thus, the prosthesis being proposed is one that would replace the computational function of damaged brain areas, and restore the transmission of that computational result to other regions of the nervous system. Such a new generation of neural prostheses would have a profound impact on the quality of life throughout society because it would offer a biomedical remedy for the cognitive and memory loss that accompanies Alzheimer's disease, the speech and language deficits that result from stroke, and the impaired ability to execute skilled movements following trauma to brain regions responsible for motor control.

Although the barriers to creating intracranial, electronic neural prostheses have seemed insurmountable in the past, the biological and engineering sciences are on the threshold of a unique opportunity to achieve such a goal. The tremendous growth in the field of neuroscience has allowed a much more detailed understanding of neurons and their physiology, particularly with respect to the dynamic and adaptive cellular and molecular mechanisms that are the basis for information processing in the brain. Likewise, there have been major breakthroughs in the mathematical modeling of nonlinear and nonstationary systems that are allowing quantitative representations of neuron and neural system functions to include the very complexity that is the basis of the remarkable computational abilities of the brain. The continuing breakthroughs in electronics and photonics offer opportunities to develop hardware implementations of biologically based models of neural systems that allow simulation of neural dynamics with true parallel processing, a fundamental characteristic of the brain, and real-time computational speed. Fundamental advances in low-power designs have provided the essential technology to minimize heat generation by semiconductor circuits, thus increasing compatibility with temperature-sensitive mechanisms of the brain. Finally, complementary achievements in materials science and molecular biology offer the possibility of designing compatible neuron/silicon interfaces to facilitate communication between silicon computational devices and the living brain.

Essential Requirements for an Implantable Neural Prosthesis

In general terms, there are six essential requirements for an implantable microchip to serve as a neural prosthesis. First, if the microchip is to replace the function of a given brain tissue, it must be truly biomimetic; that is, the neuron models incorporated in the prosthesis must have the properties of real biological neurons. This demands a fundamental understanding of the information-processing capabilities of neurons that is experimentally based. Second, a neural prosthesis is desired only when a physiological or cognitive function is detectably impaired (according to neurological or psychiatric criteria). Physiological or cognitive functions are the expression, not of single nerve cells, but of populations of neurons interacting in the context of a network of interconnections. Thus, biologically realistic neuron models must be capable of being concatenated into network models that can simulate these phenomena.

Third, the neuron and neural network models in question must be sufficiently miniaturized to be implantable, which demands their implementation in at least microchip circuitry. Given the known signaling characteristics of neurons, such an implementation will most likely involve hybrid analog-digital device designs. Fourth, the resulting microchip or multichip module must communicate with existing, living neural tissue in a bidirectional manner. Given that both electronic and neural systems generate and respond to electrical signals, this is feasible, although the region-specific, nonuniform distribution of neurons within the brain places substantial constraints on the architecture of neuron/silicon interfaces.

Fifth, the variability in phenotypic and developmental expression of both structural and functional characteristics of the brain will necessitate adaptation of each prosthetic device to the individual patient. Some provision for "personalizing" an implantable prosthesis must be anticipated and included in the neuron-network model and the device design. Finally, there is the critical issue of power required for the prosthetic device. Not only will supplying power be difficult, given implantation of a set of microchips into the depths of the brain (versus the periphery, as with a cochlear implant), but cellular and molecular mechanisms found in the brain are highly temperature sensitive, so that any solution must minimize heat generation to remain biocompatible.

We describe here an interdisciplinary, multilaboratory effort to develop such an implantable, computational prosthesis that can coexist and bidirectionally communicate with living neural tissue. We will deal with five of the requirements; only the issue of power will not be addressed here. Although the final achievement of an implantable prosthesis remains years in the future, it is nonetheless our position that the path to such a goal is now definable, allowing a solution path to be defined and followed in an incremental manner. We summarize our collective progress to date in developing the underlying science and technology that will enable the functions of specific brain regions to be replaced by multichip modules consisting of novel, hybrid analog-digital microchips. The component microchips are "neurocomputational," incorporating experimentally based mathematical models of the nonlinear dynamic and adaptive properties of real brain neurons and neural networks. The resulting hardware can perform computations supporting cognitive functions such as pattern recognition, but more generally will support any brain function for which there is sufficient experimental information.

To allow the "neurocomputational" multichip module to communicate with existing brain tissue, another novel microcircuitry element has been developed—silicon-based multielectrode arrays that are "neuromorphic," that is, designed to conform to the region-specific cytoarchitecture of the brain. When the "neurocomputational" and "neuromorphic" components are fully integrated, our vision is that the resulting prosthesis, after intracranial implantation, will receive electrical impulses from targeted subregions of the brain, process the information using the hardware model of that brain region, and communicate back to the functioning brain. The proposed prosthetic microchips also have been designed with parameters that can be optimized after implantation, allowing each prosthesis to adapt to a particular user or patient.

The System: The Hippocampus

The computational properties of the prosthesis being developed are based on the hippocampus, a cortical region of the brain involved in the formation of new long-term memories. The hippocampus lies beneath the phylogenetically more recent

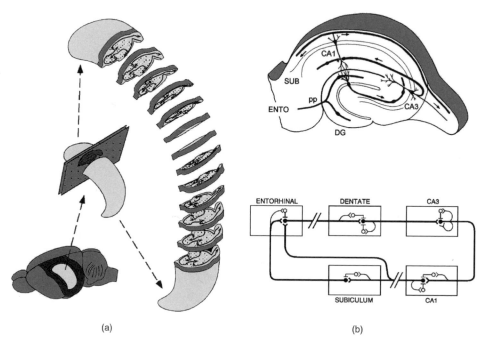

Figure 12.1
(*A*) Diagrammatic representation of the rat brain (*lower left*), showing the relative location of the hippo-campal formation on the left side of the brain (light gray); (*center*) diagrammatic representation of the left hippocampus after isolation from the brain and (*right*) slices of the hippocampus for sections transverse to the longitudinal axis. (*B*) Diagrammatic representations of a transverse slice of the hippocampus, illustrating its intrinsic organization: fibers from the entorhinal cortex (ENTO) project through the perforant path (pp) to the dentate gyrus (DG); granule cells of the dentate gyrus project to the CA3 region, which in turn projects to the CA1 region; CA1 cells project to the subiculum (SUB), which in the intact brain then projects back to the entorhinal cortex. In a slice preparation, return connections from CA1 and the subiculum are transected, creating an open-loop condition for experimental study of hippocampal neurons.

neocortex, and is composed of several different subsystems that form a closed feed-back loop (figure 12.1), with input from the neocortex entering via the entorhinal cortex, propagating through the intrinsic subregions of the hippocampus, and then returning to the neocortex. The intrinsic pathways consist of a cascade of excitatory connections organized roughly transverse to the longitudinal axis of the hippocam-pus. As such, the hippocampus can be conceived of as a set of interconnected, paral-lel circuits (Andersen et al., 1971; Amaral and Witter, 1989). The significance of this organizational feature is that after the hippocampus is removed from the brain, transverse "slices" (approximately 500 μm thick) of the structure that preserve a sub-stantial portion of the intrinsic circuitry may be maintained in vitro and thus allow detailed experimental study of its principal neurons in their open-loop condition (Berger et al., 1992, 1994).

The hippocampus is responsible for what have been called long-term "declarative" or "recognition" memories (Berger and Bassett, 1992; Eichenbaum, 1999; Shapiro and Eichenbaum, 1999; Squire and Zola-Morgan, 1998): the formation of mnemonic labels that identify a unifying collection of features (e.g., those comprising a person's face), and form relations between multiple collections of features (e.g., associating the visual features of a face with the auditory features of the name for that face). In lower species not having verbal capacity, an analogous hippocampal function is evidenced by an ability, for example, to learn and remember spatial relations among multiple, complex environmental clues in navigating and foraging for food (O'Keefe and Nadel, 1978). Major inputs to the hippocampus arise from virtually all other cortical brain regions, and transmit to the hippocampus high-level features extracted by each of the sensory systems subserved by these cortical areas.

Thus, the hippocampus processes both unimodal and multimodal features for virtually all classes of sensory input, and modifies these neural representations so that they can be associated (as in the case of forming a link between a face and a name) and stored in long-term memory in a manner that allows appropriate additional associations with previously learned information (the same face may have context-dependent names, for example, a first name in an informal, social setting and a position title in a formal or business setting), and that minimizes interference (the same name may be associated with several faces). After processing by the hippocampal system, new representations for important patterns are transmitted back to other cortical regions for long-term storage; thus, long-term memories are not stored in the hippocampus, but propagation of neural representations through its circuitry is required for a re-encoding essential for the effective transfer of short-term memory into long-term memory.

Although developing a neural model for long-term memory formation (or any other cognitive function) may initially appear somewhat daunting, there is a rational approach to the problem. Information in the hippocampus and all other parts of the brain is coded in terms of variation in the sequence of all-or-none, point-process (spike) events, or temporal pattern (for multiple neurons, variation in the spatiotemporal pattern). The essential signal-processing capability of a neuron is derived from its capacity to change an input sequence of interspike intervals into a different, output sequence of interspike intervals. The resulting input-output transformations in all brain regions are strongly nonlinear, owing to the nonlinear dynamics inherent in the molecular mechanisms that make up neurons and their synaptic connections (Magee et al., 1998). As a consequence, the output of virtually all neurons in the brain is highly dependent on the temporal properties of the input. The input-output transformations of neurons in the hippocampus and neocortex—the regions of the brain subserving pattern recognition—are the only "features" that the nervous system has to work with in constructing representations at the cortical level. Identifying the nonlinear input-output properties of neurons involved in pattern recognition is equivalent to identifying the feature models that endow the brain with its superior feature extraction capability. The input-output properties of synapses and neurons are not static, but are altered by biological learning mechanisms to achieve an optimal feature set during memory formation for a new pattern. Identifying activity-dependent forms of synaptic plasticity of the neurons involved in pattern recognition is equivalent to identifying the biological "learning rules" used in optimizing feature sets.

Biomimetic Models of Hippocampal Neuron Properties

Quantifying Input-Output Nonlinearities of Hippocampal Neurons

In order to incorporate the nonlinear dynamics of biological neurons into neuron models to develop a prosthesis, it is first necessary to measure them accurately. We have developed and applied methods for quantifying the nonlinear dynamics of hippocampal neurons (Berger et al., 1988a,b, 1991, 1992, 1994; Dalal et al., 1997) using principles of nonlinear systems theory (Lee and Schetzen, 1965; Krausz, 1975; P. Z. Marmarelis and Marmarelis, 1978; Rugh, 1981; Sclabassi et al., 1988). In this approach, properties of neurons are assessed experimentally by applying a random interval train of electrical impulses as an input and electrophysiologically recording the evoked output of the target neuron during stimulation (figure 12.2A). The input train consists of a series of impulses (as many as 4064), with interimpulse intervals varying according to a Poisson process having a mean of 500 ms and a range of 0.2–5000 ms. Thus, the input is "broadband" and stimulates the neuron over most of its operating range; that is, the statistical properties of the random train are highly consistent with the known physiological properties of hippocampal neurons.

Nonlinear response properties are expressed in terms of the relation between progressively higher-order temporal properties of a sequence of input events and the probability of neuronal output, and are modeled as the kernels of a functional power series. In the case of a third-order estimation:

$$y(t) = G_0 + G_1[h_1, x(t)] + G_2[h_2, x(t)] + G_3[h_3, x(t)] + \cdots,$$

where $y(t)$ is the output, (G_i) is a set of functionals, and (h_i) is a set of kernels that characterize the relationship between the input and output:

$$G_0(t) = h_0$$

$$G_1(t) = \int h_1(\tau) x(t - \tau) \, d\tau$$

$$G_2(t) = 2 \iint h_2(\tau, \tau + \Delta) x(t - \tau) x(t - \Delta - \tau) \, d\Delta \, d\tau$$

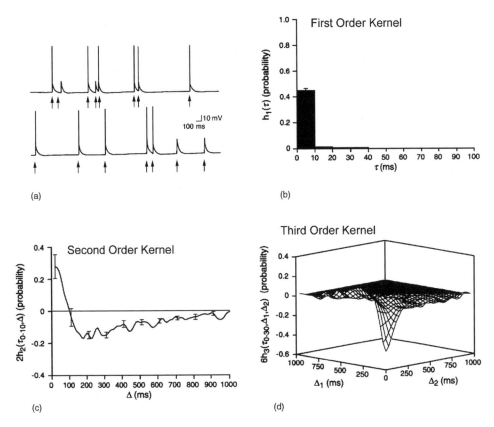

Figure 12.2
(*A*) Sample electrophysiological recording from a hippocampal granule cell during random impulse train stimulation. Each arrow indicates when an electrical impulse is applied to perforant path inputs (see figure 12.1). Large, positive-going, unitary (action potential) events indicate when an input generated an output response from the granule cell; smaller, positive-going events (e.g., to the first impulse and last two impulses) indicate when an input generated only a subthreshold response (no output). The time delay (latency) from the input event (arrow) to the granule cell response is equivalent to the parameter τ in the equations in the text (all latencies are less than 10 ms); the intervals between input events are equivalent to the parameter Δ in the equations in the text. (*B*) First-order kernel, $h_1(\tau)$, which represents the average probability of an action potential output occurring (with a latency of τ) to any input event in the train. (*C*) Second-order kernel, $h_2(\tau, \Delta)$, which represents the modulatory effect of any preceding input occurring Δ ms earlier on the most current impulse in the train. (*D*) Third-order kernel, $h_3(\tau, \Delta_1, \Delta_2)$, which represents the modulatory effects of any two preceding input events occurring Δ_1 ms and Δ_2 ms earlier on the most current impulse that are not accounted for by the first- and second-order kernels.

$$G_3(t) = 6 \iiint h_3(\tau, \tau + \Delta_1, \tau + \Delta_1 + \Delta_2) x(t - \tau) x(t - \tau - \Delta_1)$$

$$\times x(t - \tau - \Delta_1 - \Delta_2) \, d\Delta_1 \, d\Delta_2 \, d\tau$$

The train of discrete input events defined by $x(t)$ is a set of δ-functions. The first-, second-, and third-order kernels of the series are obtained using a variety of estimation procedures (Lee and Schetzen, 1965; Krausz, 1975; Marmarelis, 1990).

To clarify the interpretation of the kernels in the context of results for a typical granule cell of the hippocampus, the first-order kernel, $h_1(\tau)$, is the average probability of an action potential output occurring (with a latency of τ) to any input event in the train. The intensity of stimulation was chosen so that the first-order kernel had a probability value of 0.4–0.5 (figure 12.2B). The second-order kernel, $h_2(\tau, \Delta)$, represents the modulatory effect of any preceding input occurring Δ ms earlier on the most current impulse in the train (figure 12.2C). Second-order nonlinearities are strong: intervals in the range of 10–30 ms result in facilitation as great as 0.3–0.4 (summing the first- and second-order values, the probability of an output event is 0.8–1.0 for this range of intervals). The magnitude of second-order facilitation decreases as the interstimulus interval lengthens, with values of Δ greater than 100 ms leading to suppression; for example, interstimulus intervals in the range of 200–300 ms decrease the average probability of an output event by approximately 0.2. The third-order kernel, $h_3(\tau, \Delta_1, \Delta_2)$, represents the modulatory effects of any two preceding input events occurring Δ_1 ms and Δ_2 ms earlier on the most current impulse that are not accounted for by the first- and second-order kernels (figure 12.2D). The example third-order kernel shown is typical for hippocampal granule cells, and reveals that combinations of intervals less than approximately 150 ms lead to additional suppression of granule cell output by as much as 0.5. This third-order nonlinearity represents in part saturation of second-order facilitative effects.

Improved Kernel Estimation Methods

The output of hippocampal and other cortical neurons exhibits a dependence on the input temporal pattern that is among the greatest of any class of neuron in the brain, because of a wide variety of voltage-dependent conductances found throughout their dendritic and somatic membranes. Despite this, input-output models of the type described here provide excellent predictive models of cortical neuron behavior. Depending on the circumstances, kernels to the third order, and sometimes even to the second order alone, can account for 80–90% of the variance of hippocampal neuron output. Until recently, high-order nonlinearities have been difficult to estimate accurately; traditional kernel estimation methods (e.g., cross-correlation) are highly sensitive to noise and thus require long data sequences. To circumvent these problems, we have developed several novel methods for estimating nonlinearities that are significantly more efficient and result in substantially improved kernel estimates (Krieger et al., 1992; Marmarelis, 1990; V. Z. Marmarelis and Orme, 1993; Saglam et al., 1996; V. Z. Marmarelis and Zhao, 1997; Iatrou et al., 1999a,b; Alataris et al., 2000).

Several of the new methods involve the use of feedforward artificial neural networks (ANN). We have compared the Volterra-Wiener (cross-correlation) and ANN models in terms of their prediction ability on test data. The results showed two major advantages of the new-generation methodologies: (1) a significant reduction in the required data length (by a factor of at least 10) to achieve similar or better levels of prediction accuracy, and (2) an ability to model higher-order nonlinearities that could not be detected using traditional kernel estimation methods. In addition, we have recently developed methods capable of estimating nonstationary processes, and demonstrated their efficacy with long-term forms of hippocampal cellular plasticity (Xie et al., 1992, 1997; Thiels et al., 1994; Baudry, 1998). The ability to accurately characterize nonstationarities provides the opportunity to extend the applicability of this approach to modeling adaptive properties of hippocampal and other cortical neural systems as well.

In total, the kernel functions represent an experimentally based model that is highly accurate in describing the functional dynamics of the neuron in terms of the probability of neuron output as a function of the recent history of the input. As such, the kernels provide a mathematically "compact" representation of the resulting composite dynamics because each of the many contributing biological processes need not be represented individually, or for that matter, even be known. In addition, because of the broadband nature of the test stimulus, the model generalizes to a wide range of input conditions, even to input patterns that are not explicitly included in the random impulse train. As such, the kernels not only provide the basis for a biologically realistic neural network model, but also perhaps an ideal basis for an implantable neural prosthesis. An input-output model can be substituted for a neuron on which the model is experimentally based, without regard to the variability in neural representations that must exist from individual to individual, or the nearly infinite range of environmental stimuli that would give rise to those representations.

Neural Network Models with Biologically Realistic Dynamics

Conventional, Artificial Neural Networks
Brainlike processing is often modeled mathematically as artificial neural networks, or networks of processing elements that interact through connections. In artificial neural network models, a connection between processing elements—despite the complexity of the synaptic nonlinear dynamics described earlier—is represented as a single number to scale the amplitude of the output signal of a processing element. The

parameters of an artificial neural network can be optimized to perform a desired task by changing the strengths of connections according to what are termed learning rules, that is, algorithms for when and by how much the connection strengths are changed during optimization. This simplification of a synapse as a number results in two fundamental limitations. First, although a processing element can be connected to a large number of other processing elements, it can transmit only one, identical signal to all other elements. Second, only the connection strength can be changed during the optimization process, which amounts to merely changing the gain of the output signal of a processing element.

The "Dynamic Synapse" Neural Network Architecture

In an effort to develop more biologically realistic neural network models that include some of the temporal nonlinear signal-processing properties of neurons, we have developed the "dynamic synapse" neural network architecture (Liaw and Berger, 1996). In this scheme, processing elements are assumed to transmit information by variation in a series of point-process (i.e., all-or-none) events, and connections among processing elements are modeled as a set of linear and nonlinear processes so that the output becomes a function of the time since past input events (figure 12.3). By including these dynamic processes, each network connection transforms a sequence of input events into another sequence of output events. In the brain, it has been demonstrated that the functional properties of multiple synaptic outputs that arise from a given neuron are not identical. This characteristic of the brain also has been incorporated as a second fundamental property of dynamic synapse neural networks. Although the same essential dynamics are included in each synapse originating from a given processing unit, the precise values of time constants governing those dynamics are varied. The consequence arising from this second property is that each processing element transmits a spatiotemporal output signal, which, in principle, gives rise to an exponential growth in coding capacity.

Furthermore, we have developed a "dynamic learning algorithm" to train each dynamic synapse to perform an optimized transformation function so that the neural network can achieve highly complex tasks. Like the nonlinear dynamics described earlier and included in the dynamic synapse network models, this learning algorithm also is based on experimentally determined, adaptive properties of hippocampal cortical neurons (which cannot be reviewed here; see Xie et al., 1992, 1997; Thiels et al., 1994; Baudry, 1998), and is unique with respect to neural network modeling in that the transformation function extracts invariant features embedded in the input signal of each dynamic synapse. The combination of nonlinear dynamics and dynamic learning algorithm provides a high degree of robustness against noise, which is a major issue in processing real biological signals in the brain, as well as real-world

Conventional Neural Network

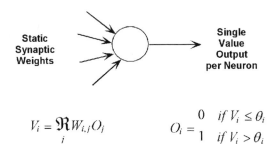

$$V_i = \mathfrak{R} W_{i,j} O_j \atop i \qquad\qquad O_i = \begin{matrix} 0 & \textit{if } V_i \leq \theta_i \\ 1 & \textit{if } V_i > \theta_i \end{matrix}$$

Dynamic Synapse Neural Network

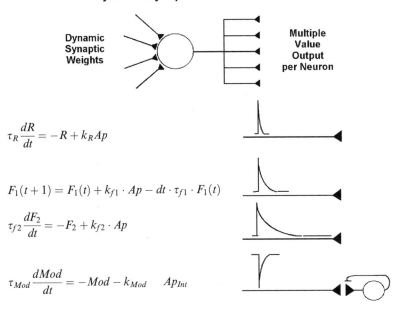

$$\tau_R \frac{dR}{dt} = -R + k_R Ap$$

$$F_1(t+1) = F_1(t) + k_{f1} \cdot Ap - dt \cdot \tau_{f1} \cdot F_1(t)$$

$$\tau_{f2}\frac{dF_2}{dt} = -F_2 + k_{f2} \cdot Ap$$

$$\tau_{Mod}\frac{dMod}{dt} = -Mod - k_{Mod} \quad Ap_{Int}$$

Figure 12.3
Properties of a processing element of a traditional artificial neural network versus properties of a processing element of a biologically realistic dynamic synapse neural network (see text for explanation).

signals, as demonstrated in our case studies of speaker-independent speech recognition described in the following paragraphs.

Application to Speech Recognition
Current state-of-the-art speech recognition technology is based on complex, multistage processing that is not biologically based. Although commercial systems can demonstrate impressive performance, they are still far from performing at the level of human listeners. To test the computational capability of the dynamic synapse neural network, two strong constraints were imposed: the network must be simple and small, and it must accomplish speech recognition in a single step, that is, with no preprocessing stages. Our system not only achieved this goal, but as will be described later, also performed better than human listeners when tested with speech signals corrupted by noise, marking the first time ever that a physical device has outperformed humans in a speech recognition task (Liaw and Berger, 1997, 1998, 1999).

Invariant Feature Extraction   Two characteristics of speech signals, variability and noise, make its recognition a difficult task. Variability refers to the fact that the same word is spoken in different ways by different speakers. Yet there exist invariant features in the speech signal, allowing the constant perception of a given word, regardless of the speaker or the manner of speaking. Our first application of the dynamic synapse neural network model to speech recognition was aimed at extracting those invariant features for a word set with very difficult discriminability, for example, "hat" versus "hut" versus "hit" (fourteen words in total), spoken by eight different speakers. The variability of two signals can be measured by how well they correlate with each other. As seen in figure 12.4 (lower left), the speech wave forms of the same word spoken by two speakers typically show a low degree of correlation; that is, they are quite different from each other. However, the dynamic synapse neural network can be trained to produce highly correlated signals for a given word (figure 12.4, lower right). Thus, the dynamic synapse neural network can extract invariant features embedded in speech signals that are inherently very difficult to discriminate, and can do so with no preprocessing of the data (only the output from a microphone was used) using a core signal-processing system that is extremely small and compact.

Robustness with Respect to White Noise   To test the robustness of the invariant features extracted by the dynamic synapse neural network, the network was first trained to recognize the words "yes" or "no" randomly drawn from a database containing utterances by some 7000 speakers with no added noise. We then evaluated the performance of the model when the speech signals not used during training were corrupted with progressively increasing amount of white noise [measured by the

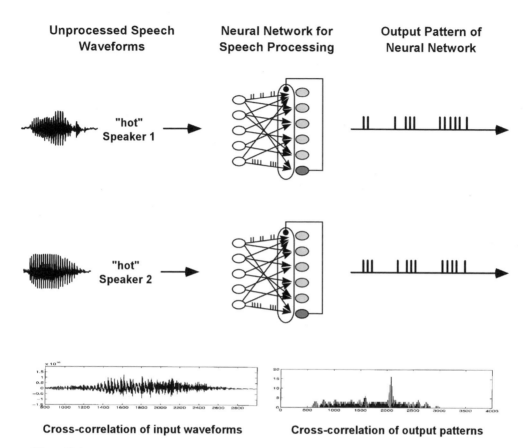

Figure 12.4

Conceptual representation of speaker-independent word recognition identification by a dynamic synapse neural network. Inputs to the network are digitized speech wave forms from different speakers for the same word, which have little similarity (low cross-correlation) because of differences in speaker vocalization. The two networks shown are intended to represent the same network on two different training or testing trials; in a real case, one network is trained with both (or more) speech wave forms. On any given trial, each speech wave form constitutes the input for all five of the input units shown in the first layer. Each unit in the first layer of the network generates a different pulse-train encoding of the speech wave form ("integrate and fire neurons" with different parameter values). The output of each synapse (arrows) to the second layer of the network is governed by four dynamic processes (see figure 12.3), with two of those processes representing second-order nonlinearities; thus, the output to the second layer neurons depends on the time since prior input events. A dynamic learning rule modifies the relative contribution of each dynamic process until the output neurons converge on a common temporal pattern in response to different input speech signals (i.e., high cross-correlation between the output patterns).

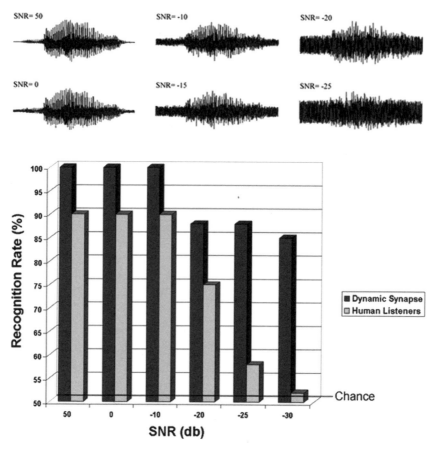

Figure 12.5
Comparison of recognition rates by the dynamic synapse neural network system (dark gray bars) and human listeners (light gray bars) for speaker-independent identification of the words "yes" and "no" when increasing amounts of white noise are added to the speech wave forms. Note that a 50% recognition rate is equivalent to chance.

signal-to-noise-ratio (SNR) in decibels]. The results showed that our model is extremely robust against noise, performing better than human listeners tested with the same speech dataset (figure 12.5). This is first time ever that a speech recognition system has outperformed human listeners, and the dynamic synapse system did so by a considerable margin.

Comparison with a State-of-the-Art Commercial Product and Robustness with Respect to Conversational Noise   The objective of this study was to compare the performance of the dynamic synapse neural network and one of the best state-of-the-art,

commercially available systems, namely, the Dragon Naturally Speaking speech recognition system. Since the Dragon system operates in a speaker-specific mode (the
system is trained specifically for one user), the speech signals consist of the words
"yes," "no," "fire," "stop" spoken by a single speaker. The Dragon system was
trained in two stages. In the first stage, the system was fully trained using the material provided by the manufacturer. In the second stage, it was further trained using
the four target words.

Once the training was complete, both the dynamic synapse neural network and the
Dragon system were tested with noise-added speech signals at various SNRs. A realistic, "conversational" type of noise was used: a recording of one female speaker and
one male speaker voice-reading newspapers simultaneously, along with the broadcast
of a news program on the radio. The same noise-added speech signals were used to
test human performance (average of five subjects). The results (figure 12.6) show that
the Dragon system is extremely sensitive to noise and performs poorly under noisy
conditions. Its performance degraded to 50% correct when the SNR was +20 dB,
whereas both the dynamic synapse neural network and human listeners retained a
100% recognition rate. The Dragon system failed to recognize any word when the
SNR was +10 dB, whereas the dynamic synapse neural network and human listeners
performed at 100 and 90% recognition rates, respectively. Furthermore, the dynamic
synapse neural network was highly robust and performed significantly better than
human listeners when the SNR dropped below +2.5 dB. For example, for an SNR
ranging from 0 to −5 dB, human performance varied from a 30 to 15% correct rate,
while the dynamic synapse neural network retained a 75% correct rate. These findings show that human listeners perform far better than the Dragon system in terms
of robustness against noise. Performance degradation under noisy conditions is well
documented for all speech recognition systems based on conventional technology,
like that used in the Dragon system. In contrast, the dynamic synapse neural network
significantly outperformed the Dragon system, demonstrating a robustness superior
to human listeners under highly noisy conditions.

The significance of these findings with respect to developing a neural prosthesis for
replacing cognitive functions is severalfold. First, the dynamic synapse neural network used in the studies described here is remarkably small: only eleven processing
units and thirty synapses. The computational power of such a small network suggests
that extremely large neural networks will not be required for developing replacement
silicon-based circuitry for the brain. Second, the speaker-independent applications of
the dynamic synapse technology were performed using an unsupervised learning algorithm, meaning that the features of the variable speech signals upon which successful word recognition were based were not identified a priori; the network was allowed
to find an optimized feature set independently. In the context of an implantable prosthesis, this is obviously a desirable advantage in the sense that it may be reasonable

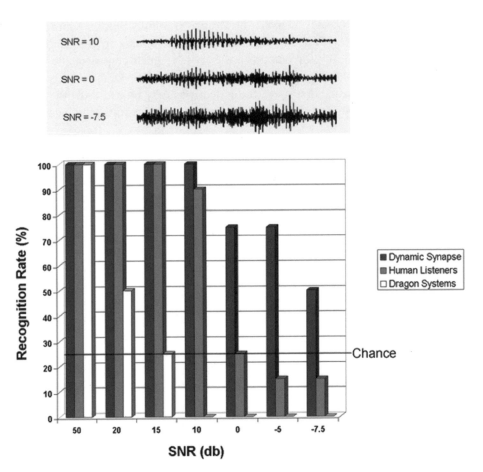

Figure 12.6
Comparison of recognition rates by the dynamic synapse neural network system (dark gray bars), human listeners (light gray bars), and the Dragon Naturally Speaking System (white bars) for speaker-specific identification of the words "yes" and "no" when increasing amounts of conversational noise (see text) are added to the speech wave forms. Note that a 25% recognition rate is equivalent to chance.

to consider devices that adapt to the host brain by optimizing a set of initial parameters. Given that we know so little about the features used in pattern recognition for many parts of the brain, having to depend on their a priori identification would represent a substantial impediment to progress. Third, the robustness of the trained dynamic synapse system clearly suggests that combining biologically based nonlinear dynamics with biologically based learning rules may provide a new paradigm for identifying algorithms of the brain for feature extraction and pattern recognition, and opens the possibility for studying radically novel feature sets that are not predictable on the basis of current theoretical frameworks.

Analog Very Large-Scale Integrated Implementations of Biologically Realistic Neural Network Models

To this point, we have addressed issues concerning the first two essential requirements for an implantable neural prosthesis. We have shown that it is possible to obtain experimentally based, biologically realistic models that accurately predict hippocampal neuron behavior for a wide range of input conditions, including those known to be physiologically relevant. In addition, we have shown that the fundamental, nonlinear dynamic properties of hippocampal neurons can provide the basis for a neural network model that can be trained according to biologically realistic learning rules to respond selectively to temporal and spatiotemporal patterns coded in the form of point-process spike trains, which are found in the brain. Moreover, patterns can be recognized by the network model even when input signals are embedded in substantial amounts of noise, a characteristic both of real-world conditions and of signaling in the brain. In the next section we address the third essential requirement, namely, the need to implement neuron and neural network models in silicon, so that miniaturization will allow intracranial implantation.

Design and Fabrication of Programmable, Second-Order, Nonlinear Neuron Models

We have designed and fabricated several generations of hardware implementations of our biologically realistic models of hippocampal neural network nonlinear dynamics using analog very large-scale integrated (VLSI) technology (Tsai et al., 1996, 1998a,b). The model expressions of the first- and second-order kernel functions describing those dynamics are computed in analog current mode instead of digital format to fully exploit massively parallel processing capability. The particular objective of the design described here was to incorporate programmable, second-order nonlinear, model-based parameters so that a flexible, generally applicable hardware model of hippocampal nonlinearities could be developed. A fabricated and tested 3×3 neural network chip is shown in figure 12.7.

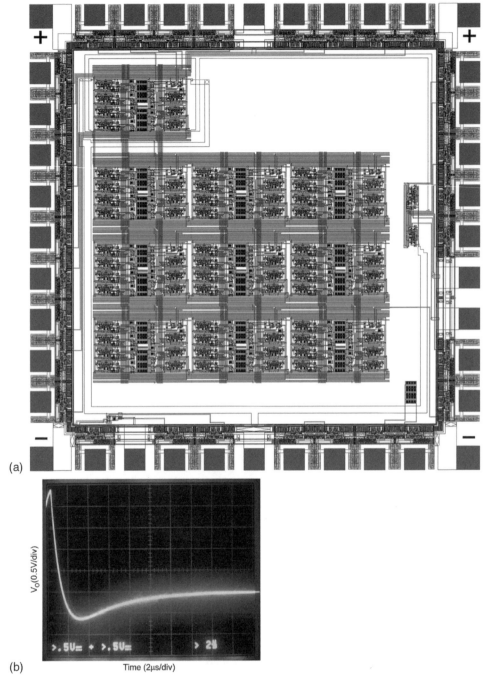

(a)

(b)

Figure 12.7
(*A*) Hybrid analog-digital VLSI implementation of a 3 × 3 network of hippocampal neuron models with second-order nonlinear properties. (*B*) A second-order kernel function generated by on-chip circuitry (compare with the second-order kernel shown in figure 12.2). The first-order kernel value and the second-order nonlinear function are programmable from off-chip circuitry.

The information transmitted among neurons is encoded in the interpulse intervals of pulse trains. Different synaptic weights can be applied to the input pulse trains. Each neuron executes the convolution of a model-based second-order kernel function as

$$h_2(\Delta) = a \times 10^{-b\Delta} - c \times 10^{-d\Delta}$$

The parameters a, b, c, d, and an h_1 offset are programmable not only so that the same design can accommodate nonlinearities characteristic of different subpopulations of hippocampal neurons, but also so that training-induced modification of nonlinearities can be accommodated.

The programmable pulse-coded neural processor for the hippocampal region was fabricated by a double-polysilicon, triple-metal process with a linear capacitor option through the Metal Oxide Semiconductor Implementation Service (MOSIS) service. Each neuron contains two input stages connected to two outputs of other neurons in the network. The exponential decay in the expression is implemented by a modified, wide-range Gilbert multiplier and a capacitor. During initialization of the chip, the initial state potentials are loaded to the state capacitors. The parameter values are stored on capacitors. These analog values are refreshed regularly by off-chip circuitry and can be changed by controlling software. Bias voltages to set the multipliers and variable resistors in the correct operational modes also are required.

When operating with a 3.3-V power supply, simulation results show a 60-dB dynamic range. Depending on the complexity of the multiplier design, the resistance can vary from 300 Ω to 300 kΩ. If the state potential is larger than the threshold when an input pulse arrives, an output pulse is generated. Testing of fabricated chips shows a reproducibility of experimentally determined input-output behavior of hippocampal neurons with a mean-square error of less than 3%.

Design of a High-Density Hippocampal Neuron Network Processor

Although it is not yet known how many silicon neurons will be needed for an effective prosthesis, the number is likely to be in the hundreds or thousands. This demands a capability to scale up the type of fundamental design described here. To accomplish this goal, we have utilized concepts of neuron sharing and asynchronized processing to complete the design of a high-density neuroprocessor array consisting of 128×128 second-order nonlinear processing elements on a single microchip (Tsai et al., 1999). Each single processor is composed of four data buffers, four indium bump flip-chip bonding pads (see later discussion), and one shared-neuron model with second-order nonlinear properties (figure 12.8). The processing procedure is as follows: (1) The input data are held in an input memory as the data arrive. (2) The input array is divided in 16 parts, with each part a 32×32 array. (3) Each part

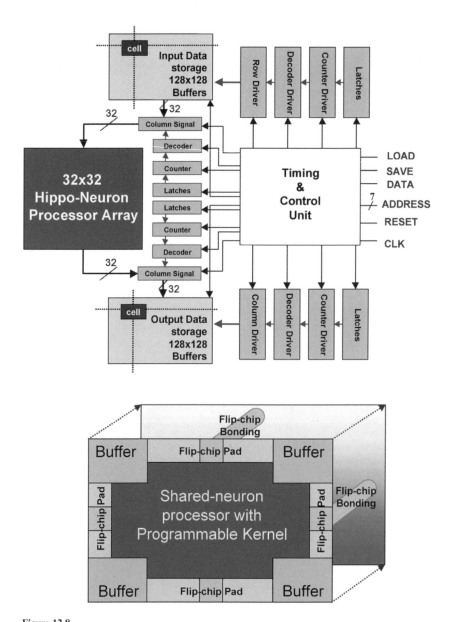

Figure 12.8
Schematic diagram for a scalable version of the programmable, second-order, nonlinear neural processor shown in figure 12.6. This layout is scalable to a 128×128 neuron model network.

of the input data is sent to the processor array, with each neuron processing four buffered data, one at a time. (4) All parameters of the kernel function are updated. (5) After all 16 data parts have been processed, the results are stored in an output buffer array.

This design not only provides programmable kernel parameters, but also incorporates indium bumps (four per processor) for flip-chip bonding to a second connectivity matrix chip. It (see figure 12.9) allows considerable connection flexibility by separating circuitry dedicated to processor dynamics from circuitry dedicated to connection architecture. With the additional technology for flip-chip bonding, the combined multichip module (not yet fabricated) will function much like a multilayer cellular neural network (CNN) structure (Chua and Yang, 1988).

VLSI Implementation of a Dynamic Synapse Neural Network

The VLSI implementation of a limited-capacity dynamic synapse neural network has been designed and fabricated using Taiwan Semiconductor Manufacturing Company (TSMC) 0.35-μm technology, as shown in figure 12.10 (Park et al., 2000). The dynamic synapse neural network chip includes six input neurons, two output neurons, one inhibitory neuron, eighteen dynamic synapses, and twenty-four input-output (I/O) pads. Each synapse consists of seven differential processing blocks, two hysteresis comparators, one AND gate, two transmission gates, and biasing circuitry. As described in the previous section, the functional properties of each synapse are determined by four dynamic processes, each having different time courses. Three of the processes are excitatory and one is inhibitory; two of the processes represent different second-order nonlinearities.

The resistor-capacitor exponential decay circuit for the dynamic processes is implemented using poly (poly1/poly2) capacitance and N-type metal-oxide semiconductor (NMOS) active registers to save chip area. The voltage-controlled active NMOS channel resistance and current source are used to achieve the programmability of parameter values of the dynamic synaptic neural network by controlling biases. Each differential equation-processing block is implemented with fully programmable voltage-controlled active resistors, poly capacitors, and a current source. Each differential processing circuit consists of two metal-oxide semiconductor field-effect transistors (MOSFETs) for active resistors, one poly capacitor, three control MOSFETs, two transmission gates, and one inverter. A novel, efficient low-power analog summation circuit was developed without using operational amplifiers, which require significant silicon area and more power consumption.

The capacity of this prototype dynamic synapse microchip is limited (because of the small number of output neurons), and not yet fully determined because the upper capacity depends in large part on the decoding scheme used to distinguish different

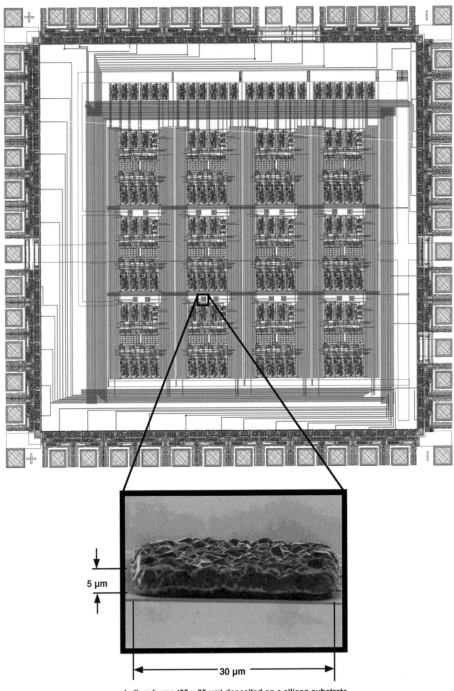

Indium bump (30 x 30 µm) deposited on a silicon substrate

temporal patterns, an issue that is still under investigation. Nonetheless, the successful implementation of this neural network model demonstrates that biologically realistic nonlinear dynamics that perform a high-level pattern recognition function can be realized in hardware. We are currently working on an expanded design that will provide for 400 dynamic synapses and on-chip implementation of the dynamic learning rule used to optimize feature extraction by the network.

What we have attempted to clarify in this section are several points relevant to a hardware implementation of biologically realistic neural network models. First, nonlinear dynamics (at least to the second order) characteristic of hippocampal and other cortical neurons can be efficiently implemented in mixed, analog-digital VLSI. The designs not only can be programmed to accommodate adaptive alterations in the dynamics of the microchip neuron models, but also can be scaled up to substantial numbers of processing elements. Considerable flexibility can be realized by separating the circuitry that implements processing element nonlinearities from the circuitry that implements the connectivity among the elements. Processing element and connectivity microchips can then be integrated as a multichip module.

Finally, a prototype of a dynamic synapse neural network capable of limited speech recognition has been designed, fabricated, and tested, demonstrating that a biomimetic neural network performing a cognitive function of neurological interest is feasible. Although the capacity of the microchips fabricated to date is admittedly not large, it is critical to distinguish between a functionality that significantly alleviates clinical symptoms and a functionality that reproduces the capabilities of an intact brain. A stroke patient who has lost all capability for speech need not be provided with a 5000-word vocabulary to substantially improve his or her quality of life; a vocabulary of even 20 words would constitute a marked recovery of function. Even the next-generation microchip neural networks will have a capacity that warrants considering their future clinical use, provided other technical barriers, such as interfacing with the living brain, can be overcome.

The Neuron/Silicon Interface

The major issues with regard to an effective neuron/silicon interface that will support bidirectional communication between the brain and an implantable neural prosthesis

Figure 12.9
Hybrid analog-digital VLSI implementation of a 4×4 network of hippocampal neuron models with second-order nonlinear properties designed using the layout scheme shown in figure 12.7. Also shown in the inset is an indium bump (two are included for each neuron model, one for input, one for output) that allows flip-chip bonding of this neuron-processing microchip to a second connectivity microchip (not shown) so that nonlinear processor properties and network connectivity properties are incorporated in different microchips of a multichip module.

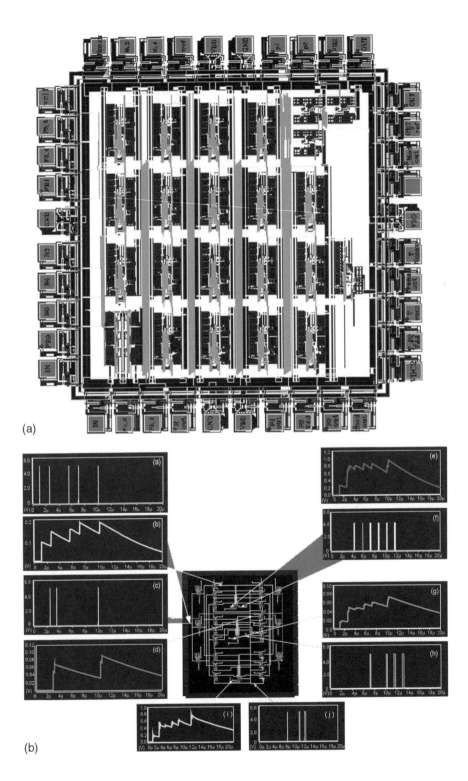

(a)

(b)

include (1) density of interconnections, (2) specificity of interconnections, and (3) bio-compatibility and long-term viability. The issue of density of interconnections refers to the fact that virtually all brain functions are mediated to a degree by a mass action of neural elements; that is, changing the activity of one neuron in a system is unlikely to have any substantial influence on the system's function, and thus on the cognitive process that depends on that function. The neuron/silicon interface must be designed so that a large number of neurons are affected by the implanted microchip.

The issue of specificity of interconnections refers to the fact that the neurons comprising a given brain region are not randomly distributed throughout the structure; most brain systems have a clear and definable "cytoarchitecture." For the hippocampus, the major features of this cytoarchitecture are a dense grouping of cell bodies into cell layers, with dendritic elements oriented perpendicular to those layers (see figure 12.1B, top). The issue of specificity also extends to the organization of intrinsic circuitry. In the case of the hippocampus, the entorhinal-to-dentate-to-CA3-to-CA1-subiculum pathway is composed of different cell populations that are spatially segregated from one another. Any neuron/silicon interface must be designed to be consistent with the cytoarchitectural constraints of the target tissue. Finally, the issue of long-term viability refers to the obvious problems of maintaining effective functional interactions between a microchip and brain tissue on a time scale of years because periodic replacement of an implant is not likely to be feasible.

Density and Specificity

With regard to density and specificity, one can either attempt to integrate these design considerations into the computational component of the prosthesis, or separate the computational and interface functions into different domains of the device and thus deal with the design constraints of each domain independently. We have chosen the latter strategy, developing silicon-based multisite electrode arrays with the capability to electrophysiologically record and stimulate living neural tissue. The fundamental technologies required for multichannel, bidirectional communication with brain tissue already exist commercially and are being developed further at a rapid rate (Egert et al., 1998; Hiroaki et al., 1999). Silicon-based, 64- and 128-electrode site recording and stimulating arrays having spatial scales consistent with the hippocampus of a mammalian animal brain (which is much smaller than that of a human) are now routinely used in our laboratory and several others (Gross et al., 1982;

Figure 12.10
(*A*) Hybrid analog-digital VLSI implementation of a six-input, two-output unit dynamic synapse neural network. The circuit design also includes one additional processing unit as part of the output layer that provides feedback to the dynamic synapses. In total, there are eighteen dynamic synapses. Network connectivity is fixed. (*B*) Results of a circuit simulation showing input and output pulse events, and analog potentials equivalent to excitatory and inhibitory synaptic events generated in the network connections.

A

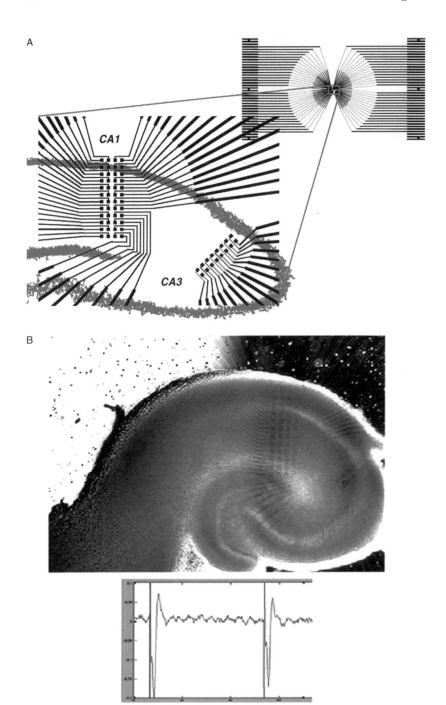

B

Wheeler and Novak, 1986; Stoppini et al., 1997; Egert et al., 1998; Stenger et al., 1998; Hiroaki et al., 1999; Berger et al., 1999; Gholmieh et al., 1999; Han et al., 2000; James et al., 2000; Shimono et al., 2000). In the near future, electrode densities sufficient to influence most of the neurons in a two-dimensional plane of a targeted brain region will be operational.

Most commercially available multisite electrode arrays have a uniform geometry, however, leaving the issue of specificity unresolved. For this reason, we have focused the greater part our research with respect to neural/silicon interfaces on designing multisite arrays in which the spatial distribution of electrode sites conforms to the cytoarchitecture of the target brain region, that is, array geometries specific to the hippocampus (Soussou et al., 1999). For example, one multisite electrode array that we have fabricated and tested was designed for CA3 inputs to the CA1 region of the rat hippocampus. Two rectangular arrays were constructed using silicon nitride and indium tin oxide (ITO): one 2×8 array of electrodes was oriented to stimulate CA3 axons that course through the dendritic region of CA1, and a second 4×12 array was positioned and oriented to record CA1 dendritic and cell body responses evoked as a consequence of stimulation through the first array (figure 12.11). This particular conformal probe had sixty-four 40×40-μm stimulating-recording pads and a 60-μm center-to-center interelectrode distance within each array.

The silicon nitride layer was deposited over the ITO electrodes, providing insulation both between the various electrodes and between each electrode and the hippocampal tissue. The layers were patterned to provide apertures only at the electrode tips. Silicon nitride films approximately 1500 Å thick were deposited using the plasma-enhanced chemical vapor deposition (PECVD) technique. Electrical characterization using a VLSI electronic probing station showed excellent insulation capability and electrical isolation, with less than a 1.8% cross-talk level on adjacent recording pads on the SiNx-insulated probes, measured over a frequency range from 100 Hz to 20 kHz with a sinusoidal wave form and 50 mV root-mean-square to 1000 mV root-mean-square signal amplitudes. Experimental testing with acutely prepared rat hippocampal slices consistently demonstrated evoked extracellular field potentials with signal-to-noise ratios greater than 10:1.

Additional mask designs that incorporate several key modifications have been successfully completed and fabricated. First, the recording-stimulating pads have been

Figure 12.11
(*A*) Schematic layout of a conformal multisite electrode array designed for electrical stimulation of CA3 inputs to the CA1 region of the hippocampus. (*B*) Photomicrograph of a hippocampal slice positioned on a conformal array fabricated on the basis of the layout shown in *A*. (*Bottom*) panel two extracellular field potential responses recorded from one of the electrode sites in the rectangular array located in CA1 following two stimulation impulses administered to two of the electrode sites (bipolar stimulation) in the rectangular array located in CA3.

resized to 30-μm diameters, a size approaching the diameter of a single neuron cell body. Combined with smaller center-to-center distances between pads, the smaller pad size will allow higher density arrays for greater spatial resolution when interfacing with a given brain region, and thus better monitoring and control of that region. Second, several new layouts have included different distributions of stimulation-recording pads that geometrically map several subregions of the hippocampus (figure 12.12). This represents the beginnings of a group of interface devices that will offer monitoring and control capabilities with respect to different subregions of the hippocampus, and ultimately other brain structures as well. In addition, more recent designs have utilized gold as the stimulation-recording electrode material to allow higher injection current densities during stimulation. Electrical characterization of the most recent generation of conformal neural probe arrays indicates, despite the higher density of electrodes, less than a 4.1% cross-talk level on adjacent recording pads.

Biocompatibility and Long-Term Viability

Many of the problems with respect to biocompatibility and long-term viability cannot be fully identified until the working prototypes of multielectrode arrays described earlier have been developed to the point that they can be tested through long-term implantation in animals. Nonetheless, we have begun to consider these issues and to develop research strategies to address them. One of the key obstacles will be maintaining close contact between the electrode sites of the interface device and the target neurons over time. We have begun investigating organic compounds that could be used to coat the surface of the interface device to increase its biocompatibility and thus promote outgrowth of neuronal processes from the host tissue and increase their adhesion to the interface materials.

Poly-D-lysine and laminin are known to be particularly effective in promoting adhesion of dissociated neuron cultures (cultures prepared from neonatal brain; neurons are prepared as a suspension and then allowed to adhere, redevelop processes, and reconnect into a network) onto inorganic materials (Stenger et al., 1998; James et al., 2000), and we have investigated their efficacy with regard to our hippocampal conformal multisite electrode arrays (Soussou et al., 1999, 2000). Poly-D-lysine and laminin were applied to the surface of the conformal arrays shown in figure 12.11, but application was limited to linear tracks aligned with the long axis of each column of electrode sites in the rectangular array. When dissociated hippocampal neurons were prepared on the surface of the array, the adhesion of cells and the extension of their processes were restricted to the treated regions; that is, hippocampal neurons were attracted, attached, and proliferated synaptic connections almost exclusively in parallel, linear tracks over the columns of electrodes (see chapter 11). Although this represents only an initial step in addressing the issues of biocompatibility, it is

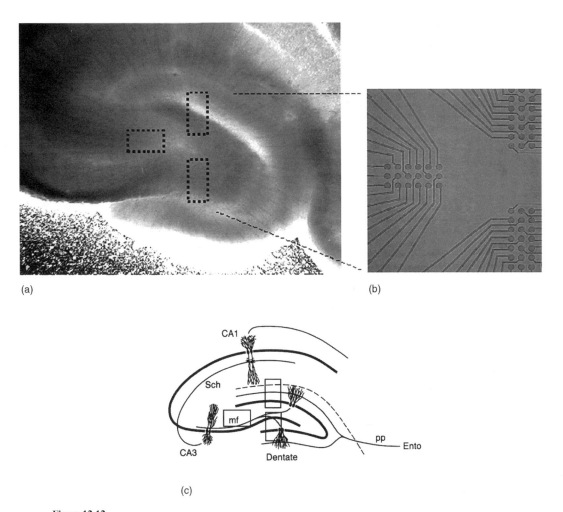

(a)

(b)

(c)

Figure 12.12
(*A*) Photomicrograph of a hippocampal slice placed over a conformal multisite electrode array designed and fabricated for stimulation and recording of activity from the dentate gyrus and CA3 regions. (*B*) Detailed visualization of the three sets of electrodes included in the dentate-CA3 array; each consists of a 3 × 6 electrode site rectangular array, with the two vertically oriented arrays designed for stimulation and recording from the dentate gyrus, and the horizontally oriented array designed for stimulation and recording from the CA3 region. (*C*) Schematic representation of a transverse section through the hippocampus illustrating the relative locations of its subfields.

through approaches such as these that we anticipate finding solutions to biocompatibility problems.

Although much of the electrophysiological testing of interfaces to date has been completed using acutely prepared hippocampal slices (which remain physiologically viable for 12–18 hr), we also have begun using hippocampal slice cultures to test the long-term viability of the neuron/silicon interface (Gholmieh et al., 1999). The latter preparations involve placing slices of hippocampus on a semipermeable membrane in contact with tissue culture media, and maintaining them long-term in a culture incubator (Stoppini et al., 1997). Slice cultures can be prepared directly onto multisite electrode arrays, which then can be taken out the incubator and tested periodically to examine the robustness of the electrophysiological interaction with the hippocampal tissue. Preliminary findings have revealed that bidirectional communication remains viable for at least several weeks, although we have yet to systematically test long-term functionality. The main point to be made here is that novel preparations like the slice culture will provide highly useful platforms for identifying and resolving viability issues.

Conclusions

The goal of this chapter was to bring into focus what we believe will be one of the premier thrusts of the emerging field of neural engineering: to develop implantable neural prostheses that can coexist and bidirectionally communicate with living brain tissue and thus substitute for a cognitive function lost as a result of damage and/or disease (figure 12.13). Because of progress in neuroscience, molecular biology, biomedical engineering, computer science, electrical engineering, and materials science, it is now reasonable to begin defining the combined theoretical and experimental pathways required to achieve this end. We have described here major progress on four of the essential requirements for an implantable neural prosthesis, achieved through a series of experimental and modeling studies using the hippocampus: biologically realistic neuron models that can effectively replace the functional properties of hippocampal cells, the concatenation of the neuron model dynamics into neural networks that can solve a pattern recognition problem of cognitive and neurological relevance, the implementation of biologically realistic neural network models in VLSI for miniaturization, and the development of silicon-based multisite electrode arrays that provide bidirectional communication with living neural tissue.

This progress does not constitute a set of final solutions to these four requirements. Additional work is needed on nonlinear models of neuron dynamics, both with respect to characterization of higher-order nonlinearities and particularly cross-input nonlinearities. All neurons receive inputs from more than one other source, and interactions among separate inputs most likely result in nonlinearities specific to

Intact Brain   Neuromorphic   Neurocomputational
                      Neuron-Silicon   Multi-Chip Module
                        Interface

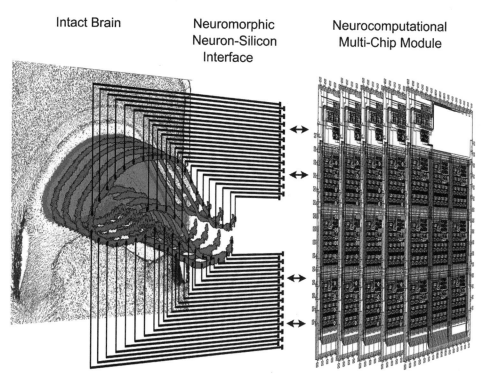

Figure 12.13
Conceptual representation of an implantable neural prosthesis for replacing lost cognitive function of higher cortical brain regions. The concept is illustrated here using a prosthesis substituting for a portion of the hippocampus. The two essential components of the prosthetic system are a "neurocomputational" multichip module that performs the computational functions of the dysfunctional or lost region of the hippocampus, and a "neuromorphic" multisite electrode array that acts as a neuron/silicon interface to allow the neurocomputational microchips to both receive input from, and send output to, the intact brain.

those interactions that cannot be characterized by our present experiments or modeling. Likewise, the dynamic synapse neural network models must be expanded both in terms of number of processing elements and numbers of network layers to begin approaching the complexity and mass action of brain subsystems for which a neural prosthesis will substitute. VLSI implementations of neural network models must be scaled up as well, and better incorporate efficient and novel interchip transmission technologies to achieve the high densities required for intracranial implantation. A critical factor is that future generations of biomimetic devices will require low-power designs to be compatible with the many temperature-sensitive biological mechanisms of the brain, an issue that our program has yet to address.

Finally, there remains much concerning organic–inorganic interactions that needs to be investigated for long-term compatibility between silicon-based technology and neural tissue. Although these problems are formidable, the rapid advances now occurring in the biological and engineering sciences promise equally rapid progress on elements of the global problem of intracranial implantable neural prostheses, particularly given the synergy that should emerge from cooperative efforts between the two sets of disciplines.

Acknowledgments

The authors gratefully acknowledge postdoctoral fellows and graduate students who made fundamental contributions to the theoretical and experimental work described here, most notably, Choi Choi, Sunil Dalal, Alireza Dibazar, Sageev George, Ghassan Gholmieh, Martin Han, T. Patrick Harty, Hassan Heidarin, Patrick Nasiatka, Walid Soussou, Dong Song, Jim Tai, Richard Tsai, Zhuo Wang, Xiaping Xie, and Mark Yeckel.

This research was supported by the Defense Advanced Research Projects Agency (DARPA) Brain Machine Interface Program (N66001-02-C-8057), Controlled Biological and Biomimetic Systems Program (grant N0001-14-98-1-0646), the DARPA Tissue-Based Biosensors Program (grant N0001-14-98-1-0825), the U.S. Office of Naval Research (grant N0001-14-98-1-0258), the National Centers for Research Resources (grant P44-RR01861), and the National Institute of Mental Health (grants MH51722 and MH00343).

References

Alataris, K., Berger, T. W., and Marmarelis, V. Z. (2000) A novel network for nonlinear modeling of neural systems with arbitrary point-process inputs. *Neural Networks* 13: 255–266.

Amaral, D. G., and Witter, M. P. (1989) The three-dimensional organization of the hippocampal formation: A review of anatomical data. *Neuroscience* 31: 571–591.

Andersen, P., Bliss, T. V. P., and Skrede, K. K. (1971) Lamellar organization of hippocampal excitatory pathways. *Exp. Brain Res.* 13: 222–238.

Baudry, M. (1998) Synaptic plasticity and learning and memory: 15 years of progress. *Neurobiol. Learning Memory* 70: 113–118.

Berger, T. W., Barrionuevo, G., Levitan, S. P., Krieger, D. N., and Sclabassi, R. J. (1991) Nonlinear systems analysis of network properties of the hippocampal formation. In J. W. Moore and M. Gabriel, eds., *Neurocomputation and Learning: Foundations of Adaptive Networks.* Cambridge, Mass.: MIT Press, pp. 283–352.

Berger, T. W., and Bassett, J. L. (1992) System properties of the hippocampus. In I. Gormezano and E. A. Wasserman, eds., *Learning and Memory: The Biological Substrates.* Hillsdale, N.J.: Lawrence Erlbaum, pp. 275–320.

Berger, T. W., Eriksson, J. L., Ciarolla, D. A., and Sclabassi, R. J. (1988a) Nonlinear systems analysis of the hippocampal perforant path-dentate projection. II. Effects of random train stimulation. *J. Neurophysiol.* 60: 1077–1094.

Berger, T. W., Eriksson, J. L., Ciarolla, D. A., and Sclabassi, R. J. (1988b) Nonlinear systems analysis of the hippocampal perforant path-dentate projection. III. Comparison of random train and paired impulse analyses. *J. Neurophysiol.* 60: 1095–1109.

Berger, T. W., Harty, T. P., Xie, X., Barrionuevo, G., and Sclabassi, R. J. (1992) Modeling of neuronal networks through experimental decomposition. *Proc. IEEE 34th Mid. Symp. Cir. Sys.*, pp. 91–97.

Berger, T. W., Chauvet, G., and Sclabassi, R. J. (1994) A biologically based model of functional properties of the hippocampus. *Neural Networks* 7: 1031–1064.

Berger, T. W., Soussou, W., Gholmieh, G., Brinton, R., and Baudry, M. (1999) Multielectrode array recordings from the hippocampus *in vitro*. *Soc. Neurosci. Abstr.* 25: 902.

Chua, L. O., and Yang, L. (1988) Cellular neural networks: Applications. *IEEE Trans. Circ. Syst.* 35(10): 1273–1290.

Dalal, S. S., Marmarelis, V. Z., and Berger, T. W. (1997) A nonlinear positive feedback model of glutamatergic synaptic transmission in dentate gyrus. In *Proceedings of the Fourth Joint Symposium on Neural Computation* 7 pp. 68–75.

Egert, U., Schlosshauer, B., Fennrich, S., Nisch, W., Fejtl, M., Knott, T., Müller, T., and Hämmerle, H. (1998) A novel organotypic long-term culture of the rat hippocampus on substrate-integrated multielectrode arrays. *Brain Res. Protoc.* 2: 229–242.

Eichenbaum, H. (1999) The hippocampus and mechanisms of declarative memory. *Behav. Brain Res.* 3: 123–133.

Gholmieh, G., Soussou, W., Brinton, R., Nordholm, A. F., Baudry, M., and Berger, T. W. (1999) Monitoring of trimethylopropane phosphate's (TMPP) neurotoxic effect on hippocampal slices and cells using multielectrode arrays. *Soc. Neurosci. Abstr.* 25: 902.

Gross, G. W., William, A. N., and Lucas, J. H. (1982) Recording of spontaneous activity with photoetched microelectrode surfaces from mouse spinal neurons in culture. *J. Neurosci. Meth.* 5: 13–22.

Han, M., Nasiatka, P., Gholmieh, G., Soussou, W., Baudry, M., Berger, T. W., and Tanguay, A. R. (2000) Conformally mapped neural probe arrays for multisite stimulation and recording. *Soc. Neurosci. Abstr.* 26: 184.

Hiroaki, O., Shimono, K., Ogawa, R., Sugihara, H., and Taketani, M. (1999) A new planar multielectrode array for extracellular recording: Application to hippocampal acute slice. *J. Neurosci. Meth.* 93: 61–67.

Humayum, M. S., de Juan Jr., E., Weiland, J. D., Dagnelie, G., Katona, S., Greenberg, R. J., and Suzuki, S. Pattern electrical stimulation of the human retina. *Vision Res.* (in press).

Iatrou, M., Berger, T. W., and Marmarelis, V. Z. (1999a) Modeling of nonlinear nonstationary dynamic systems with a novel class of artificial neural networks. *IEEE Trans. Neural Networks* 10: 327–339.

Iatrou, M., Berger, T. W., and Marmarelis, V. Z. (1999b) Application of a novel modeling method to the nonstationary properties of potentiation in the rabbit hippocampus. *Ann. Biomed. Eng.* 27: 581–591.

James, C. D., Davis, R., Meyer, M., Turner, A., Turner, S., Withers, G., Kam, L., Banker, G., Craighead, H., Isaacson, M., Turner, J., and Shain, W. (2000) Aligned microcontact printing of micrometer-scale poly-L-lysine structures for controlled growth of cultured neurons on planar microelectrode arrays. *IEEE Trans. Biomed. Eng.* 47: 17–21.

Krausz, H. (1975) Identification of nonlinear systems using random impulse train inputs. *Bio. Cyb.* 19: 217–230.

Krieger, D. N., Berger, T. W., and Sclabassi, R. J. (1992) Instantaneous characterization of time-varying nonlinear systems. *IEEE Trans. Biomed. Eng.* 39: 420–424.

Lee, Y. W., and Schetzen, M. (1965) Measurement of the kernels of a non-linear system by crosscorrelation. *Int. J. Control* 2: 237–254.

Liaw, J. S., and Berger, T. W. (1996) Dynamic synapse: A new concept of neural representation and computation. *Hippocampus* 6: 591–600.

Liaw, J. S., and Berger, T. W. (1997) Computing with dynamic synapses: A case study of speech recognition. In *Proceedings of the IEEE International Conference on Neural Networks*. New York: Institute of Electrical and Electronics Engineers, pp. 350–355.

Liaw, J. S., and Berger, T. W. (1998) Robust speech recognition with dynamic synapses. In *Proceedings of the IEEE International Conference Neural Networks*. New York: Institute of Electrical and Electronics Engineers, pp. 2175–2179.

Liaw, J. S., and Berger, T. W. (1999) Dynamic synapses: Harnessing the computing power of synaptic dynamics. *Neurocomputing* 26–27: 199–206.

Loeb, G. E. (1990) Cochlear prosthetics. *Ann. Rev. Neurosci.* 13: 357–371.

Magee, J., Hoffman, D., Colbert, C., and Johnston, D. (1998) Electrical and calcium signaling in dendrites of hippocampal pyramidal neurons. *Ann. Rev. Physiol.* 60: 327–346.

Marmarelis, V. Z. (1990) Identification of nonlinear biological systems using Laguerre expansions of kernels. *Ann. Biomed. Eng.* 21: 573–589.

Marmarelis, P. Z., and Marmarelis, V. Z. (1978) *Analysis of Physiological Systems: The White-Noise Approach.* New York: Plenum.

Marmarelis, V. Z., and Orme, M. E. (1993) Modeling of neural systems by use of neuronal modes. *IEEE Trans. Biomed. Eng.* 40: 1149–1158.

Marmarelis, V. Z., and Zhao, X. (1997) Volterra models and three-layer perceptrons. *IEEE Trans. Neural Networks* 8: 1421–1433.

Mauritz, K. H., and Peckham, H. P. (1987) Restoration of grasping functions in quadriplegic patients by functional electrical stimulation (FES), *Internat. J. Rehab. Res.* 10: 57–61.

O'Keefe, J., and Nadel, L. (1978) *The Hippocampus as a Cognitive Map.* New York: Oxford University Press.

Park, Y., Liaw, J.-S., Sheu, B. J., and Berger, T. W. (2000) Compact VLSI neural network circuit with high-capacity dynamic synapses. *Proc. IEEE Inter. Conf. Neural Networks* 4: 214–218.

Rugh, W. J. (1981) *Nonlinear Systems Theory: The Volterra/Wiener Approach.* Baltimore: John Hopkins University Press.

Saglam, M., Marmarelis, V., and Berger, T. (1996) Identification of brain systems with feedforward artificial neural networks. In *Proceedings of the World Congress on Neural Networks.* pp. 478–481.

Sclabassi, R. J., Krieger, D. N., and Berger, T. W. (1988) A systems theoretic approach to the study of CNS function. *Ann. Biomed. Eng.* 16: 17–34.

Shapiro, M. L., and Eichenbaum, H. (1999) Hippocampus as a memory map: Synaptic plasticity and memory encoding by hippocampal neurons. *Hippocampus* 9: 365–384.

Shimono, K., Brucher, F., Granger, R., Lynch, G., and Taketani, M. (2000) Origins and distribution of cholinergically induced θ rhythms in hippocampal slices. *J. Neurosci.* 20: 8462–8473.

Squire, L. R., and Zola-Morgan, S. (1998) Episodic memory, semantic memory, and amnesia. *Hippocampus* 8: 205–211.

Soussou, W., Yoon, G., Gholmieh, G., Brinton, R., and Berger, T. W. (1999) Characterization of dissociated hippocampal neurons cultured on various biochemical substrates and multielectrode arrays for the creation of neuronal networks. *Soc. Neurosci. Abstr.* 25: 903.

Soussou, W., Yoon, G., Gholmieh, G., Brinton, R., and Berger, T. W. (2000) Network responses of dissociated hippocampal neurons cultured onto multi-electrode arrays. *Soc. Neurosci. Abstr.* 26: 1699.

Stenger, D. A., Hickman, J. J., Bateman, K. E., Ravenscroft, M. S., Ma, W., Pancrazio, J. J., Shaffer, K., Schaffner, A. E., Cribbs, D. H., and Cotman, C. W. (1998) Microlithographic determination of axonal/dendritic polarity in cultured hippocampal neurons. *J. Neurosci. Meth.* 82: 167–173.

Stoppini, L., Duport, S., and Correges, P. (1997) New extracellular multirecording system for electrophysiological studies: Application to hippocampal organotypic cultures. *J. Neurosci. Meth.* 72: 23–33.

Thiels, E., Barrionuevo, G., and Berger, T. W. (1994) Induction of long-term depression in hippocampus *in vivo* requires postsynaptic inhibition. *J. Neurophysiol.* 72: 3009–3016.

Tsai, R. H., Sheu, B. J., and Berger, T. W. (1996) VLSI design for real-time signal processing based on biologically realistic neural models. *Proc. IEEE Inter. Conf. Neural Networks* 2: 676–681.

Tsai, R. H., Sheu, B. J., and Berger, T. W. (1998a) Design of a programmable pulse-coded neural processor for the hippocampus. *Proc. IEEE Inter. Conf. Neural Networks* 1: 784–789.

Tsai, R. H., Sheu, B. J., and Berger, T. W. (1998b) A VLSI neural network processor based on a model of the hippocampus. *Analog Integ. Cir. Sig. Process.* 15: 201–213.

Tsai, R. H., Tai, J. C., Sheu, B. J., Tanguay, Jr., A. R., and Berger, T. W. (1999) Design of a scalable and programmable hippocampal neural network multi-chip module. *Soc. Neurosci. Abstr.* 25: 902.

Wheeler, B. C., and Novak, J. L. (1986) Current source density estimation using microelectrode array data from the hippocampal slice preparation. *IEEE Trans. Biomed. Eng.* 33: 1204–1212.

Xie, X., Berger, T. W., and Barrionuevo, G. (1992) Isolated NMDA receptor-mediated synaptic responses express both LTP and LTD. *J. Neurophysiol.* 67: 1009–1013.

Xie, X., Liaw, J. S., Baudry, M., and Berger, T. W. (1997) Novel expression mechanism for synaptic potentiation: Alignment of presynaptic release site and postsynaptic receptor. *Proc. Natl. Acad. Sci. U.S.A.* 94: 6983–6988.

13 Brain Circuit Implementation: High-Precision Computation from Low-Precision Components

Richard Granger

Attempts to understand, let alone augment or supplant, the operation of brain circuitry rely not only on our knowledge of isolated neuron, circuit, and brain slice behavior but also on the impressive computations achieved by assemblies of these components. The variability of the constituent elements of these circuits suggests that they are arranged to operate in ways not obvious from standard engineering points of view. The quite nonstandard (and in many cases, apparently substandard) unit components of these circuit designs (synapses and cells that are probabilistic, relatively low precision, very sparsely connected, and orders of magnitude slower than the typical elements of most engineering devices) provide constraints on their possible contributions to the overall computation of neural circuits. Since the resultant brain circuits outperform extant engineering devices in many realms of crucial application ranging from recognition of complex visual or auditory signals to motoric traversal of complex terrain, our ability to imitate them can lead to two related but distinct classes of scientific advance: new and unanticipated types of hardware devices based on the unveiled engineering principles, and enabling technologies for the integration of extrinsic devices with intrinsic brain circuitry. This latter capability implies two directions of improved communication: a heightened ability to "listen to" and interpret brain activity, and a growing faculty for "talking back" to the brain, which may ameliorate impaired brain function or enhance normal function.

Background and Approach

The computations performed by human (or even rat) brains have not yet been matched by engineering approaches despite tremendous amounts of money spent on the attempts. It is not known why painstakingly developed artificial approaches continue to fall short of human performance. Even approaches that attempt to simulate complex human behaviors may well be based on descriptions of those behaviors that are incorrectly or incompletely specified. A prerequisite to replicating (let alone exceeding) human abilities may turn out to be a clear computational understanding of brain mechanisms. Among the vast body of data on brain mechanisms are a few key facts:

• The evolution of the mammalian forebrain (telencephalon) gave rise to the emergence of new circuits that do not appear in other classes (e.g., reptiles, birds). Probably the most advanced of these, thalamocortical circuits, are also by far the most numerous, accounting for an allometrically disproportionate space in mammalian brains, including the vast majority of circuits in the human brain.

• Study of the anatomical design and physiological operation of these circuits has led to the derivation of specific algorithms that these circuits may be carrying out.

• This derivation suggests that distinct brain regions carry out distinct algorithms, each contributing a different set of computations, with further composite algorithms arising from interactions among multiple brain regions.

• The key features of most telencephalic circuits include sparse connectivity among neurons ($p \leq 0.001$); low-precision synaptic connections (≤ 4 bits); simple processors (addition, multiplication); simple "learning" rules (fixed size increase or decrease); slow operation (milliseconds per operation versus nanoseconds for typical computer hardware); variable, probabilistic responses (versus the fixed, deterministic responses of engineering devices).

These characteristics should be a severe liability for brain circuits, raising the question of how they can achieve the advanced behavioral performance exhibited by organisms. Indeed, it is sometimes instead assumed that these substandard assessments of brain components are incorrect, driving an ongoing search for hidden precision in brain components, including carefully timed synchronies, as opposed to the variable synchronies underlying electroencephalograms (EEGs); precisely timed sequences of neuronal firing (spike trains), as opposed to sequences driven probabilistically (such as Poisson sequences); added topography in brain wiring, as opposed to the coexistence of topographic and highly nontopographic circuits described by much quantitative anatomical research; and complex high-precision synapses carefully arrayed on dendrites, as opposed to relatively low-precision synapses probabilistically arrayed. Typical artificial neural networks (ANNs) make use of some or all of these "improvements" in neural machinery, enabling higher-precision computation. However, owing to the costs of the higher-precision machinery used, such networks sometimes have relatively high costs in space and time complexity, resulting in systems that do not readily scale to problems of large size.

An alternative is that brain circuits do use sparse, probabilistic, slow, low-precision components to perform the rapid, high-precision computations that apparently underlie our advanced sensory and motor capabilities, via algorithms that combine these components in such a way as to enable the emergence of precision computation. Work in our laboratory in recent years has shown how these biological components, although impoverished from the viewpoint of standard engineering, nonetheless may give rise to specific useful high-precision computational methods. This research has resulted in the derivation of a range of algorithms, including hierarchical clustering (Ambros-Ingerson et al., 1990; Kilborn et al., 1996); sequence prediction (Granger et al., 1994; Aleksandrovsky et al., 1996); time dilation (Granger et al., 1994); Bayes classification (Coultrip & Granger, 1994); high-capacity storage and retrieval (Aleksandrovsky et al., 1996; Whitson, 1998; Rodriguez et al., 2004); reinforcement learning (Brucher, 2000); and novelty detection, data compression, and hash coding (Granger et al., 1994; Rodriguez et al., 2004).

If these impoverished components can carry out these advanced algorithms, then the low precision of the components becomes an advantage rather than a liability. It enables relatively cheap (sparse, slow, low-precision) components to do a job that otherwise would require much more expensive apparatus. In particular, this suggests the utility of direct hardware implementations in which low-precision components carry out these algorithms. ANNs typically require computing units with eight or more bits of precision, with relatively dense connectivity among these units, and their computations degrade in performance with reductions in either precision or connection density. A system reliant on these characteristics cannot use lower-precision components to carry out the same computations, and cannot readily be scaled to large sizes.

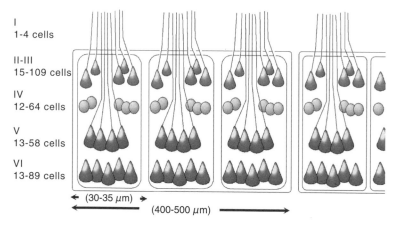

I
1-4 cells

II-III
15-109 cells

IV
12-64 cells

V
13-58 cells

VI
13-89 cells

← (30-35 μm) →

(400-500 μm)

Figure 13.1
Pyramidal cell modules (White and Peters, 1993) are anatomically organized by grouping apical dendrites of layer II, III, and V cells, and have been proposed as candidate anatomical underpinnings of vertical organizations of the cortex, such as columns (Mountcastle, 1957) that have only been described physiologically. Shown are typical ranges of numbers of neurons within each module; the variance decreases if certain less typical regions such as primary sensory and motor areas are excluded. The modules are roughly 30–35 μm in size and may be constituents of larger columnar arrangements.

Thalamocortical Circuits

Figure 13.1 illustrates the key anatomical architectural characteristics of thalamo-cortical circuits (Rodriguez et al., 2004). Neurons are vertically organized into "pyramidal cell modules" (White and Peters, 1993; Peters et al., 1994), roughly 30–35 µm across, consisting of distinct groups of layer V and layer II–III pyramidal cells whose apical dendrites are commingled. Functional "columns" that are physiologically defined in terms of receptive field properties, rather than anatomical boundaries (e.g., Mountcastle, 1957, 1978), are often described as 400–500 µm or more in extent (Jones, 1981), thus comprising perhaps 200 pyramidal cell modules apiece.

Figure 13.2 illustrates the overall architecture of the thalamocortical system. Neurons throughout the neocortex are organized into relatively stereotypical architectures. Although cortical studies describe some (subtle but potentially crucial) dif-

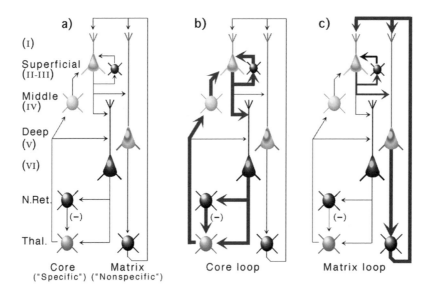

Figure 13.2
(*a*) Components and organization of the thalamocortical elements modeled. Included are features that re-cur throughout much of the neocortex, especially in polysensory and association areas. Characteristics spe-cific to primary sensory and motor areas are not modeled. (*b*) One primary loop through thalamocortical circuitry. Afferents from "core" thalamic nuclei (see text) project to layer IV and deep layer III; axons from superficial layer small pyramidal cells engage in local excitatory-inhibitory circuits as well as giving rise to collateral projections to deep layers and to adjacent cortical regions (not shown). Layer VI projects back to the thalamic core as well as to overlying nucleus reticularis (N.Ret) neurons, which send inhibitory connections to thalamic core cells. Throughout the "core" loop, the projections retain topographic rela-tions. (*c*) In the other primary thalamocortical loop, thalamic "matrix" nuclei project broadly and diffusely to layer I, contacting the apical dendrites of layer II, III, and V cells. Layer V generates both descending projections (predominantly to motor systems) and to matrix thalamic nuclei (Bourassa and Deschenes, 1995; Deschenes et al., 1998).

ferences among various cortical regions (Galuske et al., 2000; Gazzaniga, 2000), there are sufficient shared characteristics to justify attempts to identify a common basic functionality, which may be augmented by special-purpose capabilities in some regions (Lorente de No, 1938; Szentagothai, 1975; Keller and White, 1989; Castro-Alamancos and Connors, 1997; Rockel et al., 1980; Braitenberg and Schuz, 1998; Valverde, 2002). Two parallel circuit types co-occur, involving the topographic projection of certain restricted thalamic populations and broad, diffuse projection of the remaining thalamic neurons. It has been found that these two populations of thalamic cells, distinguishable by their targets and topography, can also be identified by their differential immunoreactivity to two Ca^{2+} binding proteins. The former population, called thalamic "core" regions, exhibits immunoreactivity to parvalbumin, whereas the latter, termed thalamic "matrix" nuclei, is reactive to calbindin (Molinari et al., 1995; Jones and Hendry, 1989; Jones, 1998, 2001). The topographically organized projections from the thalamic core synapse largely on layer IV and deep layer III cells; the diffuse projections form synapses predominantly in layer I, on the apical dendrites of layer II, III, and V cells. (Although the topographic afferents to middle cortical layers, for example, lateral geniculate nucleus to primary visual cortex, are often thought of as the primary input to the sensory neocortex, these fibers actually comprise only about 6% of the synapses on their primary targets (layer IV neurons), with the majority of the remaining afferents coming largely from lateral corticocortical connections (Freund et al., 1985, 1989; Peters and Payne, 1993; Peters et al., 1994; Ahmed et al., 1997).

Peripheral inputs activate thalamic core cells, which in turn participate in topographic activation of middle cortical layers; for example, ear → cochlea → auditory brainstem nuclei → ventral subdivision of medial geniculate nucleus (MGv) → A1. In contrast, matrix nuclei are most strongly driven by corticothalamic feedback (Bender, 1983; Diamond et al., 1992a,b), supporting a system in which peripheral afferents first activate core nuclei, which in turn activate the cortex (via a stereotypical vertically organized pattern: middle layers → superficial layers → deep layers), which then activate both core and matrix nuclei via corticothalamic projections (Mountcastle, 1957; Hubel and Wiesel, 1977; Di et al., 1990; Kenan-Vaknin and Teyler, 1994).

Three primary modes of activity have typically been reported for thalamic neurons: tonic, rhythmic, and arrhythmic bursting. The latter appears predominantly during non-rapid eye movement (REM) sleep whereas the first two appear during waking behavior (McCarley et al., 1983; Steriade and Llinás, 1988; McCormick and Feeser, 1990; Steriade et al., 1990; McCormick and Bal, 1994; Steriade and Contreras, 1995). There is strong evidence for ascending influences (e.g., basal forebrain) affecting the probability of response of excitatory cells during the peaks and troughs of such "clocked" inhibitory cycles. The most excitable cells will tend to fire in response to even slight afferent activity, whereas less excitable neurons will only be activated in response to stronger input; this excitability gradient selectively determines the order in which neurons will be recruited to respond to inputs of any given intensity.

Axons of inhibitory interneurons densely terminate preferentially on the bodies, initial axon segments, and proximal apical dendrites of excitatory pyramidal cells in the cortex, and thus are well situated to exert powerful control over the activity of target excitatory neurons. When a field of excitatory neurons receives afferent stimulation, those that are most responsive will activate the local inhibitory cells in their neighborhood, which will in turn inhibit local excitatory cells. The typical time course of an excitatory (depolarizing) postsynaptic potential (PSP) at normal resting potential, in vivo, is brief (15–20 ms), whereas corresponding GABAergic (γ-aminobutyricacid) inhibitory PSPs last roughly an order of magnitude longer (80–150 ms) (Castro-Alamancos and Connors, 1997). Thus excitation tends to be brief, sparse, and curtailed by longer and stronger lateral inhibitory feedback (Coultrip et al., 1992).

Based on the biological regularities specified, a greatly simplified set of operations has been posited (Rodriguez et al., 2004). Distinct algorithms arise from simulation and analysis of core versus matrix loops (see figure 13.2).

Thalamocortical "Core" Circuits
In the core loop, simulated superficial cells that initially respond to a particular input pattern become increasingly responsive not only to that input but also to a range of similar inputs (inputs that share many active lines, for example, small Hamming distances from each other), so that similar but distinguishable inputs will come to elicit identical patterns of output from layer II–III cells, even though these inputs would have given rise to slightly different output patterns before synaptic potentiation. These effects can be described in terms of the mathematical operation of clustering, in which sufficiently similar inputs are placed into a single category or cluster. This can yield useful generalization properties, but somewhat counterintuitively, it prevents the system from making fine distinctions among members of a cluster. For instance, four similar inputs may initially elicit four slightly different patterns of cell firing activity in layer II–III cells, but after repeated learning and synaptic potentiation episodes, all four inputs may elicit identical activation patterns. Results of this kind have been obtained in a number of different models with related characteristics (von der Malsburg, 1973; Grossberg, 1976; Rumelhart and Zipster, 1985; Coultrip et al., 1992).

Superficial layer responses activate deep layers. Output from layer VI initiates feedback activation of the nucleus reticularis (NRt) (Liu and Jones, 1999), which in turn inhibits the core thalamic nucleus (Ct). Since, as described, topography is preserved throughout this sequence of projections, the portions of Ct that become inhibited will correspond topographically to those portions of layer II–III that were active. On the next cycle of thalamocortical activity, the input will arrive at Ct against the background of the inhibitory feedback from NRt, which has been shown to last for hundreds of milliseconds (Huguenard and Prince, 1994; Cox et al., 1997; Zhang et al., 1997). Thus it is hypothesized that the predominant component of the next input to the cortex is only the uninhibited remainder of the input, whereupon the same operations as before are performed. The result is that the second cortical response will consist of a set of neurons quite distinct from those of the initial response, since many of the input components giving rise to that first response are now inhibited relative to their neighbors. Analysis of the second (and ensuing) responses in computational models has shown successive subclustering of an input: The first cycle of response identifies the input's membership in a general category of similar objects (e.g., flowers); the next response (a fraction of a second later) identifies its membership in a particular subcluster (e.g., thin flowers, flowers missing a petal), then the next sub-subcluster, etc. Thus the system repetitively samples across time, differentially activating specific target neurons at a series of successive time points, to discriminate among inputs.

An initial version of this derived algorithm arose from studies of feedforward excitation and feedback inhibition in the olfactory paleocortex and bulb, and was readily generalized to nonolfactory modalities (vision, audition) whose superficial layers are closely related to those of the olfactory cortex, evolutionarily and structurally. The method can be cast in the form of an algorithm (see table 13.1) whose costs compare favorably with those in the (extensive) literature on such methods (Ambros-Ingerson et al., 1990; Granger and Lynch, 1991; Gluck and Granger, 1993; Kilborn et al., 1996; Rodriguez et al., 2004). Elaboration of the algorithm has given rise to families of computational signal-processing methods whose performance on complex signal

Table 13.1
Formalization of core circuit operation

---

for input X
   for $C \in \text{win}(X, W)$
      $W_j \Leftarrow W_j + k(X - C)$
   end_for
$X \Leftarrow X - \text{mean}[\text{win}(X, W)]$
end_for

where
X = input activity pattern (vector)
W = layer I synaptic weight matrix
C = responding superficial layer cells (column vector)
k = learning rate parameter
$\text{win}(X, W)$ = column vector in W most responsive to X before lateral inhibition [e.g., $\forall j, \max(X \times W_j)$]

Source: Rodriguez et al. (2004).

classification tasks has consistently equaled or exceeded the performance of competing methods (Coultrip and Granger, 1994; Kowtha et al., 1994; Granger et al., 1997; Benvenuto et al., 2002).

Analysis demonstrates good time and space costs for the derived algorithm. The three time costs for the processing of a given input X are (1) summation of inputs on dendrites, (2) computation of "winning" (responding) cells C, and (3) synaptic weight modifications. For n learned inputs each of dimensionality N, in a serial processor summation can be performed in $O(nN)$ time; computation of winners takes $O(n)$ time; and modification of weights is $O(N \log n)$. When carried out with appropriate parallel hardware, these three times reduce to $O(\log N), O(\log n)$, and constant times, respectively, that is, better than linear time. Space costs are similarly calculated: given a weight matrix W, to achieve complete separability of n cues, the bottom of the constructed hierarchy must contain at least n units as the leaves of a tree consisting of log Bn hierarchical layers, if B is the average branching factor at each level. Thus the complete hierarchy will contain $\sim n[B/(B-1)]$ units, and the space required to learn n cues of dimensionality N will be linear, or $O(nN)$ time (Ambros-Ingerson et al., 1990; Kilborn et al., 1996; Rodriguez et al., 2004).

Thalamocortical "Matrix" Circuits

In contrast to the topography-preserving projections in the "core" loop between Ct and the cortex, the diffuse projections from L.V to the matrix thalamic nucleus (Mt) and from Mt back to cortex in the "matrix" loop are modeled as sparsifying and orthogonalizing their inputs, so that any structural relationships that may obtain among inputs are not retained in the resulting projections. Thus input patterns in Mt or in L.V that are similar may result in very different output patterns, and vice versa. As has been shown in previously published studies, owing to the nontopographic nature of layer V and Mt, synapses in L.V are very sparsely selected to potentiate; that is, relatively few storage locations (synapses) are used per storage or learning event (Granger et al., 1994; Aleksandrovsky et al., 1996; Whitson, 1998; Rodriguez et al., 2004). For purposes of analysis, synapses are assumed to be binary (i.e., assume the lowest possible precision, that synapses are either naive or potentiated). A sequence of length L elicits a pattern of response according to the algorithm given here for superficial layer cells. Each activated superficial cell C in turn activates deep layer cells. Feedforward activity from the matrix thalamic nucleus also activates L.V. Synapses on cells receiving activation from both sources (the intersection of the two inputs) become potentiated, and the activity pattern in layer V is fed back to Mt. The loop repeats for each of the L items in the sequence, with the input activity from each item interacting with the activity in Mt from the previous step (see Rodriguez et al., 2004).

The activation of layer V in rapid sequence via superficial layers (in response to an element of a sequence) and via Mt (corresponding to feedback from a previous element in a sequence) sparsely selects responding cells from the most activated cells in the layer (Coultrip et al., 1992) and sparsely selects synapses on those cells as a function of the sequential pattern of inputs arriving at the cells. Thus the synapses potentiated at a given step in L.V correspond to both the input occurring at that time step and the orthogonalized feedback arising from the input just prior to that time step. The overall effect is "chaining" of elements in the input sequence via the "links" created as a result of coincident layer V activity corresponding to current and prior input elements. As in the operating rule described by Granger et al. (1994), the sparse synaptic potentiation enables L.V cells to act as a novelty detector, selectively responding to those sequential strings that have previously been presented. The implicit data structures created by the operation of this system are trees in which initial sequence elements branch to their multiple possible continuations ("tries," Knuth, 1997). Sufficient information therefore exists in the stored memories to permit completion of arbitrarily long sequences from prefixes that uniquely identify the sequence. Thus the sequence "Once upon a time" may elicit (or "prime") many possible continuations, whereas "Four score and seven" elicits a specific continuation.

The resulting algorithm (see table 13.2) can be characterized in terms of computational storage methods that are used when the actual items that occur are far fewer than those that in principle could occur. The number of possible eight-letter sequences in English is 268, yet the eight-letter words that actually occur in English number less than 10,000, that is, less than one ten-millionth of the possible words. The method belongs to the family of widely used and well-studied data storage techniques of "scatter storage" or "hash" functions, known for the ability to store large amounts of data with extreme efficiency. Both analytical results and empirical studies have found that the derived matrix loop method requires an average of less than two bits (e.g., just two low-precision synapses) per complex item of information stored.

Table 13.2
Formalization of matrix circuit operation

---

for input sequence $X(L)$
   for $C \in$ TopographicSuperficialResponse $[X(L)]$
     for $V(s) \in C \cap NNt$Response $[X(L-1)]$
       Potentiate $[V(s)]$
       $NNt(L) \Leftarrow$ NontopographicDeepResponse (V)
     end_for
   end_for
end_for

(where
L = length of the input sequence
C = columnar modules activated at step $X(L)$
$V(s)$ = the synaptic vector of responding layer V cell
$NNt(L)$ = response of nonspecific thalamic nucleus to feedback from layer V)

Source: Rodriguez et al. (2004).

The method exhibits storage and successful retrieval of very large amounts of information at this rate of storage requirement, leading to extremely high estimates of the storage capacity of even small regions of cortex. Moreover, the space complexity of the algorithm is linear, or $O(nN)$ for n input strings of dimensionality N; that is, the required storage grows linearly with the number of strings to be stored (Granger et al., 1994; Aleksandrovsky et al., 1996; Whitson, 1998; Rodriguez et al., 2004).

Circuits of the Striatal Complex

The basal ganglia, or striatal complex, is a collection of disparate but interacting structures including the caudate-putamen, globus pallidus, subthalamic nucleus, and substantia nigra pars compacta (SNc). It is the second largest telencephalic component after thalamocortical circuits, phylogenetically predating the mammals and operating as the primary brain engine for reptiles. In reptiles, and in mammals with relatively small brain-to-body size ratios, the primary anatomical efferents of the striatal complex descend to the brainstem nuclei, presumably driving complex sequential motor movements, including species-specific behaviors (e.g., stalking, grooming). In all mammals, the striatal complex is tightly linked to the anterior neocortex. As brain size grows allometrically larger, a number of fundamental relationships between the neocortex and the striatal complex are altered, predominantly as a result of the disproportionate growth of the anterior neocortex:

• Fascicular growth: the connection pathways between the anterior and posterior neocortex grow, greatly increasing the relative size of the large axon bundles (fasciculi) connecting them.

• Corticostriatal loop growth: the dual efferent pathways from the striatal complex, one descending to the brainstem nuclei and one ascending to the anterior neocortex (via the ventral thalamus), change in relative size; the cortical outputs grow far larger than the descending outputs.

• Pyramidal tract growth: descending outputs from the anterior cortex to motor systems grow disproportionately larger than the descending striatal motor outputs.

These changes in anatomical design are illustrated in figure 13.3; the elements discussed grow disproportionately with increases in brain-to-body size ratios, becoming most notable in humans. In relatively small-brained mammals such as mice, the primary motor area of the neocortex is an adjunct to the striatally driven motor system. Whereas damage to the motor cortex in mice causes subtle impairments in motor behavior, damage to the motor cortex in humans causes paralysis. In this example of encephalization of function (Jackson, 1925; Ferrier, 1876; Karten, 1991; Aboitiz, 1993), motor operations are increasingly "taken over" by the cortex as the size of the pyramidal tract overtakes that of the descending striatal system. The role of the stria-

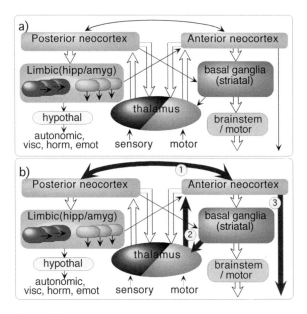

Figure 13.3
Primary constituents of mammalian telencephalon and subcortical connections. (*a*) The posterior neocortex makes strong reciprocal connections with dorsal thalamic nuclei, as well as with the limbic system, which in turn provides descending projections to hypothalamic regulatory systems. The anterior neocortex, with corresponding strong reciprocal connections to ventral thalamic nuclei, also projects to the basal ganglia (striatal complex), which in turn projects to brainstem nuclei. (*b*) In mammals with larger brain-to-body size ratios, a number of allometric changes occur, of which three of the largest are highlighted: (1) growth of the fascicular connections between the posterior and anterior cortices, (2) growth of efferent pathways from the striatal complex to the cortex via the ventral thalamus and concomitant reduction of the relative size of the descending projections from the striatal complex, and (3) an increase in size of the descending pyramidal tract projections from the cortex to motor systems, as though in compensation for the reduced descending striatal pathway.

tal complex in mammals with large brain-to-body ratios is presumably altered to reflect the fact that its primary inputs and outputs are now to the anterior neocortex; in other words, it is now primarily a tool or "subroutine" available for query by the anterior cortex. Its operations then are most profitably viewed in light of its dual utility either as an organizer of complex motor sequences (in small-brained mammals) or as an informant to the anterior cortex (in large-brained mammals).

Figure 13.4 schematically illustrates the primary components of the striatal complex. Striking differences from the circuitry of the thalamocortical system include the very different, apparently specialized designs of these components: matrisomes (matrix), striosomes (patch), globus pallidus, pars interna and externa (pallidum), tonically active cholinergic neurons (TACs), and substantia nigra pars compacta (SNc). In contrast with the thalamocortical system, which is dominated by glutamatergic and local GABAergic neurotransmitter systems, the striatal complex depends

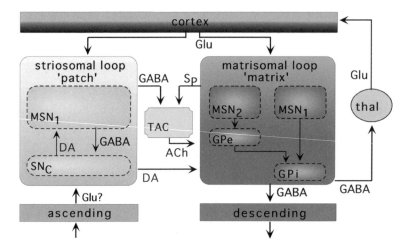

Figure 13.4
Schematic illustration of the striatal complex (basal ganglia). Glutamatergic cortical afferents activate both matrisomal (matrix) and striosomal (patch) targets. Two GABAergic matrix pathways from medium spiny neurons (MSN) through the pallidum project to brainstem motor systems, and back to cortical targets via the thalamus. The patch projects GABAergically to the substantia nigra pars compacta (SNc) and to tonically active cholinergic neurons (TACs), which in turn make cholinergic projections to the matrix. Both patch and matrix receive dopaminergic input from the SNc, which in turn receives ascending information conveying external "reward" and "punishment."

on a broad variety of different neurotransmitter pathways, including GABA, glutamate (Glu), dopamine (DA), acetylcholine (ACh), and substance P (Sp) among others.

The two pathways from the cortex through the matrix components of the striatal complex involve different subpopulations of cells in matrisomes (matrix): (1) MSN1 neurons, which express dopamine D1 receptors, project to the globus pallidus pars interna (GPi), which in turn projects to the ventral thalamus and back to the cortex; (2) MSN2 neurons, which express D2 receptors, project to the globus pallidus pars externa (GPe), which in turn projects to the GPi (and thence to the thalamus and cortex). Unlike thalamocortical circuits, in which long axon projections are glutamatergic, the MSN and GP projections are GABAergic, inhibiting their targets. Thus cortical glutamatergic activation of MSN1 cells causes inhibition of GPi cells, which otherwise inhibit thalamic and brainstem targets; hence MSN1 cell activation disinhibits, or enhances, thalamic activation of the cortex and striatal activation of brainstem nuclei. In contrast, an extra GABAergic link is intercalated in the pathway from MSN2 neurons to the output stages of the matrix. It can be seen that activation of MSN2 neurons decreases thalamic activation of the cortex and striatal activation of brainstem nuclei. The two pathways from MSN1 and MSN2 neurons are thus termed "go" and "stop" pathways respectively, for their opposing effects on their ultimate motor targets. A complex combination of activated ("go") and withheld ("stop") muscle responses (e.g., to stand, walk, throw) can be created by coordinated operation over time of these pathways.

Two primary afferents to the striosomes are cortical and ascending inputs. The former are the same as the inputs to the matrix (despite the schematized depiction in the figure, patch components are distributed throughout, and colocalized with, matrix). The ascending inputs to the patch denote "reward" and "punishment" information and have been shown to up- and downregulate dopamine responses from the SNc (as well as other dopaminergic sites) in response to external stimuli carrying innate or learned valences (e.g., water to a thirsty organism). A cortically triggered action, followed by an ascending DA reward signal from the SNc to the patch, selectively enhances active cortical glutamatergic synapses onto both matrix and patch targets. Patch output back to the SNc then inhibits a DA response, so that increased cortical activation of the patch (via enhanced synaptic contacts) will come to limit the DA input from the SNc. On any given trial, then, the size of the DA signal from the SNc comes to reflect the size of the actual ascending DA input (i.e., the reward signal) that occurred over previous trials. Thus with repeated experience, adaptive changes occur in both matrix and patch. Initially random matrix responses to a cortical input become increasingly selected for responses that produce reward, and initial naive striosomal responses will become increasingly good "predictors" of the size of the reward (or punishment) expected to ensue as a result of the action (Brucher, 2000).

Tonically active cholinergic neurons represent a small fraction (<5%) of the number of cells in the striatal complex, yet densely contact cells throughout the matrix; thus they most likely play a modulatory role rather than conveying specific information. The GABAergic inhibition of these cells by the patch will come to increase for those patch responses that lead to reward, since in these instances the cortical drivers of these patch responses become synaptically enhanced. Thus in those circumstances where cortical inputs lead to the expected reward, TAC cells will tend to have less excitatory effect on the matrix. Since the TAC afferents to matrix are dense and nontopographic, they represent a random "background noise" input, which can increase the variance in selected matrix responses to cortical inputs, making the striatally selected motor response to a cortical input somewhat nondeterministic. The resulting behavior should appear "exploratory," involving a range of different responses to a given stimulus. With repeated exposure to the stimulus, as some responses differentially lead to reward, the corresponding synapses in both matrix and patch will be enhanced, leading to the increased probability of the selected responses (via matrix) and increasingly accurate "prediction" of reward size (via the patch), as stated. An additional effect of a synaptic increase in the patch is that the afferent patch stimulation of TAC cells will increase, inhibiting TAC activity and diminishing the breadth of the exploratory variability in the response just described. Thus as rewards occur, not only will reward-associated responses be increasingly selected by the matrix, the variability among those responses will decrease.

Applications and Implementations

The coordinated activity of simulated thalamocortical and corticostriatal loops has yielded computational methods applicable to a variety of domains with surprising efficacy. Analysis of military signals showed these brain circuit-derived methods specifically outperforming not only standard statistical approaches such as Bayesian nets but also methods based on typical artificial neural network approaches such as backpropagation (Kowtha et al., 1995). Analyses of electroencephalographic information in populations of Alzheimer's patients and matched control populations have demonstrated that these brain circuit methods outperform even advanced statistical approaches (projection pursuit). The resulting analyses, applied to the task of classifying the subjects by diagnostic category (Alzheimer's versus normal) proved significantly more effective than competing approaches (Benvenuto et al., 2002). These and related brain circuit algorithms are currently under development for a range of additional applications.

The simplifying constraints that led to derivation of these novel algorithms implies added efficiencies from direct hardware implementations. Figure 13.5 illustrates candidate designs for three constituent elements of thalamocortical circuitry: (a) a "ladder" circuit that determines which cells in a thalamic nucleus will respond in terms of their order of excitability; (b) a "winner-take-all" circuit that implements the effects of lateral inhibition in a typical cortical layer, selecting the most responsive excitatory unit(s) and suppressing responses from others; and (c) a sparse, random synaptic matrix connecting input axons (e.g., from thalamic matrix nuclei) to dendrites in neocortical layer I, via synaptic elements of various designs (e.g., floating gates; see Mead, 1989; Hasler et al., 1995; Shoemaker et al., 1992, 1996).

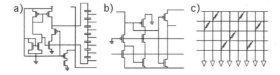

Figure 13.5
Designs for three constituents of thalamocortical circuitry. (*a*) A "ladder" circuit determining the order of cell response by the order of excitability. (*b*) A competitive or "winner-take-all" circuit implementing the effects of lateral inhibition in typical cortical local circuits (see text). (*c*) Sparse, random synaptic matrix connecting input axons (horizontal) with cortical dendrites (vertical) in nontopographic connectivity layers such as neocortical layer I.

Tasks that remain unsolved by current approaches range from complex visual processing (even simple static images, let alone complex movies) and auditory tasks (unconstrained voice recognition and speech processing) to broadened medical applications (increased diagnostic use as well as utility for amelioration and treatment of neurological impairments). Algorithms constrained by the simplicities and weaknesses of actual brain circuits and their constituents (Ambros-Ingerson et al., 1990; Anton et al., 1991; Coultrip et al., 1992; Coultrip and Granger, 1994; Granger et al., 1994; Aleksandrovsky et al., 1996; Kilborn et al., 1996; Shimono et al., 2000; Granger, 2002; Benvenuto et al., 2002; Rodriguez et al., 2004) have been shown to have powerful computational properties and good costs in terms of space and time complexity, indicating their ability to be scaled to large size, and have given rise to novel systems for analyzing complex time-varying signals in military, commercial, and medical applications.

Current work is focused on the use of these findings for novel circuit designs, new approaches to medical signal processing, and enhancement of the two-way communication between brain systems and extrinsic systems. Although initial visual face and character recognition systems exist, these are kept from widespread use by their shortcomings, such as high false-alarm rates. Similarly, current voice-processing systems (e.g., automated telephone operators) can process only simple and very brief utterances, and remain limited by their inability to operate on extended speech streams. The development of these and related systems will not only advance our scientific understanding of mammalian telencephalic operation and provide novel device designs applicable to a broad variety of commercial, military, and medical task domains, it will also increasingly enable two-way communication between brain circuits and extrinsic systems, with concomitant medical and scientific benefits.

References

Aboitiz, F. (1993) Further comments on the evolutionary origin of mammalian brain. *Med. Hypoth.* 41: 409–418.

Ahmed, B., Anderson, J. C., Martin, K. A. C., and Nelson, J. C. (1997) Map of the synapses onto layer 4 basket cells of the primary visual cortex of the cat. *J. Comp. Neurol.* 380: 230–242.

Aleksandrovsky, B., Whitson, J., Garzotto, A., Lynch, G., and Granger, R. (1996) An algorithm derived from thalamocortical circuitry stores and retrieves temporal sequences. In *IEEE International Conference on Pattern Recognition*, IEEE Computer Society Press, Los Alamitos, Ca. vol. 4, pp. 550–554.

Ambros-Ingerson, J., Granger, R., and Lynch, G. (1990) Simulation of paleocortex performs hierarchical clustering. *Science* 247: 1344–1348.

Anton, P. S., Lynch, G., and Granger, R. (1991) Computation of frequency-to-spatial transform by olfactory bulb glomeruli. *Biol. Cybern.* 65: 407–414.

Bender, D. B. (1983) Visual activation of neurons in the primate pulvinar depends on cortex but not colliculus. *Brain Res.* 279: 258–261.

Benvenuto, J., Jin, Y., Casale, M., Lynch, G., and Granger, R. (2002) Identification of diagnostic evoked response potential segments in Alzheimer's disease. *Exper. Neurol.* 176: 269–276.

Bourassa, J., and Deschenes, M. (1995) Corticothalamic projections from the primary visual cortex in rats: A single fiber study using biocytin as an anterograde tracer. *Neuroscience* 66: 253–263.

Braitenberg, V., and Schüz, A. (1998) *Cortex: Statistics and geometry of neuronal connectivity*. New York: Springer-Verlag.

Brucher, F. (2000) Unpublished dissertation, University of California.

Castro-Alamancos, M., and Connors, B. (1997) Thalamocortical synapses. *Prog. Neurobiol.* 51: 581–606.

Coultrip, R., and Granger, R. (1994) LTP learning rules in sparse networks approximate Bayes classifiers via Parzen's method. *Neural Networks* 7: 463–476.

Coultrip, R., Granger, R., and Lynch, G. (1992) A cortical model of winner-take-all competition via lateral inhibition. *Neural Networks* 5: 47–54.

Cox, C. L., Huguenard, J. R., and Prince, D. A. (1997) Nucleus reticularis neurons mediate diverse inhibitory effects in thalamus. *Proc. Natl. Acad. Sci. U.S.A.* 94: 8854–8859.

Deschenes, M., Veinante, P., and Zhang, Z. W. (1998) The organization of corticothalamic projections: Reciprocity versus parity. *Brain Res. Brain Res. Rev.* 28: 286–308.

Di, S., Baumgartner, C., and Barth, D. S. (1990) Laminar analysis of extracellular field potentials in rat vibrissa/barrel cortex. *J. Neurophysiol.* 63: 832–840.

Diamond, M., Armstrong-James, M., and Ebner, F. (1992a) Somatic sensory responses in the rostral sector of the posterior group (POm) and in the ventral posterior medial nucleus (VPM) of the rat thalamus. *J. Comp. Neurol.* 318: 462–476.

Diamond, M., Armstrong-James, M., Budway, M., and Ebner, F. (1992b) Somatic sensory responses in the rostral sector of the posterior group (POm) and ventral posterior medial nucleus (VPM) of rat thalamus. *J. Comp. Neurol.* 319: 66–84.

Ferrier, D. (1876) *The Functions of the Brain*. London: Smith, Elder.

Freund, T. F., Martin, K. A., and Whitteridge, D. (1985) Innervation of cat visual areas 17 and 18 by physiologically identified X- and Y-type thalamic afferents. I. Arborization patterns and quantitative distribution of postsynaptic elements. *J. Comp. Neurol.* 242: 263–274.

Freund, T. F., Martin, K. A., Soltesz, I., Somogyi, P., and Whitteridge, D. (1989) Arborisation pattern and postsynaptic targets of physiologically identified thalamocortical afferents in striate cortex of the macaque monkey. *J. Comp. Neurol.* 289: 315–336.

Galuske, R. A., Schlote, W., Bratzke, H., and Singer, W. (2000) Interhemispheric asymmetries of the modular structure in human temporal cortex. *Science* 289: 1946–1949.

Gazzaniga, M. S. (2000) Regional differences in cortical organization. *Science* 289: 1887–1888.

Gluck, M., and Granger, R. (1993) Computational models of the neural bases of learning and memory. *Ann. Rev. Neurosci.* 16: 667–706.

Granger, R. (2002) Neural computation: Olfactory cortex as a model for telencephalic processing. In J. Byrne, ed., *Learning and Memory*, pp. 445–450. New York: Macmillian.

Granger, R., and Lynch, G. (1991) Higher olfactory processes: Perceptual learning and memory. *Curr. Opin. Neurobiol.* 1: 209–214.

Granger, R., Whitson, J., Larson, J., and Lynch, G. (1994) Non-Hebbian properties of long-term potentiation enable high-capacity encoding of temporal sequences. *Proc. Natl. Acad. Sci. U.S.A.* 91: 10104–10108.

Granger, R., Wiebe, S., Taketani, M., Ambros-Ingerson, J., and Lynch, G. (1997) Distinct memory circuits comprising the hippocampal region. *Hippocampus* 6: 567–578.

Grossberg, S. (1976) Adaptive pattern classification and universal recoding: I. Parallel development and coding of neural feature detectors. *Biol. Cybern.* 23: 121–134.

Hasler, P., Diori, C., Minch, B., and Mead, C. (1995) Single transistor learning synapses. *Adv. Neural Inf. Proc. Sys.* 7: 817–824.

Hubel, D., and Wiesel, T. (1977) Functional architecture of macaque monkey visual cortex. *Proc. R. Soc. Lond. B.* 198: 1–59.

Huguenard, J. R., and Prince, D. A. (1994) Clonazepam suppresses GABAB-mediated inhibition in thalamic relay neurons through effects in nucleus reticularis. *J. Neurophysiol.* 71: 2576–2581.

Jackson, J. H. (1925) *Neurological Fragments.* London: Oxford University Press.

Jones, E. (1981) Functional subdivision and synaptic organization of mammalian thalamus. *Int. Rev. Phys.* 25: 173–245.

Jones, E. (1998) A new view of specific and nonspecific thalamocortical connections. *Adv. Neurol.* 77: 49–71.

Jones, E. (2001) The thalamic matrix and thalamocortical synchrony. *Trends Neurosci.* 24: 595–601.

Jones, E., and Hendry, S. (1989) Differential calcium binding protein immunoreactivity distinguishes classes of relay neurons in monkey thalamic nuclei. *Eur. J. Neurosci.* 1: 222–246.

Karten, H. (1991) Homology and evolutionary origins of 'neocortex'. *Brain Behav. Evol.* 38: 264–272.

Keller, A., and White, E. (1989) Triads: A synaptic network component in cerebral cortex. *Brain Res.* 496: 105–112.

Kenan-Vaknin, G., and Teyler, T. (1994) Laminar pattern of synaptic activity in rat primary visual cortex: Comparison of in vivo and in vitro studies employing current source density analysis. *Brain Res.* 635: 37–48.

Kilborn, K., Granger, R., and Lynch, G. (1996) Effects of LTP on response selectivity of simulated cortical neurons. *J. Cog. Neurosci.* 8: 338–353.

Knuth, D. (1997) *The Art of Computer Programming.* Reading, Mass.: Addison-Wesley.

Kowtha, V., Satyanarayana, P., Granger, R., and Stenger, D. (1995) Learning and classification in a noisy environment by a simulated cortical network. In Proceedings of the Third Annual Computation and Neural Systems Conference, ed. Bower, J. M. Boston: Kluwer, pp. 245–250.

Liu, X., and Jones, E. (1999) Predominance of corticothalamic synaptic inputs to thalamic reticular nucleus neurons in the rat. *J. Comp. Neurol.* 414: 67–79.

Lorente de No, R. (1938) Cerebral cortex: Architecture, intracortical connections, motor projections. In J. Fulton, ed., *Physiology of the Nervous System.* London: Oxford, pp. 291–340.

McCarley, R., Winkelman, J., and Duffy, F. (1983) Human cerebral potentials associated with REM sleep rapid eye movements: Links to PGO waves and waking potentials. *Brain Res.* 274: 359–364.

McCormick, D., and Bal, T. (1994) Sensory gating mechanisms of the thalamus. *Curr. Opin. Neurol.* 4: 550–556.

McCormick, D., and Feeser, H. (1990) Functional implications of burst firing and single spike activity in lateral geniculate relay neurons. *Neuroscience* 39: 103–113.

Mead, C. (1989) *Analog VLSI and Neural Systems.* New York: Addison-Wesley.

Molinari, M., Dell'Anna, M., Rausell, E., Leggio, M., Hashikawa, T., and Jones, E. (1995) Auditory thalamocortical pathways defined in monkeys by calcium-binding protein immunoreactivity. *J. Comp. Neurol.* 362: 171–194.

Mountcastle, V. (1957) Modality and topographic properties of single neurons of cat's somatic sensory cortex. *J. Neurophysiol.* 20: 408–434.

Mountcastle, V. (1978) Brain mechanisms for directed attention. *J. Roy. Soc. Med.* 71: 14–28.

Peters, A., and Payne, B. (1993) Numerical relationships between geniculocortical afferents and pyramidal cell modules in cat primary visual cortex. *Cerebral Cortex* 3: 69–78.

Peters, A., Payne, B., and Budd, J. (1994) A numerical analysis of the geniculocortical input to striate cortex in the monkey. *Cerebral Cortex* 4: 215–229.

Rockel, A. J., Hiorns, R. W., and Powell, T. P. S. (1980) Basic uniformity in structure of the neocortex. *Brain* 103: 221–244.

Rodriguez, A., Whiston, J., Granger, R. (2004) Derivation and analysis of basic computational operations of thalamocortical circuits. *J. Log. Neurosci.* 16: 856–877.

Rumelhart, D., and Zipser, D. (1985) Feature discovery by competitive learning. *Cognitive Sci.* 9: 75–112.

Shimono, K., Brucher, F., Granger, R., Lynch, G., and Taketani, M. (2000) Origins and distribution of cholinergically induced beta rhythms in hippocampal slices. *J. Neurosci.* 20: 8462–8473.

Shoemaker, P., Hutchens, C., and Patil, S. (1992) Hierarchical clustering network based on a model of olfactory processing. *Analog Integr. Circ. Signal Proc.* 2: 297–311.

Shoemaker, P., Hutchens, C., Copper, J., and Lagnado, I. (1996) Floating-gate synapse in thinfilm SOS and its application to a learning neural network chip. *Analog Integr. Circ. Signal Proc.* 5: 104–110.

Steriade, M., and Contreras, D. (1995) Relations between cortical and thalamic cellular events during transition from sleep patterns to paroxysmal activity. *J. Neurosci.* 15: 623–642.

Steriade, M., and Llinás, R. (1988) The functional states of thalamus and associated neuronal interplay. *Phys. Rev.* 68: 649–742.

Steriade, M., Datta, S., Pare, D., Oakson, G., and Curro, R. (1990) Neuronal activities in brainstem cholinergic nuclei related to tonic activation processes in thalamocortical systems. *J. Neurosci.* 10: 2541–2559.

Szentagothai, J. (1975) The "module-concept" in cerebral cortex architecture. *Brain Res.* 95: 475–496.

Valverde, F. (2002) Structure of the cerebral cortex. Intrinsic organization and comparative analysis of the neocortex. *Rev. Neurol.* 34: 758–780.

von der Malsburg, C. (1973) Self-organization of orientation sensitive cells in striate cortex. *Kybernetik* 14: 85–100.

White, E., and Peters, A. (1993) Cortical modules in the posteromedial barrel subfield (Sml) of the mouse. *J. Comp. Neurol.* 334: 86–96.

Whitson, J. (1998) Derivation and analysis of high capacity fault tolerant circuit designs from mammalian telencephalon. Unpublished dissertation, Irvine University of California.

Zhang, S., Huguenard, J., and Prince, D. (1997) GABAa receptor mediated Cl⁻ currents in rat thalamic reticular and relay neurons. *J. Neurophysiol.* 78: 2280–2286.

14 Hybrid Electronic/Photonic Multichip Modules for Vision and Neural Prosthetic Applications

Armand R. Tanguay, Jr. and B. Keith Jenkins

In this chapter we describe one possible approach to the development of neural prosthetic devices. This approach is based on the design and fabrication of compact modules containing multiple silicon very-large-scale integrated (VLSI) chips that implement neural or neural-like functionality, including dense weighted (synapse-like) interconnections among arrays of neuron-like units. These modules would be designed for surgical implantation at the site of a diseased or lesioned brain region, with interfaces to active brain tissue that would allow bidirectional transmittance of signals between a layer of extant biological neurons and one or more surfaces of the implanted module.

Our current efforts toward eventual implementation of these modules are in large part based on a parallel effort in which we have attempted to leverage recent advances in VLSI electronics, optics, and photonics to develop semiautonomous adaptive vision sensors. These vision sensors are designed to provide advanced object recognition functions for robotic vision applications (among others), and involve the mapping of biologically inspired vision models onto a combination of specific VLSI circuitry and dense fan-out/fan-in interconnection patterns. Although these adaptive vision modules are not intended for application as implant devices, the basic principles of this approach potentially allow the development of implantable modules with modifications in the specific devices and architectures employed. Also, due attention must be paid to the problem of interfacing an implanted neural prosthetic device to living nerve tissue.

As a direct result of the vision-based focus of our research to date, the types of neuron-like units (hereinafter referred to as "neuron units") and interconnectivity patterns that we are currently investigating are potentially most appropriate for implantation in specific regions of the visual cortex, which comprises the largest volume fraction of mammalian brains. Other types of neuron units as well as modified interconnectivity patterns that are specifically emulative of their biological counterparts could in principle be incorporated in modules of this type to allow implantation in other functional regions of the brain. For example, hippocampal neuron units, along with their associated dense interconnections, might be incorporated to provide modules that either imitate or emulate specific interconnected regions within the hippocampus, and hence perform memory-related brain functions.

Our treatment of these emerging compact multiple-chip (so-called multichip) modules in this chapter will use to a great extent the implementation of autonomous visual functionality as a vehicle to describe the potential capabilities and technical hurdles associated with this approach to the development of large-scale neural prostheses with inherent complex functionality. Generalization of the approach to other regions of the brain will be included as appropriate.

We now briefly describe several observations that guide our research on an autonomous vision sensor, and on the constraints that specifically characterize vision applications and hence define key performance requirements. As we will show later, the applicability of our vision sensor research to neural prostheses rests to a large degree on the observation that many key performance requirements are common to the two applications, so that a synthetic approach designed and fabricated within a common technology base seems viable.

The recent emergence of such a common technology base has in large part been enabled by significant advances in the psychology and physiology of vision, in computational neurobiology, in hybrid analog/digital VLSI technology and parallel processing systems, in micro-optics, in photonic technology, and in hybrid electronic/photonic packaging over the past decade. This technology convergence has in turn made the long-sought goal of an adaptive vision sensor appear feasible (Jenkins and Tanguay, 1992; Tanguay et al., 2000; Veldkamp, 1993; Tanguay and Jenkins, 1996). The development of both a generic theoretical understanding of, and a technology implementation platform for, adaptive vision sensors could enable the development of a wide range of advanced smart camera and smart display systems. In addition, the rapid emergence of multimedia applications has both created a critical need for advanced vision sensors and generated increased interest in both hybrid analog/digital approaches and hybrid electronic/photonic systems implementations.

In parallel with these advances, adaptive vision applications that involve rapid identification of objects, tracking of moving objects, and estimation of pose (the spatial orientation of an object), such as those envisioned for augmented reality systems, place stringent upper bounds on the computational throughput required to accomplish the desired visual task in times significantly less than those characteristic of human perception and/or reaction. In many such applications, several hierarchical stages of processing must be completed within this stringent time limit, including (for example) image acquisition, image preprocessing, feature extraction, object recognition, extraction of image orientation with respect to environmental coordinates, determination of course of action, and (in some cases) precise registration of computer animation and/or graphics with respect to structured or natural environments.

In addition to the requirement for rapid processing within a given time limit, many emerging vision models and algorithms involve operations that are parallel in nature, nonlinear in functionality, and both local and nonlocal in structure. The resulting computational complexity places correspondingly complex demands on any envisioned hardware implementations.

In order to satisfy these requirements, we are investigating a hybrid electronic/photonic multichip module (PMCM) architecture based on multiple layers of silicon VLSI detection and processing circuitry (Jenkins and Tanguay, 1992; Tanguay et al., 2000) comprising arrays of neuron-like signal-processing units that are coupled (in the layer-to-layer dimension) with dense photonic fan-out/fan-in interconnections (Tanguay et al., 1995, 2000; Tanguay and Jenkins, 1996, 1999; Tanguay and Kyriakakis, 1995). These interconnections are implemented by two-dimensional (2-D) arrays of either multiple quantum well (MQW) modulators (illuminated by an integrated optical power bus) or vertical cavity surface-emitting lasers (VCSELs) that are flip-chip bonded on a pixel-by-pixel basis to the silicon VLSI detector/processor array, in conjunction with proximity-coupled diffractive optical element and microlens arrays that implement 2-D weighted space-invariant or space-variant fan-out patterns, as described in more detail in a succeeding section. As a consequence of the layer-to-layer fan-out, the effective projective field of a given input pixel (picture element) increases with the number of following layers. Likewise, the effective receptive field of a given neuron unit increases with the number of preceding layers.

This layered, densely interconnected architecture is inspired by, but not directly emulative of, biological vision systems (as well as many, if not all, functional regions of the mammalian brain) in which multiple concatenated nonlinear operations are interspersed with the weighted interlayer fan-out and fan-in of information. For example, biological vision systems commonly exhibit high spatial complexity but also relatively high layer-to-layer processing and signal propagation delays, whereas photonic multichip modules are expected to exhibit more modest spatial complexities in conjunction with much lower layer-to-layer delays. In order to effectively map emerging vision models and algorithms onto this hardware platform, we have investigated several approaches for using this intrinsic space-bandwidth tradeoff to advantage.

In this chapter we describe the results of our multidisciplinary research effort to date, which has focused on an analysis of the biological imperative for layering throughout the mammalian visual system; the mapping of biologically inspired vision models and algorithms onto the emerging hybrid electronic/photonic multichip module platform; the incorporation of spatial and temporal multiplexing approaches to implement computationally complex operations; and the design, fabrication, testing, and integration of the corresponding hardware components.

A

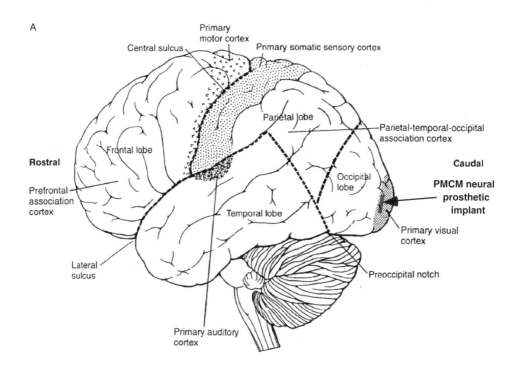

B

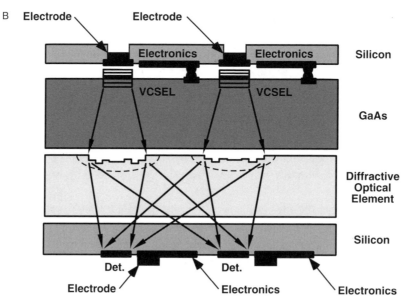

We begin by outlining several of the key functionality requirements for neural prosthetic multichip modules that apply (to first order, at least) irrespective of the technology base of implementation, and hence set the performance parameters that must be met before any given technology can be applied to neural prosthetic devices. Next we describe the envisioned architecture and implementation strategy of the multichip modules. Several general principles extracted from neurobiological systems are then described, particularly as they apply to the general problem of efficiently imitating or emulating the functionality of a biological system. The hierarchical organization and mapping of various computational models onto the emerging hardware platform are presented next, with specific focus on the mapping of biologically inspired vision models and the extraction of a generalizable "toolbox" of mappable functions. Tradeoffs between spatial and temporal complexity (multiplexing techniques) are discussed in the following section, based on the fact that mammalian wetware and hybrid electronic/photonic hardware have vastly different performance characteristics and limitations. The circuits and devices that comprise the emerging hardware platform are then described individually, and the section concludes with a discussion of the integration issues that are associated with the incorporation of such devices in three-dimensional (3-D) photonic multichip modules. Projected performance metrics for such modules are described next from the perspective of a comparison with somewhat-idealized biological neural networks. In the final section we analyze the fundamental scientific and technological issues that affect the further development of densely interconnected neural implants.

Functionality Requirements for Neural Prosthetic Multichip Modules

The set of functionality requirements for prospective implantable neural prostheses is, from the technological implementation perspective, at the very least a bit daunting. First, any candidate neural prosthetic multichip module must provide for a viable interface with the living biological tissue surrounding the implant site, as shown schematically in figure 14.1. This biotic/abiotic interface should optimally be three-dimensional and therefore cover much of the external surface of the implanted module. In addition, the interface should incorporate a high density of interconnection sites (electrodes) at an electrode spacing (pitch) that corresponds to the mean neuron

Figure 14.1
(*a*) Conceptual diagram of a hybrid electronic/photonic multichip module (PMCM) surgically implanted in a given brain region as a neural prosthesis, interfaced to living neural tissue and implementing both fixed and adaptive functionality (after Kandel et al., 1991, figure 19-4, p. 278). (*b*) Expanded view of the neural prosthetic device, showing a thinned and counteretched silicon substrate with electrodes on the front (top) face of the prosthetic device, as well as additional electrodes on the rear (bottom) face, to allow direct contact with neural tissue. In this case, only a two-layer structure is shown for illustration. Det., detector; VCSEL, vertical cavity surface-emitting laser; GaAs, gallium arsenide.

spacing in the adjacent living neural tissue, with the potential for penetration of the interfacial connections through an intervening layer of damaged tissue. Optimally, these interfacial arrays should reflect the local cytoarchitecture (functional layout) of the implanted region, and in that sense instantiate "conformal" mappings (Berger et al., 2001). Neural connections throughout the brain often project far beyond the nearest neurons, with interconnection patterns that are determined both ontogenetically (by "nature") as well as adaptively (by "nurture"). Thus a viable neural prosthesis will optimally contain an interface or set of interface devices that allow some combination of 3-D interconnectivity as well as adaptivity under retraining for (presumably lost) behavioral functionality.

One possible method for developing flexible 3-D interconnections at the neural tissue/prosthesis interface is shown in figure 14.2, which depicts once-dissociated neonatal rat hippocampal neurons that have self-organized on a two-dimensional array of aluminum electrodes, which in turn have been deposited on an insulating layer of silicon dioxide (SiO_2) thermally grown on a silicon (Si) substrate (Berger et al., 2001). Initial clustering of multiple neurons on a given electrode is followed by self-organized interconnections among neuron clusters that develop via axonal and dendritic projections. These projections appear in the microscope to be highly directive in that they grow with high selectivity toward other nearby neural clusters. These features provide the prospect of incorporating once-dissociated biological cellular arrays on the surface of an implantable neural prosthesis, which then provide self-generated (and perhaps adaptively directed) 3-D interconnections with adjoining healthy tissue.

Neural prosthetic modules must, at least within the first few layers of the module at any prosthesis/tissue interface, be capable of interacting with biological signal representations (such as spiking behavior) that are characteristic of the local brain tissue. Some neural prostheses may prove to be successful with instantiations of this signal representation alone throughout all of the interconnected layers of the device. On the other hand, many neural prostheses will most likely contain multiple signal representations, biological in nature near the interface but with progressive transformations of representation farther from the surface in order to make effective use of the key technological characteristics of silicon VLSI electronics, optical elements, and photonic devices. For example, in certain regions of the brain it may prove advantageous to progress from neural spike encoding to a pure analog representation, with bidirectional translation back and forth between the two primary signal representations.

The equivalent computational capacity (and complexity) associated with a neural prosthesis is likely to be considerable, depending on the particular brain region in which it is implanted as well as the degree of lost functionality. This computational complexity can to some degree be usefully expressed in neural network terms as the

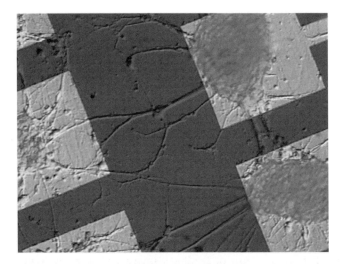

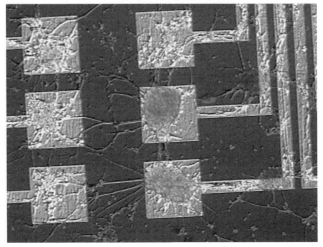

Figure 14.2
Optical photomicrographs of a silicon very-large-scale integrated (VLSI) chip with an aluminum electrode pattern (150-μm × 150-μm electrodes, with 50-μm separations between adjacent electrodes and 30-μm wide interconnection lines), on which dissociated neonatal rat hippocampal cells have self-associated and self-organized to provide a potential prosthetic interface for subsequent projection into living neural tissue at a given lesion site.

number of connections per second that can be implemented, or adaptively in terms of the number of connection updates per second that can be accomplished. The form of this computational complexity must take into account the fact that most "operations" performed throughout the brain involve nonlinear, nonlocal, adaptive, complex, and hierarchical characteristics that must be "captured" in the prosthetic device in some form or other. To first order, the computational complexity in a neural prosthesis will scale with the number of neuron units that can be instantiated within a given physical layer, the number of physical layers that can be interconnected, and the degree of fan-out and fan-in that can be incorporated between pairs of such physical layers.

Beyond computational capacity and complexity, the temporal bounds on any functional implementation must satisfy strict latency constraints (the time from the initiation of a given event, such as presynaptic reception of a set of spike trains at the prosthesis/tissue interface, to the completion of any intervening signal processing and signal transmission in either feedforward or feedback interconnections to living tissue). Signals within the brain are believed to be well contained within a bandwidth of 10 kHz or so, which therefore yields a first-order response-time requirement of about 100 μs for interactions at or near a prosthesis/tissue interface, and perhaps 1–100 ms for completion of significant (higher level) prosthetic functional interactions. Although these are seemingly tight time constraints, they actually allow considerable temporal multiplexing on the artificial prosthetic side, as discussed further in a succeeding section.

These concomitant requirements of low latency (low processing delay) and high computational complexity, combined with associated biocompatibility restrictions on size, power dissipation, weight, and reliability (longevity) are unlikely to be satisfied by conventional systems approaches based on microprocessor and digital signal processor (DSP) chips. To satisfy these requirements, we are investigating the implementation architecture and associated technology based on the hybrid electronic/photonic multichip module approach introduced above, and described in detail in the next section.

Envisioned Architecture and Implementation Strategy

A conceptual diagram of the 3-D integrated electronic/photonic multichip module (PMCM) structure is shown in figure 14.3. Multiple layers of pixellated silicon VLSI chips (chips that are divided into arrays of nearly identical devices or functional regions) are densely interconnected by a combination of electronic, optical, and photonic devices to produce either a space-invariant or space-variant degree of fan-out and fan-in to each pixel (neuron unit, or processing node). These weighted fan-out/fan-in interconnections are suggestive of the axonal projections, synapses,

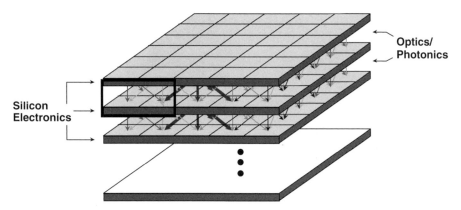

Figure 14.3
Conceptual diagram of a three-dimensional (3-D) PMCM providing both emulative and nonemulative neural-like functionality, and showing silicon analog/digital VLSI chips aligned in layers and interfaced in the vertical (layer-to-layer) dimension with dense fan-out/fan-in optical interconnections.

and dendritic tree structures that characterize biological organisms. The use of optical and photonic devices in particular allows the implementation of such dense weighted fan-out/fan-in interconnection patterns between adjacent physical layers within the stack of chips without significant cross-talk, thus eliminating the need for electrical connections that must penetrate through each chip. The incorporation of these optical and photonic devices further provides for fan-out from one terminal on a given chip to many terminals on the adjacent chip (with individual weights on each connection).

In one such implementation (Tanguay et al., 1995, 2000; Tanguay and Jenkins, 1996, 1999; Tanguay and Kyriakakis, 1995), shown schematically in figure 14.4, two-dimensional arrays of inverted cavity indium gallium arsenide/aluminum gallium arsenide (InGaAs/AlGaAs) multiple quantum well modulators fabricated on a gallium arsenide (GaAs) substrate provide optical outputs from a given integrated layer of the structure. These MQW modulator arrays are flip-chip bonded on a pixel-by-pixel basis to the silicon VLSI chips, which typically incorporate local optical detectors (for optical inputs from the previous layer), processors (either acting alone or in concert with electrical inputs from nearest and next nearest neighbors within the plane), memory elements (in the analog or digital domain), and modulator drivers. Alternatively, the detectors can be co-integrated with the modulator elements on the GaAs substrate, but at the cost of twice as many bump bonds per pixel. In this modulator-based implementation, an optical power bus provides the requisite illumination to the modulator elements, which act as an array of electrically driven reflecting elements with varying reflectivities to incident light. The optical power bus principally consists of an array of one-dimensional (1-D) rib waveguides with a 2-D

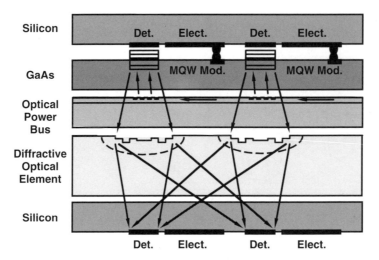

Figure 14.4
Schematic diagram of one possible implementation of a multilayer hybrid electronic/photonic computa-
tion/interconnection element within the PMCM, showing a novel optical power bus and a diffractive optical element array. Only two elements within an N × N or other conformal geometry array, as well as only
two (of M) silicon chip layers are shown. MQW mod., multiple quantum well modulator.

array of outcoupling gratings spaced to match the pitch of the modulator array, and
is powered by a semiconductor laser source or source array to provide the required
uniform 2-D array modulator readout beams. Proximity-coupled diffractive optical
element (DOE) arrays, designed to incorporate both focal power (lens) and weighted
fan-out functions, are used to establish interconnections that are modulated (temporally varied) in intensity by each modulator element and its associated Si driver circuit. Alternative versions of this combined focusing and fan-out DOE array element
can be employed, such as either combined refractive/diffractive elements or separate
concatenated DOE and microlens arrays.

In another such implementation (Tanguay et al., 1995, 2000; Tanguay and Kyriakakis, 1995; Tanguay and Jenkins, 1999), shown schematically in figure 14.5, 2-D
arrays of bottom-emitting vertical cavity surface-emitting lasers are flip-chip bonded
on a pixel-by-pixel basis to the silicon VLSI chips, which act in this case as VCSEL
drivers in addition to the functions described in the modulator case. This replacement
of the modulator array with a VCSEL array has the simplification of eliminating the
requirement for the optical power bus, provided the power dissipation of the VCSEL
array can be made low enough to allow for the requisite (aggregate) operational
bandwidth.

For the specific case of adaptive vision sensors, the design of the individual Si
VLSI chips, and in particular the use of spatiotemporal multiplexing techniques for
network implementation and signal-processing functions, is motivated by the recent

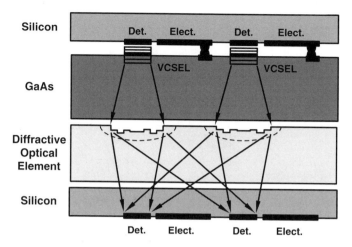

Figure 14.5
Schematic diagram of a second possible implementation of a multilayer hybrid electronic/photonic computation/interconnection element within the PMCM, showing VCSEL and diffractive optical element arrays. Only two elements within an N × N array or other conformal geometry array, as well as only two (of M) silicon chip layers are shown.

development of several promising biologically inspired vision algorithms that can potentially be mapped into the emerging 3-D PMCM platform. Software-based implementations of these vision algorithms, which collectively include low-level, mid-level, and high-level visual processing functions, have in a number of cases been directly tested against human (and in some cases trained human) observers, with the result that the recognition rates and even confusion matrices are surprisingly well correlated (Biederman and Kalocsai, 1997).

As the level of representation extends from low-level vision through mid-level vision to high-level vision operations, interconnections tend to become both more sparse and more global; in some cases, particularly between functionally partitioned vision-processing modules, dense global interconnections may be required. Both local and global interconnection cases can be accommodated within the PMCM architecture by incorporating novel stratified volume diffractive optical elements (SVDOEs) (Tanguay et al., 1995, 2000; Tanguay and Jenkins, 1996, 1999; Tanguay and Kyriakakis, 1995; Chambers and Nordin, 1999), as shown schematically in figure 14.6 (as "volume holographic optical elements"), which consist of multiple layers of proximity-coupled and aligned DOEs that implement either space-variant or space-invariant interconnection patterns with properties characteristic of volume holograms. These new devices offer the advantages of planar fabrication methods compatible with VLSI design rules, and thus could circumvent the difficulties inherent in optical recording of traditional volume holograms.

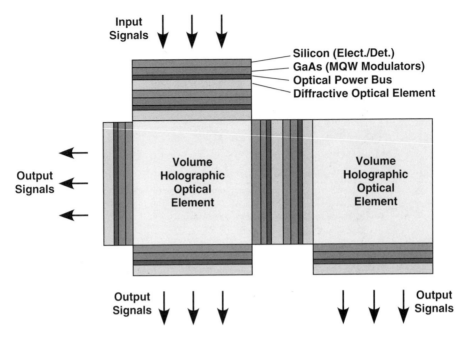

Figure 14.6
Densely interconnected 3-D hybrid electronic/photonic computational module, showing both local (diffractive optical element) and global (volume holographic optical element) optical interconnections.

The extension of this envisioned architecture to the case of neural prostheses involves replacing the neuron units in the interfacial layers with artificial neuron units that emulate the key functionality of adjacent biological neurons, while providing dense fan-out/fan-in interconnectivity patterns characteristic of the specific brain region within which the prosthetic device is implanted.

General Principles Extracted from Neurobiological Systems

The development of a viable neural prosthetic technology base will require the co-development of a "toolbox" of implementable functions and architectures that can be flexibly employed to mimic as closely as possible the cytoarchitecture of the implanted region. Thus it is worth reviewing key general principles that can be extracted from neurobiological systems and then crafted in hybrid electronic/photonic form, a base technology substrate that differs in many respects from human wetware (Mead, 1989). Although the following discussion is both based on and framed within the human visual system (including the retina through the early visual cortex), these architectural principles to a large extent apply throughout the mammalian brain.

Biological vision systems exhibit a number of common themes, including (1) a propensity for layering of the processing architecture (Hubel, 1988; Wandell, 1995), (2) the employment of massive parallelism with simple local processing units and minimal (if any) local storage within each processing unit, (3) the use of a multiplicity of neuron unit types and associated fan-out and fan-in patterns (which gives rise to a set of interpenetrating neural network topologies), (4) the incorporation of dense interconnections at all scales (from local to global, among multiple brain regions; Zeki, 1993) with a high degree of fan-out and fan-in at each processing node within the visual cortex, (5) adaptivity on multiple time scales as exhibited by both short-term and long-term plasticity, (6) distributed storage of information as exemplified by the plasticity of neuronal interconnection weights at individual synapses, (7) an associative memory organizational construct, (8) the potential importance of temporal correlations for both synaptic plasticity and neuron activation (von der Malsburg, 1981), and (9) the incorporation of more complex synaptic behavior, such as adaptive temporal dynamics within each synapse (Liaw and Berger, 1996, 1999) (giving rise to nonlinear dynamical system properties throughout). This latter feature may prove key to understanding the responsivity of the vision system to continuous rather than framed motion, as well as speech and sound recognition in the auditory system.

Primate visual systems, for example, use dense layers of photoreceptors and neurons at the lowest levels of vision processing, with primarily local, fixed, weighted interconnections among multiple preprocessing layers within the retina (Dowling, 1992). The density of photoreceptors can be extremely high, ranging from about 1×10^7 to 3×10^7 cm^{-2} in the fovea (corresponding to a cone diameter on the order of 1 μm) to 4×10^6 cm^{-2} in the periphery (Wandell, 1995) (with a mixture of 4 to 10-μm-diameter cones separated by a much higher density of 1-μm-diameter rods). This density can be instructively compared with the current pixel densities of solid-state imaging sensor arrays [including focal plane arrays in the visible, infrared (IR), and ultraviolet (UV); charge-coupled device (CCD) arrays; and active pixel sensor (APS) arrays], which range from about 1×10^6 cm^{-2} to 4×10^6 cm^{-2}. Current smart pixel arrays do not come close to achieving even these densities as a result of the incorporation of local processing circuitry within each pixel of the array.

For the stages of early vision implemented within the retina and the lateral geniculate nucleus, and extending into the lowest level of the visual cortex (region V1), the interconnection mappings tend to be local (restricted neighborhoods), highly regular (retinotopic), and only partially adaptive. Higher up the biological processing stream (within the primate visual cortex), interconnections tend to become gradually less local, less regular, and more adaptive, with a degree of interconnectivity (fan-out from and fan-in to a given neuron) that is typically 10^3 to 10^4 (Hubel, 1988; Wandell, 1995; Dowling, 1992). Throughout the biological vision system, color information is merged and remerged with spatial information (Wandell, 1995), as well as with inputs from other sensory modalities (beyond a certain stage of the visual system). This variety and degree of interconnectivity is difficult if not impossible to achieve in a current VLSI implementation within a given plane, as a result of limitations both in the number of metallization layers allowed in a given process (five to seven) and in the number of following devices that can be driven from a given device without intervening buffers and signal amplifiers.

Since the extension of VLSI chip implementations of smart cameras and biologically inspired vision systems from single-chip 2-D arrays to 3-D hybrid electronic/photonic multichip modules is a principal focus of our technical approach, it is of considerable interest to examine the biological imperative for layering. In primate visual systems, layered structures provide a number of important functions. (1) The existence of a layered structure provides a convenient mechanism for the implementation of multiple concatenated operations that include nonlinearities and weighted fan-out/fan-in functions. The latter operation can be viewed as the convolution of a 2-D input function with a set of 2-D kernels (weighting functions), and provides the basis for implementing both space-invariant and space-variant nonlocal operations across multiple spatial scales. The separation of a given complex operation into several sequential steps of nonlinearity/convolution also allows access to intermediate-scale results for both feedforward and feedback connections that project beyond intervening layers, as observed throughout biological vision systems. (2) Layering also enables the implementation of higher-order complexity (hierarchical) operations that can be derived from simple primitives implemented over multiple spatial scales. (3) Layering naturally provides for the hierarchical buildup of the size of the receptive field, so that nonlocal operations such as contrast enhancement and color constancy can be implemented such that they are independent of the size of the object. (4) Finally, layering carries with it the potential for increased algorithmic efficiency, in that certain operations (e.g., even certain linearly decomposable convolutions at a given kernel size) can be performed in multiple layers with less cost in computational resources (e.g., fan-out from neurons via axons, synapses, and dendrites; total number of equivalent primitive operations; computational energy).

From a systems perspective, an unresolved question of considerable interest is the overall efficiency of *representation* in biological vision systems, as defined by the efficiency with which higher-level representations are generated from the input visual field through the use of lower-level primitives. Key to understanding this question is the related efficiency of representation from the perspective of memory organization (storage and recall). These two interrelated efficiencies are crucial to the effective design of a biologically inspired vision system, particularly one implemented in a technology base with capabilities and characteristics vastly different from those provided by biological wetware.

The Hierarchical Organization and Mapping of Neurobiological Models

In this section we focus on the development of appropriate hierarchical organization models for the implementation of neurobiological or neurobiologically inspired functionality in neural prosthetic devices, and describe our current strategies for mapping such models onto the emerging hybrid electronic/photonic multichip module platform. As such, we again rely on the visual system as an applicable paradigm for generalization to other brain regions.

To date, the majority of attempts to develop artificial systems capable of vision-related tasks are software based, implemented on digital computer hardware, and rely on some combination of computational vision algorithms to perform functions such as image processing, image segmentation, texture discrimination, pattern recognition, stereopsis, motion detection, object recognition, and object tracking. In current implementations, these computational vision algorithms employ synthetic techniques (e.g., graphical, statistical, or decision theoretic in nature) to solve vision tasks that are confined to limited problem domains.

Computational vision algorithms that work well in the real world are (usually severely) constrained by the computational power available. As computational resources improve in the future, both the sizes of the problem domains and the generality of the algorithms will increase. One approach that may enable such continued progress is threefold: (1) an emphasis on biologically inspired algorithms; (2) the development of special-purpose hardware and appropriate system architectures that are to a degree biologically inspired as well, but that at the same time respect the technological constraints imposed by the hardware; and (3) a reductionist (and therefore generalizable) approach to mapping algorithms onto the hardware. Such a reductionist approach involves the use of tools for implementing basic operations that are common to vision models and algorithms. The differences among vision models and algorithms tend to reduce or even dissolve when viewed from the standpoint of the basic operations needed to implement them. When developed from a biologically inspired viewpoint, these basic operations are more likely to be efficiently implementable on special-purpose hardware that is highly parallel in structure and amenable to the direct mapping of biologically inspired algorithms, such as the photonic multichip module described in this chapter.

Consider, for example, three key yet complementary biologically inspired vision models: recognition of highly disparate objects based on their constituent primitive features [Mel's SEEMORE object/scene recognition system and its variants, based on taking selected combinations (conjunctions and disjunctions) of extracted primitive features (Mel, 1997; Mel and Fiser, 2000)]; robust recognition and evaluation of the similarities and differences of related objects (e.g., faces) based on elastic graph matching [von der Malsburg's Dynamic Link Architecture, based on wavelet

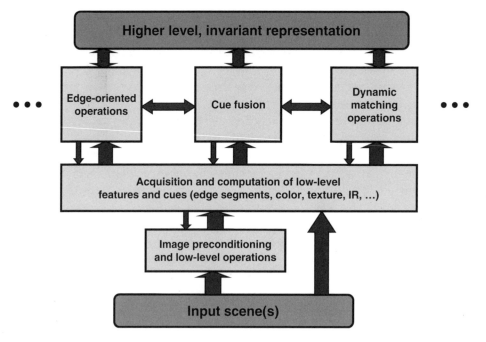

Figure 14.7
Overview of a vision system employing aspects of three complementary biologically inspired vision models
(all levels).

decomposition (Lades et al., 1993; Wiskott et al., 1998; Phillips, 1997)]; and recognition based on features that are invariant over 3-D transformations [Biederman's Recognition by Components, based on the extraction of geometrically simple 3-D components, or geons (Hummel and Biederman, 1992; Biederman and Gerhardstein, 1993; Biederman, 1995; Bar and Biederman, 1998; Biederman and Kalocsai, 1998; Kalocsai and Biederman, 1998)]. Together, these three models exhibit the potential for invariance not only to scale and orientation but also to object deformations and 3-D viewpoints. A schematic depiction of the key features of these three complementary models as they might be combined in a hierarchical vision system is shown in figures 14.7 to 14.9. This conceptual system spans representational levels from the input scene(s) to a higher-level invariant representation that can be used by a subsequent processor for decision making, initiation of actions, and storage in an associative memory, or passed on to processing modules that perform specialized functions.

From this viewpoint, the process of mapping a given vision algorithm onto the hardware architecture can be divided into a sequence of two steps. The first step, algorithm modeling, represents the original algorithm (such as object recognition as

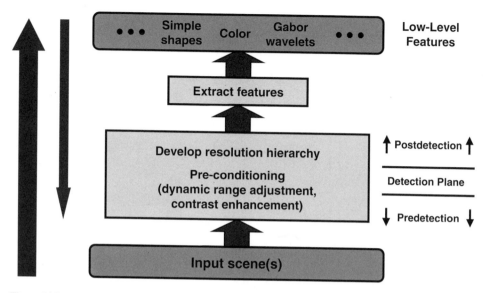

Figure 14.8
Expanded overview of a vision system employing aspects of three complementary biologically inspired vision models (lower levels).

implemented in SEEMORE, wavelet transformation, or elastic graph matching) as a set of lower-level operations (such as repeated comparisons, inner products, and point nonlinearities). The second step, which uses implementation tools, converts these to a physical representation (such as forms of optical interconnection patterns, interconnection weights, and electronic shift registers). Because this step begins with low-level operations, in a sense it is blind to the vision algorithm being implemented and therefore is generalizable across vision algorithms that can be decomposed into appropriate lower-level operations. Its function is to map these low-level operations onto the hardware in a way that is inherently parallel, provides sufficiently low latency, and is reasonably hardware efficient. As an illustration of the issues that arise in the mapping of vision (or other brain function) models onto the photonic multichip module hardware, the possible synergistic combination of biologically inspired spatial multiplexing with electronic- and photonic-technology-inspired temporal multiplexing is described in the next section.

The Incorporation of Temporal Multiplexing Approaches

The envisioned hybrid electronic/photonic hardware platform is in some ways biologically inspired (with its capability for weighted fan-out/fan-in interconnections, layered structure, and parallelism), and in some ways not (with its much higher

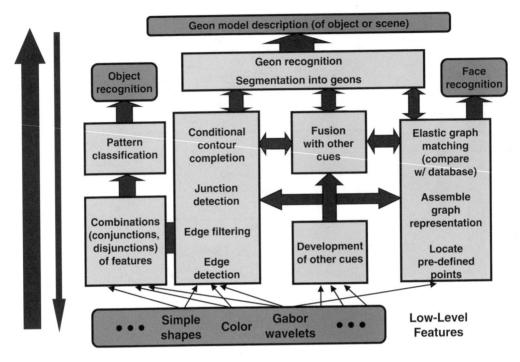

Figure 14.9
Expanded overview of a vision system employing aspects of three complementary biologically inspired vision models (higher levels).

anticipated temporal bandwidth and much lower anticipated spatial parallelism, compared with biological systems). These characteristics beg for some form of temporal multiplexing that can make use of both the parallel nature of the algorithms and the spatiotemporal nature (Wang et al., 1993) of the hardware (Jenkins and Wang, 1991). The need for multiplexing is also apparent in applications for which the first hardware layer receives an input image from the physical world, as shown at the top of figure 14.10. For these applications, a large mismatch in bandwidth exists between the input image stream ($\sim$100-Hz frame rate in the biological vision context) and the available processing rate that can be achieved in subsequent layers ($\sim$50 to 100 MHz analog bandwidth; $\sim$200 to 500 MHz digital synchronous clock rate or asynchronous operation rate; $\sim$1 to 100 MHz layer-to-layer interconnection bandwidth per pixel). Similar bandwidth mismatches are likely to occur at or near the neural tissue/prosthesis interfaces in the case of implanted devices. Again, some form of spatiotemporal multiplexing is desirable in subsequent (interior) layers to make use of the available hardware processing capabilities.

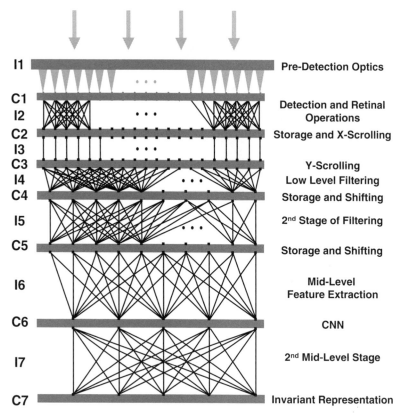

I1 — Pre-Detection Optics

C1
I2 — Detection and Retinal Operations

C2
I3 — Storage and X-Scrolling

C3
I4 — Y-Scrolling Low Level Filtering

C4 — Storage and Shifting

I5 — 2nd Stage of Filtering

C5 — Storage and Shifting

I6 — Mid-Level Feature Extraction

C6 — CNN

I7 — 2nd Mid-Level Stage

C7 — Invariant Representation

Figure 14.10
Example optoelectronic eye-and-vision processor layout, shown in cross-section, and depicting different functionalities implemented in each layer, as well as a hierarchical architecture with layer-to-layer variations in the degree of fan-out and fan-in employed. CNN, cellular neural network.

It should be noted that the availability of temporal multiplexing capability represents an advantage for hybrid electronic/photonic hardware platforms but, as always, such advantages have associated costs. In general, higher bandwidths imply higher power dissipation, an undesirable feature for any reasonably compact implanted device. Thus many versions of neural prostheses based on this type of hardware platform may not make full use of the available processing or communication bandwidths in order to conserve power.

Because of their biological inspiration, the vision algorithms we have described in this chapter (as well as many other possible vision or other brain-like functional algorithms) are likely to be most efficiently implemented using some weighted interconnections that are fixed and some that are adaptive when implemented using

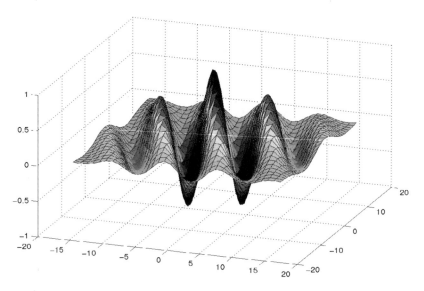

Figure 14.11
Example Gabor wavelet kernel plotted in two orthogonal spatial coordinates (e.g., x and y).

parallel hardware. The hardware described in this chapter currently employs optical (physical) interconnection weights that are designed a priori and fixed once fabricated, while the in-plane electronic interconnections (nearest neighbor or next nearest neighbor) can be either fixed or adaptive. Thus the multilayered network depicted schematically in figure 14.10 can be represented as a set of interpenetrating network topologies, with both fixed and adaptive weights. At this point, it is an open question as to whether or not this combined topology contains sufficient adaptive capability for the full range of envisioned applications. Consequently, temporal multiplexing techniques could be used to provide additional means for effectively achieving adaptive or programmable interconnection weights at the functional level, even for the layer-to-layer interconnections.

As an example, consider the Gabor wavelet transform (Lades et al., 1993; Wiskott et al., 1998) mentioned in a previous section. This transform can be modeled as a set of convolutions, each with a kernel of the type shown in figure 14.11, but at different scales and orientations. (For example, the Dynamic Link Architecture [Lades et al., 1993] typically uses eight different orientations and five different scales, yielding forty different kernels.) Once the transform is so modeled, a variety of physical implementations are possible. One such implementation uses a "direct mapping" approach that involves representing the input image data in analog form, laid out spatially (topographically, or retinotopically) in a first hardware plane. Each convolution kernel is then laid out as an optical weighted interconnection, that is, as a fan-in pat-

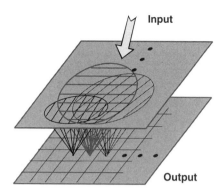

Figure 14.12
Direct parallel mapping of Gabor wavelet decomposition, showing fan-in patterns for three kernels.

tern to a processing element (pixel) in a second, or receiving, hardware plane. (The use of bipolar or complex numbers and arithmetic, if desired, can be handled by employing any of a variety of known representations.) Neighboring processing elements (pixels) in the receiving plane correspond to different kernels (three kernels are depicted in figure 14.12), so that an $n \times m$ region is used to implement all nm kernels. The $n \times m$ array of fan-in kernels is repeated across the array. Thus, the transform is performed in one time step as the data set moves from one plane through the interconnections (kernels) and is summed optically at the detectors (for example) as it is received in the subsequent plane. Although one processing element in the receiving plane corresponds to just one kernel, mappings of this type can be sampled sufficiently to avoid any loss of meaningful information.

While this direct mapping approach uses space efficiently, it may result in inefficient use of the temporal domain (because one useful time step may be followed by a series of idle ones). A second technique can be implemented with a similar set of $n \times m$ fan-in patterns, but repeated more sparsely across the array. Interconnections for other operations are implemented in the interleaving regions. Upon operation, the input image data set is shifted across the first plane in time (Goldstein and Jenkins, 1996; Goldstein, 1997); viewed from a given interconnection kernel (and therefore from a given processing element in the second plane), different portions of the input image data are input to this interconnection kernel at different instances in time. After a sufficient number of time shifts, each (and every) kernel has operated on the entire input image. This technique allows multiple operations to be performed (for example, Gabor wavelet decomposition, and matching to a variety of small templates for primitive feature extraction) in a single layer. These operations are multiplexed partially in time and partially in space, resulting in a more efficient utilization of the hardware-processing capability available.

Temporal multiplexing techniques could also be used to significant advantage in implementing adaptive functionality. For example, the incorporation of a cellular neural network (CNN) layer (depicted schematically as layer C6 in figure 14.10) naturally allows the implementation of programmable flexibility through the array of distributed mixed analog/digital processing units that comprise the CNN. Furthermore, to the extent that the image shifting or scrolling functions are programmable, the operations performed can be sequenced or altered in time. Because the resulting data are spatiotemporally multiplexed, appropriate design techniques must be used to ensure layer-to-layer compatibility of the data format.

Finally, spatiotemporal multiplexing techniques may prove useful for transforming signal representations from the pure biological (spike train-based) substrate to the hybrid analog/digital neural prosthesis, as described in a previous section.

Integration of the Photonic Multichip Module Components

Considerable prior research has focused on the development of both biologically inspired and biologically emulative vision chips that implement one or more functions characteristic of biological vision systems, such as dynamic range compression, edge enhancement, and motion sensing (see, for example, Mead, 1989), and that are fabricated using VLSI semiconductor processing techniques. In each case, considerable functionality has been achieved within the constraints imposed by limited lateral connectivity and the inherent 2-D nature of the single-chip substrate. However, in nearly every case, these 2-D implementation strategies are not amenable to generalization to the full 3-D interconnection problem that is characteristic of viable neural prosthetic devices. For example, the chip real estate required to form the neural tissue/prosthesis interface itself is likely to consume a large fraction of the surface of the outermost chip layer. If only one chip is used, little if any surface area will be available for the implementation of neuron unit arrays and their interconnections. In addition, the extension to large-scale arrays of neuron units is compromised by a single-chip approach, particularly insofar as the neural network architecture implements multiple layers with high degrees of connectivity between and among layers. As a result, we have focused on the problem of densely interconnecting multiple hybrid analog/digital silicon (Si) VLSI chips in the third (out-of-plane) dimension, in order to provide additional flexibility and functionality.

As in the algorithm and architecture development effort outlined in previous sections, the principal goal of the hardware integration effort is to develop a flexible toolbox of component technologies that can be used to implement a wide variety of smart cameras and artificial vision systems, as well as implantable neural prostheses. In the subsections that follow, we describe the basic functionality required and the results achieved to date in each of the component technologies that constitute the

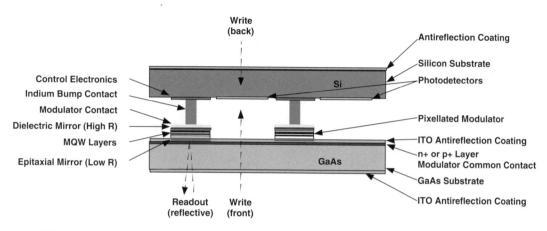

Figure 14.13
Schematic diagram of multilayer hybrid electronic/photonic computation/interconnection element, depicting flip-chip bonding of silicon photodetector/driver chip and gallium arsenide (GaAs) multiple quantum well (MQW) modulator array.

hardware integration platform of the photonic multichip module, as well as efforts to achieve PMCM integration. Fabrication and performance details of several of the components have been reported in part elsewhere, as noted in the references where appropriate.

Silicon VLSI Detector/Processor Arrays

As shown schematically in figures 14.3 to 14.6, silicon VLSI chips are incorporated in each submodule (layer) primarily to implement as-designed processing functions [such as logarithmic transformations, sigmoidal (thresholding) transformations, differencing operations, sample-and-hold, as well as temporal integration and differentiation; neuron emulation functions can also be directly incorporated, as described by Berger et al. (2001) and in chapter 12]. In some implementations, the Si chips also carry photodetection capability (for example, in the input image plane) as well as device drivers for III–V compound semiconductor modulators or vertical cavity surface-emitting lasers, as shown in figures 14.4, 14.5, and 14.13. In other implementations, the photodetection functions and/or III–V device drivers can be co-integrated with the modulators or VCSELs.

For vision-related applications, we have focused to date on the implementation of a test chip that implements a nonlinear sigmoidal input/output transformation (Jenkins and Tanguay, 1992; Tanguay et al., 1995, 2000; Tanguay and Jenkins, 1996, 1999; Tanguay and Kyriakakis, 1995; Cartland et al., 1995). The current Si chip design consists of a 16×16 array of neuron units placed on a 100-μm pitch; figure 14.14 displays a photomicrograph of a single neuron unit. Each neuron unit contains

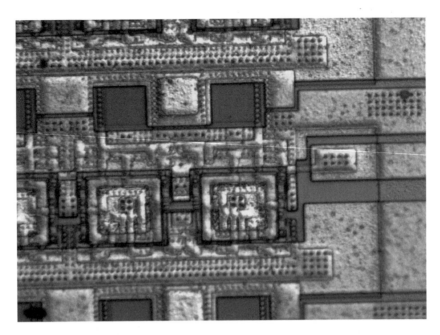

Figure 14.14
Photograph of a portion of the 16 × 16 array of neuron units. Shown is a single sigmoidal neuron unit that incorporates dual photodetectors (to instantiate both excitatory-like and inhibitory-like inputs), active control circuitry and device drivers, and dual output bonding pads for flip-chip bonding.

silicon complementary metal oxide semiconductor (CMOS) control electronics, two Si vertical photodiode detectors, and three bonding pads to allow vertical interconnection to two multiple quantum well modulators or VCSELs and an electrical ground. The control circuitry provides a −2 to −9-V nonlinear sigmoidal response to the difference in light intensity incident on the two photodetectors. A separate sigmoidal response characteristic is provided for each signed difference, thereby allowing the representation of both excitatory-like and inhibitory-like inputs as intensity values.

The analog 16 × 16 array test chip was fabricated through the Metal Oxide Semiconductor Implementation Service (MOSIS) foundry using the 1.2-μm Hewlett-Packard scalable CMOS n-well process. The large-signal sigmoidal response characteristic has been demonstrated at frequencies up to 100 kHz, with a small-signal response in excess of 1 MHz (test equipment limited); SPICE simulations (a software package for simulating circuit functionality based on a schematic diagram and definition of key parametric values) indicate a small-signal response in excess of 4 MHz. The estimated chip power dissipation is 2 mW per pixel or about 0.5 W per chip. Significantly higher bandwidths can most likely be achieved as these chips are re-designed in smaller minimum-feature-size processes.

Inverted-Cavity MQW Modulator Arrays

In the PMCM configuration shown in figures 14.4 and 14.13, 2-D arrays of inverted-cavity multiple-quantum-well modulators (Cartland et al., 1995; Hu et al., 1991a,b; Karim et al., 1994, 1995; Karim, 1993; Kyriakakis, 1993) are incorporated to provide an electrical-to-optical conversion function, thereby producing a signal-encoded array of output beams that can be individually fanned out with weights that are implemented by proximity-coupled diffractive optical elements.

The inverted asymmetric Fabry-Perot cavity modulator arrays were fabricated by molecular beam epitaxy (MBE) on III–V compound semiconductor gallium arsenide (GaAs) substrates, and consist of a *p-i-n* (*p*-type semiconductor, intrinsic semiconductor, *n*-type semiconductor) InGaAs/AlGaAs MQW region (35 quantum wells) sandwiched between an MBE-grown low-reflectance aluminum arsenide/ gallium arsenide (AlAs/GaAs) distributed-Bragg-reflector front mirror and an ex situ-deposited high-reflectivity multilayer dielectric back mirror (Karim et al., 1994, 1995; Karim, 1993). The 2-D array of InGaAs/AlGaAs MQW modulators operates at a central wavelength of 980 ± 1 nm in the near-infrared region of the spectrum (with a 2-D uniformity of ± 0.3 nm), and exhibits an average contrast ratio of 13:1 at -9 V applied bias (the saturation value of the Si chip sigmoidal output channels) (Cartland et al., 1995). This operational wavelength has been chosen to allow relatively low-loss transmission through the GaAs substrate and the following (thinned) Si substrate, as well as for acceptable Si photodetector quantum efficiency, while retaining the high uniformity and state of technological advancement characteristic of the InGaAs/AlGaAs modulator system.

Flip-Chip Bonding of Si and GaAs Chips

A cold-weld indium bump flip-chip bonding process has been developed and used for the hybrid integration of the Si photodetection/control/driver chips and the GaAs MQW modulator arrays, as shown schematically in figure 14.13. In this process, approximately 8-μm-high indium bumps are deposited on the mating electrode pads of both chips and patterned by a lift-off photolithographic process. The thermal or electron-beam deposition parameters are set to achieve a roughened ("velcro") surface on both indium bumps, which significantly improves both adhesion and contact resistance by providing enhanced surface penetration when the two bumps are brought into contact using a visible flip-chip aligner-bonder. Figure 14.15 shows a scanning electron microscope (SEM) photomicrograph of the resulting bump surfaces and bump uniformity.

The flip-chip bonding process is based on a near-room-temperature cold-weld procedure that avoids significant heating of the modulator and Si substrates. Measurements of MQW modulator reflectivity as a function of wavelength both before and after flip-chip bonding show no significant degradation in performance (figure 14.16).

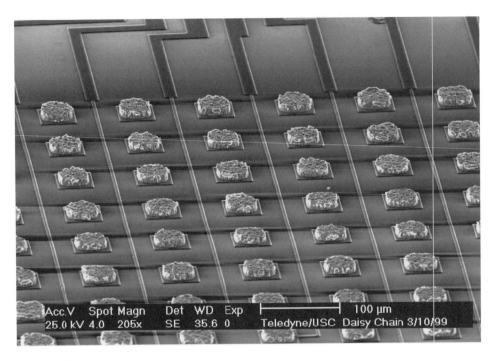

Figure 14.15
Large-scale scanning electron microscope photomicrograph illustrating the thermally evaporated indium bump uniformity achieved in the flip-chip bonding process.

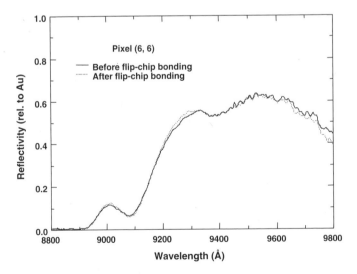

Figure 14.16
Measurement of both pre- and post-flip-chip-bonded modulator reflectivities, showing relatively minor perturbations induced by the flip-chip bonding process.

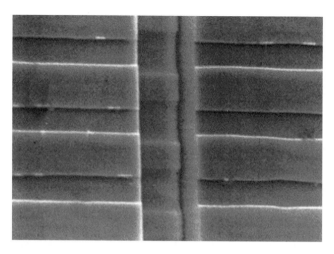

Figure 14.17
Photomicrograph of one section of an optical power bus fabricated on an aluminum gallium arsenide/
gallium arsenide (AlGaAs/GaAs) multilayered substrate consisting of 660 individual rib waveguides, each
8 μm wide and 1 cm long, with 2-μm gaps; and with an integrated, continuous, 1-μm feature (2-μm pitch,
or period) outcoupling grating on top of each waveguide. In the PMCM implementation shown in figure
14.4, the outcoupling gratings are discrete and colocated with each modulator element associated with
each pixel within the array.

Optical Power Bus

For the modulator implementations of the PMCM described in previous sections and
in figures 14.4 and 14.13, reflective readout of the 2-D MQW modulator array must
be provided in a highly compact manner. This function is performed by an optical
power bus, which consists of a 2-D array of 1-D rib waveguides with superimposed
outcoupling gratings. Optical intensity provided to the set of rib waveguides from
an edge-mounted semiconductor laser diode or diode array propagates along each
rib waveguide, confined in the lateral and vertical dimensions. Outcoupling gratings
are provided at each location that corresponds to an individual modulator element,
so that light is coupled out of the plane of the optical power bus, impinges on a given
modulator element within the array, and is thereby both modulated in intensity and
reflected back through the optical power bus toward the proximity-coupled diffractive optical element (see figure 14.4). The outcoupling gratings are designed to operate in the very low diffraction efficiency limit (approximately 10^{-3}), so that only a
very small fraction of the light propagating in the waveguide is outcoupled below
each modulator element, thereby providing uniform illumination along the length of
each rib waveguide and minimizing any recoupling back into the waveguide.

Optical power buses have been fabricated to date in titanium indiffused lithium
niobate (LiNbO$_3$) waveguides, as well as in AlGaAs/GaAs waveguides, as shown in
figure 14.17 (Rastani, 1988; De Mars, 1995). Similar outcoupling grating arrays

have also been fabricated in polymer waveguides (Tang et al., 2000). In the case of AlGaAs/GaAs, we have fabricated arrays of up to 660 individual 1-cm long, 8-μm wide ribs with 2-μm gaps. Outcoupling gratings of both 2-μm (shown in the SEM photomicrograph in figure 14.17) and 4-μm pitch have been successfully fabricated by a double photolithographic and ion beam milling process, with good output uniformity (De Mars, 1995).

Vertical Cavity Surface Emitting Laser Arrays

The use of VCSEL arrays for the electrical-to-optical conversion function described previously (as shown schematically in figure 14.5) promises increased simplicity for photonic multichip module implementation because both the optical modulator array and optical power buses would be replaced with a single component and at least one additional (critical) alignment step would be eliminated. At the relatively low operational bandwidths envisioned for these hybrid analog/digital PMCMs, however, power dissipation considerations currently favor the use of optical modulator arrays. With continued progress in ultra-low threshold VCSEL arrays, such arrays could be employed to advantage in future PMCMs.

In both the optical modulator and the VCSEL cases, co-integration of III–V compound semiconductor photodetectors can provide natural wavelength compatibility between the emitters or modulators on the one hand, and the detectors on the other. This potential modification allows more flexibility in choice of operational wavelength, provided sufficient space can be allocated for the additional bump bonds required within each pixel to connect the photodetector outputs back to the Si control circuitry.

Diffractive Optical Element Arrays

The PMCM architectures shown schematically in figures 14.4 and 14.5 incorporate diffractive optical element (DOE) arrays to implement dense 3-D fan-out/fan-in interconnections with fixed (nonadaptive) interconnection weights. The DOE arrays can be designed to provide either space-invariant or space-variant convolution kernels, depending on the layer-to-layer functionality required. For this application, the DOE designs minimize the distribution of undesired diffracted orders (Huang et al., 1998; Huang, 1997), not only to reduce the semiconductor laser diode power requirements and overall PMCM power dissipation, but also to avoid illumination of light-sensitive components that are distributed throughout the PMCM stack.

Diffractive optical element arrays that implement a number of different fan-out and fan-in patterns have been designed and fabricated. For example, a computer-calculated reconstruction pattern of a DOE that performs a 4:2:1 fan-out function (Huang, 1997) (Gaussian-like, with a 4:2:1 ratio of intensities diffracted to the vertically displaced center pixel, four nearest-neighbor pixels, and four next-nearest-neighbor pixels, respectively) is shown in figure 14.18 alongside the experimental re-construction pattern. This commercially fabricated quartz substrate DOE (QPS, Inc., Dorval, Canada) had a design etch depth of 192 nm and a measured etch depth of 197.8 nm, and exhibited a root-mean-square (rms) diffracted-spot intensity error of approximately 5%. Extensive analysis of fabrication tolerances and errors across multiple fabrication runs of identical DOE arrays has shown that such arrays can be produced with minimal run-to-run variances in performance (Shoop et al., 1999).

The 4:2:1 DOE has been tested for fan-in accuracy as well, by employing two vertical cavity lasers within a VCSEL array for illumination of the DOE (through a pair of relay lenses), with the results shown in figure 14.19. The two DOE reconstruction patterns were displaced diagonally along the next-nearest-neighbor direction, producing overlapping diffracted spot intensities in the central four spots, with an rms error of approximately 9%. This result demonstrates both the fan-out and fan-in capabilities of the interconnection system, which will be further tested in a proximity-coupled geometry with multiple elements within a DOE array.

In a multichip module such as that described in this chapter, the number of optical surfaces is considerable, and antireflection (AR) coating techniques must be employed carefully. We have previously developed low-reflectivity indium tin oxide (ITO) antireflection coatings for high-index compound semiconductor substrates (Karim, 1993; Kyriakakis, 1993), and have recently used them for AR coating of DOEs fabricated in GaAs. An example of an AR-coated GaAs DOE that provides a 3×3 weighted fan-out is shown in figure 14.20. Experimental measurements of the diffracted order intensities both before and after AR coating demonstrated not only the expected large improvement in optical throughput efficiency, but also a reduction in rms diffracted-spot error from 15% to 6%. The use of stratified volume diffractive optical elements (Tanguay et al., 1995, 2000; Tanguay and Jenkins, 1996, 1999; Tanguay and Kyriakakis, 1995; Chambers and Nordin, 1999) for highly nonlocal to global interconnection functions, as described in a previous section, carries with it a similar AR coating issue, particularly in view of the large number of additional optical surfaces involved in this case. Minimization of fabrication errors is important for successful implementation of the overall SVDOE interconnection function (Jung, 1994).

Photonic Multichip Module Integration Issues
Given the emergence of functional components as described in this chapter, a wide range of issues pertain to the successful integration of photonic multichip modules that contain both hybrid substrates and mixed analog/digital representations. These issues include the computational complexity implemented per unit power dissipation; the analog accuracy achievable within each processing stage as well as overall after multiple stages; the total power consumption, with resultant thermal dissipation and

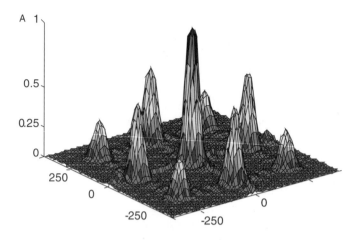

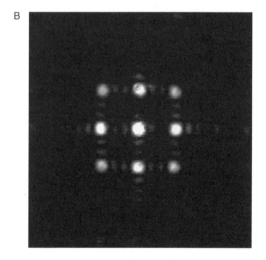

Figure 14.18
(*a*) Computer-calculated reconstruction and (*b*) experimental reconstruction of a diffractive optical element that implements a weighted 3 × 3 fan-out interconnection pattern, with relative intensities of 4:2:1.

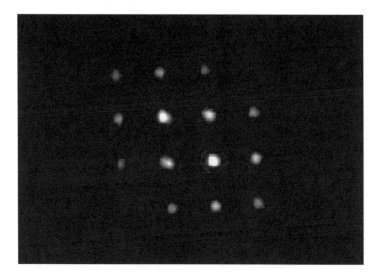

Figure 14.19
Reconstruction of a single diffractive optical element by two proximately placed vertical cavity surface-emitting lasers, showing both individual fan-out interconnection patterns as well as the resulting (summed) fan-in pattern.

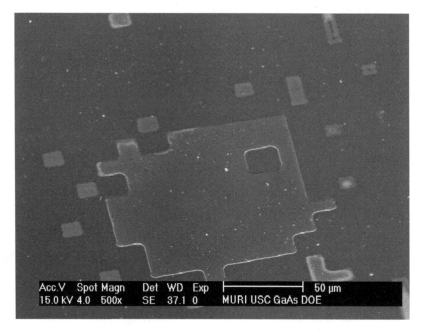

Figure 14.20
Antireflection-coated gallium arsenide diffractive optical element (DOE) that provides a weighted 3×3 fan-out interconnection pattern.

uniformity; the manufacturability and fabrication tolerances of hybrid-integration alignment techniques; the development of integrated computer-aided design (CAD) techniques for hybrid electronic/photonic systems; and the assessment of inherent design tradeoffs.

Projected Performance Metrics for PMCMs

The assessment of projected performance for any computational device inherently depends on the intended application. The hybrid electronic/photonic multichip modules that we envision for incorporation in neural prosthetic devices can be configured in a wide range of architectures, and can conceivably include various combinations of analog, digital, and hybrid computational components.

Perhaps one generic means of assessing the potential computational capacity of such multichip modules is to estimate the total number of processing elements that can be included with current state-of-the-art fabrication design rules, the mean connectivities that can be implemented using the combined optical elements and photonic components described previously, and the operational bandwidth of the key elements of the structure. These characteristics in turn allow an estimate of the total number of connections per second (CPS) that can be envisioned for PMCMs, in direct analogy with a common neural network implementation metric.

Table 14.1 contains estimates of each of these performance characteristics, assuming a PMCM $1 \times 1 \times 1$ cm in size. Within this 1-cm^3 volume, approximately eight layers can be included, allowing a layer thickness of 1.25 mm (including the Si substrate, the GaAs substrate, an optical power bus if modulators are employed, the diffractive optical element array, a microlens array if not included in the DOE array, and sufficient propagation distance within the DOE or microlens array substrates to allow diffractive separation of the interconnection beams). If the neuron unit (processor) area is set initially at 100×100 μm, then about forty transistors can be included, along with the requisite interconnection pads for flip-chip bonding to the

Table 14.1
Characteristics of hybrid electronic/photonic multichip modules

	No. of Processing Elements (or Neurons)	Mean Connectivity	Temporal Bandwidth	Aggregate Connection Rate
Photonic Multichip Module (1 cm^3 active volume)	8×10^4	25	50 MHz	1×10^{14} connections/ second
Human Visual System (simplified)	5×10^{10}	10^3	100 Hz	5×10^{15} connections/ second

GaAs substrate using 0.85-μm minimum feature sizes in the VLSI semiconductor manufacturing process. Currently, several 0.5- to 0.3-μm processes are available for hybrid analog/digital circuits, and 0.3- to 0.18-μm processes can be employed for repetitive geometry structures (such as dynamic [DRAM] and static [SRAM] random access memory). Although these processes will allow more circuit complexity, they are unlikely to affect the pixel (neuron unit) size significantly because the photodetector and interconnection pad sizes occupy most of the pixel area at present. This pixel size yields a total of 8×10^4 processing elements integrated over the eight layers of the assumed PMCM structure.

Consideration of the physics of diffraction, as well as signal-to-noise and cross-talk minimization requirements at each detector location, yields approximately 25 as a modest estimate of the fan-out (5×5) that can be expected from each DOE within the array (Huang et al., 1998; Huang, 1997; Shoop et al., 1999). By symmetry, this also implies a fan-in of 25 at each photodetector location within the neuron unit arrays. Although provision is made for dual inputs and dual outputs from each neuron unit as currently implemented and described in a previous section, we have not included this factor of two in the performance estimate.

At present, digital VLSI circuitry can be configured to operate at clock speeds greater than 1 GHz (commercially available personal computers in some cases have clock speeds in excess of 3 GHz midway through 2005). However, the hybrid analog/digital circuitry described here has additional constraints, primarily arising from the analog circuitry components, that currently limit the bandwidth to 50 MHz or so. These constraints derive from a number of sources, including the requirement to maintain linearity (or a specific nonlinearity) over the entire range of operational frequencies, the incorporation of large-scale device drivers (particularly for the case of vertical cavity surface-emitting lasers), and the necessity of limiting the total power dissipation within each physical layer of the photonic multichip module to approximately 1 W to avoid significant thermal effects within the module. It should be noted that the latter constraint is much more stringent than is typical in Si VLSI implementations of microprocessors and digital signal processors, which involve only a single physical chip (layer) that can be proximity-coupled to an efficient heat sink on the back surface to allow power dissipation budgets of up to 100 W/cm^2.

The combination of these estimates yields an aggregate connection rate of 1×10^{14} CPS. This performance parameter indicates the total number of full-scale variations that can be accommodated in all of the weighted interconnections throughout the photonic multichip module per unit of time. Since the PMCM was assumed to occupy a 1-cm^3 volume, the aggregate connection rate density is 1×10^{14} CPS/cm^3. To provide an appropriate context for this estimate, table 14.1 contains typical values for the human visual system (including the primary visual cortex and other visual processing areas within the neocortex), as estimated from neurobiological studies and averaged over numerous sources (Mead, 1989; Hubel, 1988; Wandell, 1995, esp. pp. 153–193 and cover sheets; Kandel et al., 1991; Churchland and Sejnowski, 1992; Arbib, 1995; Dowling, 1992, pp. 31, 376; Palmer, 1999). The total number of neurons that comprise the human visual system is a large fraction of the total number of neurons in the brain, and is conservatively taken here as approximately 5×10^{10}. The mean connectivity of neurons throughout the brain is on the order of 10^3, and the combined temporal bandwidth of the electrical activity of neurons, axons, dendrites, and synapses in the brain is on the order of 100 Hz. Therefore the aggregate electrical connection rate of the human visual system, from a highly simplified neural network viewpoint, is likely to be on the order of 5×10^{15} CPS, plus or minus perhaps an order of magnitude or so.

This comparison is only suggestive because no comprehensive computational model of the brain (or even the human visual system) has been proposed so far, and we have of course left out all chemical (e.g., neurotransmitter) interactions in our estimate, as well as the computational intricacies associated with spike train encoding. The comparison is illuminating nonetheless from the perspective provided in an earlier section on the need for efficient use of temporal multiplexing techniques within PMCMs. The volume of the human visual system is much larger than the volume assumed for the PMCMs analyzed in this chapter, but even given this disparity and further reductions in device sizes with corresponding advances in semiconductor VLSI and photonic technologies, the sheer density of neuron units will most likely always favor biological brain structures over any form of envisioned neural prosthesis. Likewise, the interconnection density of living neurons is difficult to achieve in any current technological implementation of a prosthetic device. The temporal bandwidth parameter, however, weighs heavily in favor of PMCM structures, provided that it can be employed efficiently and to advantage. If so, PMCM structures may be able to supply prosthetic functionality in local brain regions without significant mismatches in this performance metric on a per unit-volume basis.

Neural Prosthetic Multichip Modules: Fundamental Scientific and Technological Issues

We conclude this chapter by briefly addressing a number of the fundamental scientific and technological challenges that must be met before hybrid electronic/photonic multichip modules can form the basis of a viable neural prosthetic device. These issues include bidirectionality, adaptivity, scalability, the neural tissue/prosthesis prosthetic interface, biocompatibility, power consumption, and supply of electrical power.

As described in a previous section, the PMCM modules under current development incorporate signal feedforward from layer to layer, with explicit provision for feedback only locally (e.g., nearest neighbor, next-nearest neighbor) within each layer. This lack of layer-to-layer bidirectionality strongly limits the types of neural network architectures that can be implemented. Bidirectionality of signal propagation can be included locally if a combination of both top-emitting and bottom-emitting VCSELs is employed in the GaAs layer, provided that the surface area on the associated silicon driver chip is devoid of both circuitry and bonding pads directly above the top-emitting (feedback) VCSELs, at the cost of increasing the pixel (neuron unit) size to provide this chip real estate. Alternatively, bidirectionality can be included nonlocally for each layer by laterally transferring aggregate information to the chip edges, where these signals could be used to drive additional chip stacks arrayed at the PMCM perimeter and oriented in the reverse signal propagation direction. In this latter case, the form of feedback will necessarily be spatially integrative, as a result of topological signal routing constraints.

The potential incorporation of adaptivity in the weighted interconnection patterns is an issue of considerable importance for prosthetic device applications because it is highly unlikely that sophisticated multilayer devices can be programmed a priori to function in the living brain without significant behavioral retraining. The combinations of optical and photonic interconnections described in previous sections provide significant capabilities for dense fan-out/fan-in connectivity between layers, but are not easily amenable to adaptation. As such, these interconnections constitute a "nature-like" architectural component that can provide a general interconnection structure from layer to layer that instantiates, for example, center-surround connections. The "nurture-like" architectural component can conceivably be incorporated in weighted lateral connections among neighboring neuron units within a given chip (physical layer) that include the nearest neighbors as well as potentially the next nearest neighbors. Further lateral interconnectivity among neuron units is limited by the number of metal interconnection layers (five to seven) available in current or envisioned semiconductor VLSI technology, as well as by the additional chip real estate required to implement adaptively programmable weights. Should these types of adaptive lateral connections be incorporated, one fundamental scientific question that arises is how best to structure the architecture to make optimal use of this unusual nature/nurture admixture, in which two separate interpenetrating network topologies separately implement the a priori and a posteriori weights. A second fundamental question relates to the optimal training algorithm to employ, and how best to map it onto the available hardware.

A neural prosthetic device technology must be inherently scalable to large numbers of densely interconnected neuron units if the complexities and potential impairment associated with surgical implantation are to be offset by the functionality sought and regained. Ideally, the neuron unit and interconnection densities should approximate those characteristic of human wetware, although as pointed out earlier, this goal is perhaps not feasible in the near future. As a result, some combination of signal transformation and temporal multiplexing within the prosthetic device are most likely required to offset displaced neuron density. Photonic multichip modules configured as described in this chapter will be limited to local fan-outs (and hence fan-ins) of 25 or so from (and to) each neuron unit within the array, and to interconnections between adjacent layers only. The scientific and technological limitations that currently proscribe the degree of fan-out should be carefully evaluated to see if alternative implementations are feasible with enhanced fan-out capabilities (see, e.g., figure 14.6). In addition, the current architectural limit of only adjacent layer connectivity should be examined to develop methods that allow layer-to-layer connectivity to project through and to multiple layers.

The issue of providing a flexible, adaptive, and potentially self-organizing neural tissue/prosthetic device interface has been discussed extensively in this chapter. Several fundamental issues obtain here in addition to those discussed previously, including the key issue of providing a functional interface over as much of the surface area of the neural prosthetic device as possible. To this end, it should be noted that if fewer layers are incorporated, the aspect ratio of the resultant module can be biased toward planarity, thereby allowing implantation within highly layered brain regions with viable top and bottom interfacial layers only, assuming a parallel orientation of the as-implanted module, and assuming further that a viable means for incorporating signal bidirectionality can be implemented as described in this section. This interface issue is in many ways related to the issue of overall biocompatibility, which involves the exclusion of all potentially toxic components from the as-implanted device, the provision for surgical and treatment methodologies that obviate rejection processes, the essential guarantee of performance over a given patient's lifetime, and the adequate encapsulation of semiconductor and photonic components in biocompatible as well as inorganic-material-compatible sheaths.

The total power consumption of any viable neural prosthetic device must be kept as low as possible, both to provide an acceptable equilibrium temperature for the interior of the module and the neural tissue/prosthetic device interfaces, and to require minimal external power resources. The current PMCM implementations are designed with an upper bound of 1 W per physical layer, which corresponds to a total of 8 W in an assumed eight-layer, 1-cm^3 module. It is still to be determined whether this level of power dissipation, even spread over the approximately 6-cm^2 surface area (approximately 1.3 W/cm^2) can be accommodated in the surrounding neural tissue without compromising cellular functionality or longevity. If full-bandwidth operation cannot be accommodated, it is possible that reduced bandwidth operation (with an associated reduction in power dissipation) could still provide adequate prosthetic functionality.

Associated with the issue of total power consumption (or dissipation) is the key issue of providing electrical power to the implanted module. Stand-alone batteries are not likely to provide adequate power for the operational periods desired (limited by the total energy capacity of the battery), and the inclusion of batteries adds topological compromise as well. A more likely power source is the external transmission into the cranium of convertible power signals, received by a compact power conversion device that might be incorporated at either the module or single-chip level. The ultimate challenge will be the development of electrical power cells capable of tapping into the electrochemistry of the brain itself, so that efficient electrical conversion can be provided at the implant site using only local metabolic processes.

In conclusion, one may hope that none of the challenges outlined in this chapter will have to be met, in that advances in medical science may either provide therapeutic means for stimulating neural repair mechanisms or develop stem (or otherwise cytologically specific) cell injections or implants that can transform and interconnect as necessary to replace lost neural functionality. Should these developments not prove feasible, the artificial neural prosthetic devices described in this chapter may provide a nonoptimal but useful solution.

Acknowledgments

The authors are pleased to acknowledge their many collaborators in this research effort, including Christoph von der Malsburg, Bartlett Mel, Gary Holt, John O'Brien, Irving Biederman, Anupam Madhukar, P. Daniel Dapkus, Theodore W. Berger, Michel Baudry, Roberta D. Brinton, Vasilis Marmarelis, Jim-Shih Liaw, Nicholas George (University of Rochester, Institute of Optics), Gregory P. Nordin (University of Alabama, Huntsville), Mandyam Srinivasan (Australian National University), Chris Kyriakakis, Zaheed S. Karim, Scott DeMars, Kasra Rastani, Jong-Je Jung, Ke-Zhong Hu, Kartik Ananthanarayanan, Ching-Chu Huang, Charles Kuznia, Adam A. Goldstein, Ladan Shams, Suresh Subramaniam, Moshe Bar, Robert Cartland, Jaeyoun Cho, Hsing-Hua Fan, Martin Han, Yunsong Huang, Hung-Min Jen, Po-Tsung Lee, Jaw-Chyng (Lormen) Lue, Patrick Nasiatka, Nankyung Suh, and Dennis Su.

Research on adaptive vision sensors at the University of Southern California is supported in part by the FY 98 Multidisciplinary University Research Initiative (MURI), Adaptive Optoelectronic Eyes: Hybrid Sensor/Processor Architectures, Office of the Undersecretary of Defense (DDR&E), administered through the Army Research Office; in part by an FY 99 Defense University Research Instrumentation Program (DURIP) grant, also administered through the Army Research Office; in part by the Defense Advanced Research Projects Agency research program on Dense

3-D Integrated Photonic Multichip Modules for Adaptive Spatial and Spectral Image Processing Applications within the Photonic Wavelength and Spectral Signal Processing (PWASSP) initiative; and in part by Teledyne Electronic Technologies, the Eastman Kodak Company, Xerox Corporation, and the TRW Foundation. One of us (ART) gratefully acknowledges the significant hospitality, collegiality, and resources afforded to him during both a sabbatical leave and ongoing visiting faculty appointments at the California Institute of Technology and the University of Rochester, Institute of Optics.

References

Arbib, M. A., ed. (1995) *The Handbook of Brain Theory and Neural Networks.* Cambridge, Mass.: MIT Press, pp. 4–11.

Bar, M., and Biederman, I. (1998) Subliminal visual priming. *Psychol. Sci.* 9: 464–469.

Berger, T. W., Baudry, M., Brinton, R. D., Liaw, J.-S., Marmarelis, V., Park, A. Y., Sheu, B. J., and Tanguay, A. R., Jr. (2001) Brain-implantable biomimetic electronics as the next era in neural prosthetics. *Proc. IEEE* 89(7): 993–1012.

Biederman, I. (1995) Visual object recognition. In S. G. Kosslyn and D. N. Osherson, eds., *An Invitation to Cognitive Science*, 2nd ed., chap. 4, Cambridge, Mass.: MIT Press, pp. 121–165.

Biederman, I., and Gerhardstein, P. C. (1993) Recognizing depth-rotated objects: Evidence and conditions for three-dimensional viewpoint invariance. *J. Exp. Psychol.* 19: 1162–1182.

Biederman, I., and Kalocsai, P. (1997) Neurocomputational bases of object and face recognition. *Phil. Trans. R. Soc. Lond.* B 352: 1203–1219.

Biederman, I., and Kalocsai, P. (1998) Neural and psychophysical analysis of object and face recognition. In H. Wechsler, P. J. Phillips, V. Bruce, F. F. Soulie, and T. Huang, eds., *Face Recognition: From Theory to Applications*, NATO ASI Series F. Heidelberg: Springer-Verlag, pp. 3–25.

Cartland, R. F., Madhukar, A., Ananthanarayanan, K., Nasiatka, P., Su, D., and Tanguay, A. R., Jr. (1995) Hybrid electronic/photonic 2-D neural array using InGaAs/AlGaAs multiple quantum well modulators flip-chip bonded to a CMOS Si analog control chip. In *Trends in Optics and Photonics*, vol. 14, Washington, D.C.: Optical Society of America, pp. 51–56.

Chambers, D. M., and Nordin, G. P. (1999) Stratified volume diffractive optical elements as high-efficiency gratings. *J. Opt. Soc. Am. A* 16(5): 1184–1193.

Churchland, P. S., and Sejnowski, T. J. (1992) *The Computational Brain.* Cambridge, Mass.: MIT Press, pp. 48–60.

De Mars, S. (1995) Advanced hybrid bulk/integrated optical signal processing modules. Ph.D. thesis, University of Southern California, Los Angeles.

Dowling, J. E. (1992) *Neurons and Networks: An Introduction to Neuroscience.* Cambridge, Mass.: Harvard University Press.

Goldstein, A. A. (1997) Scalable photonic neural networks for real-time pattern classification. Ph.D. thesis, University of Southern California, Los Angeles. SIPI Report No. 307, Signal and Image Processing Institute, Department of Electrical Engineering-Systems.

Goldstein, A. A., and Jenkins, B. K. (1996) Neural-network object recognition algorithm for real-time implementation on 3-D photonic multichip modules. Paper presented at the Annual Meeting of the Optical Society of America, paper ThKK2, Optical Society of America, Washington, D.C.

Hu, K., Chen, L., Madhukar, A., Chen, P., Rajkumar, K. C., Kaviani, K., Karim, Z., Kyriakakis, C., and Tanguay, A. R., Jr. (1991a) High contrast ratio asymmetric Fabry-Perot reflection light modulator based on GaAs/InGaAs multiple quantum wells. *Appl. Phys. Lett.* 59(9): 1108–1110.

Hu, K., Chen, L., Madhukar, A., Chen, P., Kyriakakis, C., Karim, Z., and Tanguay, A. R., Jr. (1991b) Inverted cavity GaAs/InGaAs asymmetric Fabry-Perot reflection modulator. *Appl. Phys. Lett.* 59(14): 1664–1666.

Huang, C.-C. (1997) Diffractive optical elements for space-variant interconnections in three-dimensional computation structures. Ph.D. thesis, University of Southern California, Los Angeles. SIPI Report No. 314, Signal and Image Processing Institute, Department of Electrical Engineering-Systems.

Huang, C.-C., Jenkins, B. K., and Kuznia, C. B. (1998) Space-variant interconnections based on diffractive optical elements for neural networks: Architectures and cross-talk reduction. *Appl. Opt.* 37(5): 889–911.

Hubel, D. H. (1988) *Eye, Brain, and Vision*. New York: Scientific American Library Series (No. 22), distributed by W. H. Freeman.

Hummel, J. E., and Biederman, I. (1992) Dynamic binding in a neural network for shape recognition. *Psychol. Rev.* 99(3): 480–517.

Jenkins, B. K., and Tanguay, A. R., Jr. (1992) Photonic implementations of neural networks. In B. Kosko, ed., *Neural Networks for Signal Processing*, chap. 9. England Cliffs, N.J.: Prentice-Hall, pp. 287–382.

Jenkins, B. K., and Wang, C. H. (1991) Use of optics in neural vision models. *Optical Society of America Annual Meeting Technical Digest 1991*, vol. 17, Washington, D.C.: Optical Society of America, p. 22.

Jung, J.-J. (1994) Stratified volume holographic optical elements: Analysis of diffraction behavior and implementation using InGaAs/GaAs multiple quantum well structures. Ph.D. thesis, University of Southern California, Los Angeles.

Kalocsai, P., and Biederman, I. (1998) Differences of face and object recognition in utilizing early visual information. In H. Wechsler, P. J. Phillips, V. Bruce, F. F. Soulie, and T. Huang, eds., *Face Recognition: From Theory to Applications*. NATO ASI Series F. Heidelberg: Springer-Verlag, pp. 492–502.

Kandel, E. R., Schwartz, J. H., and Jessell, T. M. (1991) *Principles of Neural Science*, 3rd ed. Norwalk, Conn.: Appleton & Lange, pp. 121, 283.

Karim, Z. (1993) Thin-film coatings for optical information processing and computing applications. Ph.D. thesis, University of Southern California, Los Angeles.

Karim, Z., Kyriakakis, C., Tanguay, A. R., Jr., Hu, K., Chen, L., and Madhukar, A. (1994) Externally deposited phase-compensating dielectric mirrors for asymmetric Fabry-Perot cavity tuning. *Appl. Phys. Lett.* 64(22): 2913–2915.

Karim, Z., Kyriakakis, C., Tanguay, A. R., Jr., Cartland, R. F., Hu, K., Chen, L., and Madhukar, A. (1995) Post-growth tuning of inverted cavity InGaAs/GaAs spatial light modulators using phase-compensating dielectric mirrors. *Appl. Phys. Lett.* 66(21): 2774–2776.

Kyriakakis, C. (1993) Fundamental and technological limitations in optical processing and computing: Algorithms, architectures, and devices. Ph.D. thesis, University of Southern California, Los Angeles.

Lades, M., Vorbrueggen, J. C., Buhmann, J., Lange, J., von der Malsburg, C., Wuertz, R. P., and Konen W. (1993) Distortion invariant object recognition in the dynamic link architecture. *IEEE Trans. Comp.* 42: 300–311.

Liaw, J.-S., and Berger, T. W. (1996) The dynamic synapse: A new concept for neural representation and computation. *Hippocampus* 6: 591–600.

Liaw, J.-S., and Berger, T. W. (1999) Dynamic synapse: Harnessing the computing power of synaptic dynamics. *Neurocomputing* 26–27: 199–206.

Mead, C. (1989) *Analog VLSI and Neural Systems*. Reading, Mass.: Addison-Wesley.

Mel, B. W. (1997) SEEMORE: Combining color, shape, and texture histogramming in a neurally inspired approach to visual object recognition. *Neural Comput.* 9: 777–804.

Mel, B. W., and Fiser, J. (2000) Minimizing binding errors using learned conjunctive features. *Neural Comput.* 12: 247–278.

Palmer, S. E. (1999) *Vision Science: Photons to Phenomenology*. Cambridge, Mass.: MIT Press, p. 24.

Phillips, P. J. (1997) The face recognition technology (FERET) program. Paper presented at the CTAC International Technology Symposium, Chicago, Illinois, August 18–22.

Rastani, K. (1988) Advanced integrated optical signal processing components. Ph.D. thesis, University of Southern California, Los Angeles.

Shoop, B. L., Wagner, T. D., Mait, J. N., Kilby, G. R., and Ressler, E. K. (1999) Design and analysis of a diffractive optical filter for use in an optoelectronic error-diffusion neural network. *Appl. Opt.* (special issue on diffractive optics and micro-optics, J. N. Mait and H. P. Herzig, eds.), 38(14): 3077–3088.

Tang, S. R., Chen, T., Li, B., and Foshee, J. (2000) Waveguides take to the sky. *IEEE Circ. Dev.* 16(1): 10–16.

Tanguay, A. R., Jr., and Jenkins, B. K. (1996) Modulator-based photonic chip-to-chip interconnections for dense three-dimensional multichip module integration. U.S. Patent 5,568,574. Issued October 22.

Tanguay, A. R., Jr., and Jenkins, B. K. (1999) Emerging smart camera technologies: Toward an adaptive optoelectronic eye. Paper presented at Winter Conference on Synaptic Plasticity, Workshop on Hardware Implementations of Neural Networks.

Tanguay, A. R., Jr., and Kyriakakis, C. (1995) Hybrid electronic/photonic packaging using flip-chip bonding. Paper presented to Research Working Group on Multiple Modules and Input/Output, 9th Biennial Workshop on Superconductive Electronics: Devices, Circuits, and Systems.

Tanguay, A. R., Jr., Jenkins, B. K., and Madhukar, A. (1995) Photonic implementations of neural networks. *1995 Technical Digest Series*, vol. 10. Washington, D.C.: Optical Society of America, pp. 128–130.

Tanguay, A. R., Jr., Jenkins, B. K., von der Malsburg, C., Mel, B., Holt, G., O'Brien, J., Biederman, I., Madhukar, A., Nasiatka, P., and Huang, Y. (2000) Vertically integrated photonic multichip module architecture for vision applications. *Proc. SPIE* 4089: 584–600.

Veldkamp, W. B. (1993) Wireless focal planes "on the road to amacronic sensors." *IEEE J. Quant. Electron.* 29(2): 801–813.

von der Malsburg, C. (1981) The Correlation Theory of Brain Function. Internal Report No. 81-2, Max Planck Institute for Biophysical Chemistry, Department of Neurobiology, Gottingen, Germany.

Wandell, B. A. (1995) *Foundations of Vision*. Sunderland, Mass.: Sinauer Associates.

Wang, C.-H., Jenkins, B. K., and Wang, J. M. (1993) Visual cortex operations and their implementation using the incoherent optical neuron model. *Appl. Opt.* 32(11): 1876–1887.

Wiskott, L., Fellous, J.-M., Krueger, N., and von der Malsburg, C. (1998) Face recognition by elastic graph matching. *IEEE Trans. Pattern Anal. Machine Intell.* 19(7): 775–779.

Zeki, S. (1993) *A Vision of the Brain*. Oxford: Blackwell Scientific.

15 Reconfigurable Processors for Neural Prostheses

Jose Mumbru, Krishna V. Shenoy, George Panotopoulos, Suat Ay, Xin An, Fai Mok, and Demetri Psaltis

The prospect of helping paralyzed patients by translating neural activity from the brain into control signals for prosthetic devices has improved greatly in recent years (Wolpaw et al., 2000; Barinaga, 1999; Fetz, 1999). This improvement has been fueled by discoveries in systems neuroscience and by the rapid advance of microelectromechanical systems (MEMS) and computational technologies. However, potential barriers to continued progress in neural prosthetic systems exist. These barriers include our modest understanding of neural coding, fairly short-lived neural interfaces, and the relatively limited computational power available for mobile real-time processing of neural signals. As we have seen in other chapters, systems neuroscientists and MEMS engineers are rapidly lowering the first two barriers by elucidating the fundamental mechanisms of information processing in the brain and by designing sophisticated micromachined neural probes (Lee et al., 1998; Si et al., 1998; Hatsopoulos et al., 1998; Schmidt et al., 1999). In this chapter we address the third potential barrier by proposing the use of reconfigurable processors to meet the computational challenges of neural prosthetic systems.

In broad terms, neural prosthetic systems or brain/computer interfaces aim to provide disabled patients with new options for interacting with the world (Wolpaw et al., 2000). Sensory prostheses, such as cochlear implants or artificial vision, encode information from the environment and deliver it to the nervous system by appropriate electrical stimulation. Motor prostheses work in reverse, by translating neural activity into control signals for prosthetic devices, to assist patients with upper spinal cord injuries, neurodegenerative diseases, or amputations (Lauer et al., 2000; Chapin et al., 2000; Isaacs et al., 2000; Shenoy et al., 1999). Communication systems, such as cortically controlled computer cursors for locked-in brainstem stroke or amyotrophic lateral sclerosis (ALS) patients, are closely related (Kennedy et al., 2000). Finally, "intracentral nervous system" (intra-CNS) prosthetic systems interact with neural processing by stimulating brain regions (e.g., chronic thalamic stimulation to suppress tremor for Parkinson's and essential-tremor patients (Benabid et al., 1996)) or by recording from one region and stimulating another region (e.g., proposed sense or disrupt systems for epilepsy or cortical bypass systems for stoke).

Despite the great variety of sensors and actuators needed to address the dysfunctions mentioned here, sensory, motor, and intra-CNS prosthetic systems have many computational requirements in common. From a computational perspective, these systems will most likely grow to look even more alike as, for example, motor prosthetic systems evolve to include supplementary sensory feedback to the nervous system, and all prosthetic systems incorporate learning and adaptation to contend with, and take advantage of, neural plasticity. The anticipated similarities among these systems, as well as the demanding requirements imposed by mobile real-time processing of neural and/or sensory data, prompt the development of a processor optimized for neural prosthetic systems.

In the following two sections we review the principles of reconfigurable processing and discuss its potential role in neural prosthetic systems. We suggest that reconfigurable processors are well suited for neural prostheses for three principal reasons. First, neural prosthetic systems require many diverse computations, and a single processor capable of being "rewired" rapidly can efficiently perform a wide range of calculations. Second, neural prosthetic systems run in real time, and reconfigurable processors can meet these real-time demands by being "wired" nearly optimally for any given task, which often includes a parallel-processing topology. Finally, neural prosthetic systems are likely to require greater computational resources as, for example, the number and variety of sensors (e.g., electrodes) used to collect information from across neural representations expands. Reconfigurable processors, as with other high-speed electronic systems, are likely to scale well as the number of recorded neural signals increases, owing to the relatively slower time scale of the biological system, which allows time-multiplexing schemes to absorb the increasing computational demands. We conclude by briefly describing how a reconfigurable processor for a neural prothesis could function in a motor prosthetic system.

An Example of a Neural Prosthetic System

Before proceeding, however, it is useful to introduce a specific example of a neural prosthetic system so that the relevance and potential merits of reconfigurable processing can be seen more easily. We use a motor prosthetic system for this purpose, but the principles are not specific to this class of system. Figure 15.1 is a block diagram of a system that translates cortical activity into control signals for stimulating the musculature in a paralyzed arm. A person typically sees (senses) an object that he or she wishes to reach toward, forms a mental plan for where and how to move the arm, and finally sequences through the movement commands. Different attributes of this movement are found in different regions of cortex, with any one attribute (e.g., reach location) encoded across numerous neurons. This neural activity can be sensed in many ways, typically with permanently implanted electrodes. It is thought that

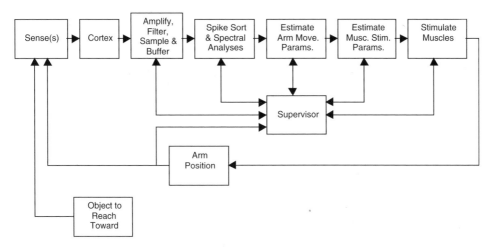

Figure 15.1
Block diagram of a motor prosthetic system (a prosthetic arm system). Each element is described in the text. Lines indicate information flow, with arrows indicating the direction of this flow. Information can be transmitted down subcutaneous wires or with telemetry, in which case additional transmit and receive circuitry is required.

tens to hundreds of electrodes, implanted in several cortical areas, will eventually be needed to harvest enough detail of the motor plan (i.e., information transmission rate) to accurately reconstruct the desired movement in real time. Therefore numerous neural signal channels need to be amplified, filtered, and digitized for subsequent processing, and much of this circuitry may eventually be integrated with or near the recording electrodes. After passing through this front end, a digitized signal stream from each electrode must be processed to associate action potentials (spikes) with particular neurons, to estimate spectral power density, and to estimate other spatiotemporal signal features that researchers are continuing to relate to movement parameters. These signals can then be compared with each neuron's (and electrode's) previously characterized responses to arrive at a moment-by-moment estimate of the desired movement parameter, such as the direction of an arm movement or location of an end point. Common estimation methods include maximum likelihood and neural networks.

Once the movement parameters of interest have been decoded from the neural measurements, the neural prosthetic system must generate estimates for muscle-stimulation parameters (i.e., inverse kinematics). In this particular example, the goal is to electrically stimulate the paralyzed arm's musculature to achieve arm movements. This prosthetic arm system is controlled through negative feedback by visually comparing the arm's new position with the desired location and iterating as necessary. It is important to note that even with careful calibration of the entire system, so that a person's desired arm movements are executed accurately, the system will change with time and experience. As time passes, recording quality changes as a result of electrode drift and the death of neurons, and the efficacy of muscle stimulation can also change. As users gain more experience, neurons will almost certainly adapt (plasticity) in order to improve the performance of the system, as the brain does whenever it is presented with a demanding new task. Unless the neural prosthetic system also adapts to contend with and take advantage of these changes, system performance will eventually deteriorate to the point of being useless.

A supervisor could monitor these time-dependent and experience-dependent changes, and adjust the system accordingly. For example, if one of the neurons controlling the system drifts out of recording range or even dies, the supervisor could remove this neuron from the database, thereby making performance robust against such events. Then, if a new neuron becomes detectable, the supervisor could monitor the neuron's response to ongoing prosthetic arm movements in order to learn this new neuron's encoding characteristics. After a certain level of confidence is reached, this neuron would be entered into the database of neurons whose activity is controlling movement. The supervisor could similarly evolve the system's model for how each neuron responds to account for neural plasticity effects.

Reconfigurable Processing

The level of computational complexity in a neural prosthetic system, beyond what an implanted or autonomous system would ideally have, requires a solution that allows reusing some limited amount of hardware resources. Moreover, the need for some kind of supervising intelligence able to correct the system for neuronal changes suggests a reconfigurable prosthetic processor as a solution.

Reconfigurable processors bring a new computational paradigm in which the processor modifies its structure to suit a given application, rather than having to modify the application to fit the device. The reconfigurability makes it possible for these processors to use their resources more efficiently by adjusting themselves, depending on the characteristics of the input or on unsatisfactory previous results, to better implement the target task.

Given an application such as pattern recognition in figure 15.2, the reconfigurable processor can be customized to deal with a specific class of objects, but with enough flexibility that, if at a later time the salient class of objects becomes a different one, the device can be reprogrammed to deal with the new problem without degradation of its performance. Furthermore, the processor can adapt itself in order to be robust to changes in orientation or illumination of the input object. By reprogramming, the same hardware can be time multiplexed to sequentially carry out several tasks on the same input, or perform different tasks for different parts of the same input image.

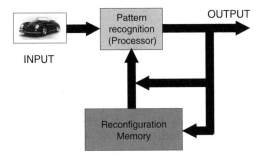

Figure 15.2
Reconfigurable processor applied to pattern recognition. The external memory stores the configuration templates that define the functionality of the processor. Using reconfiguration, the same processor can perform different tasks on the same input image.

Reconfiguration also makes it possible to implement learning by allowing the processor to evolve in a controlled manner in order to learn the function that needs to be computed.

In other applications, where it is necessary to implement different concurrent tasks by partitioning the hardware resources among them, a reconfigurable processor can outperform a nonreconfigurable solution by dynamically reallocating the hardware of idle tasks to those that are temporarily overloaded. This feature, called spatial multiplexing, becomes very attractive when partial rather than global reconfiguration is possible because it allows part of the device to be reprogrammed without halting execution in the rest of it.

Field-Programmable Gate Arrays
A field-programmable gate array (FPGA) is a device in which this idea of reconfigurable hardware can be implemented. They emerged as a new technology for the implementation of digital logic circuits during the mid-1980's. The basic architecture of an FPGA consists of a large number of configurable logic blocks (CLBs) and a programmable mesh of interconnections. Both the function performed by the logic blocks and the interconnection pattern can be specified by the circuit designer. In the beginning FPGAs were mostly viewed as large programmable logic devices (PLDs) and they were usually employed for the implementation of the "glue-logic" used to tie together complex very large-scale integrated (VLSI) chips like the microprocessors and memories used to build general-purpose computers.

While several FPGAs were configured by static random access memory (SRAM) cells, this was generally considered a limitation by users concerned about the chip's volatility. For this reason, fuse-based FPGAs were also developed and for many applications were much more attractive, both because they were faster and smaller

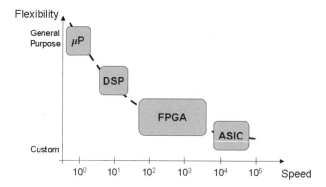

Figure 15.3
Tradeoff comparison of flexibility versus speed for different hardware implementations: microprocessors (µP), digital signal processors (DSP), field-programmable gate arrays (FPGA), and application-specific integrated circuits (ASIC).

owing to less programming overhead, and because there was no volatility in their configuration since this had been burned into the chip. Not until the late 1980s and early 1990s did it become clear that the volatility of SRAM-based FPGAs was not a liability, but could open an entirely new spectrum of applications, since the programming of such FPGAs could be changed electrically at almost any point during operation.

These devices have gained popularity because they are between a software-oriented solution, such as a microprocessor running a program stored in memory, and a hardware-oriented solution, such as an application-specific integrated circuit (ASIC) (figure 15.3). The FPGA-based solution is faster than a microprocessor or digital signal processor (DSP) because the FPGA is conceived as a large array of small logic blocks working in parallel and operating at the bit level, exactly where general-purpose processors are most inefficient. Even though microprocessors have more capabilities, in order to keep their generality, they are still designed to operate with fixed data formats (8, 16, 32, 64 bits ...). Therefore they perform poorly when they need to deal with problems where data have "nonstandard" lengths. On the other hand, the fine granularity of the computing blocks of the FPGA allows the user to better map the hardware resources of the chip to meet the demands of the problem. Using FPGA platforms, speedups of several orders of magnitude have been achieved for some applications (Stogiannos et al., 2000; Benedetti and Perona, 1998; Jean et al., 2000; Kaps and Paar, 1999). Most of the time the ASIC solution provides the optimal implementation both in terms of speed and silicon area requirement; however, it has the drawback of being a single-purpose processor. Compared with ASICs, FPGAs are much more flexible since they contain some hardware resources that can be programmed by the user to implement a given task and, by

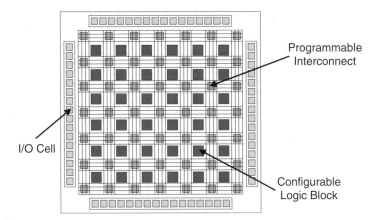

Figure 15.4
Architecture of a typical FPGA. A symmetric array of configurable logic blocks (CLBs) is surrounded by a mesh of buses and matrices of programmable interconnects that provide connectivity among the CLBs, as well as with the input-output (I/O) cells.

changing that configuration, the same hardware can be used to carry out something totally different with minimal development time and cost.

Although FPGA architecture design is a field of important research in the FPGA community, and many different implementations have already become commercially available, it is beyond the scope of this chapter to describe all of them. To illustrate the common features of their internal structure, one of the most widely used designs, the symmetric array (Brown et al., 1992), will be analyzed (figure 15.4). In this case, the CLBs are arranged in a two-dimensional array and interleaved with vertical and horizontal buses used to establish connectivity among them. Segments in two different buses can also be connected by programmable interconnects in switching matrices. Finally, on the periphery of the chip, there are some input-output cells.

The basic functional unit of the FPGA is the configurable logic block, which implements an elementary Boolean operation. Despite the fact that there are CLBs based on multiplexors or OR-AND arrays, the use of look-up tables (LUTs) to synthesize logic functions provides much greater flexibility (Brown et al., 1992). An LUT can be seen as a small memory bank in which the inputs encode the address of a position that stores the result of a preprogrammed logic function of the inputs. By changing the bits stored in the LUT, the computed function can be altered.

A simple example, like the majority rule function, can be used to illustrate how an LUT operates. In this case, the operation to be implemented has to produce an output "1" if at least two of the three input bits are "1," and output "0" otherwise. This function could be implemented using only a three-input LUT. The LUT needs to store the result of the computation for each of the eight possible input sequences

Table 15.1
LUT definition for the majority rule function

Input	Output
000	0
001	0
010	0
011	1
100	0
101	1
110	1
111	1

from "000" to "111." Therefore the LUT holds logic "1" for the sequences "011," "101," "110," and "111," and logic "0" for "000," "001," "010," and "100," so table 15.1 is generated.

Since all possible input states are accounted for in the table, every time an instance is presented, the FPGA processor only needs to look up the result. Despite the simplicity of the problem, a general-purpose microprocessor would already perform worse than the FPGA since the microprocessor needs to retrieve the input data and then sequentially compare it with each one of the sequences containing at least two logic "1"; or alternatively, summing the three inputs and comparing the result with the value 2, which is also slower.

In the same way as in the example, more interesting functions such as a 1-bit full adder can be mapped in an LUT. Arbitrarily large adders and multipliers are implemented by cascading several 1-bit full adders together with shift registers. Higher-level functions, such as filters or correlators, are then synthesized by combining adders and multipliers.

Figure 15.5 shows the schematic of an LUT-based CLB. In this case, two sets of inputs, on the left-hand side, feed two independent four-input LUTs. A third LUT has the ability to combine the results of the LUTs from the previous stage, increasing the functionality of the CLB to implement more complex logic functions. The two outputs of the CLB are on the right-hand side and can be buffered if necessary by flip-flops. These registers allow sequential logic to be implemented in the CLB.

FPGAs have traditionally been successfully used as accelerators in many applications, such as signal processing (Stogiannos et al., 2000), image filtering (Benedetti and Perona, 1998), automated target recognition (Jean et al., 2000), or cryptography (Kaps and Paar, 1999). In a typical arrangement, as shown in figure 15.6, the FPGA is set up as a coprocessor that is controlled by the microprocessor. For a given application, if there is some task that is computationally very expensive, the microprocessor

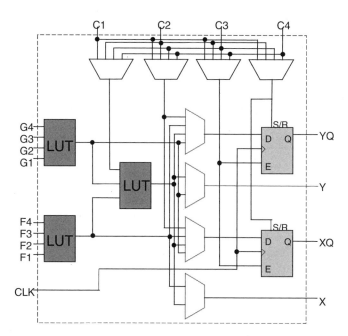

Figure 15.5
Schematic of a look-up table (LUT)-based CLB. Two independent sets of inputs F[1–4] and G[1–4] feed the LUTs on the left of the figure. The outputs of the LUTs can be combined using an additional LUT for more complex Boolean functions. The control signals C[1–4] define the way the results of the LUTs are routed to the output of the CLB by the multiplexers. This output can be buffered, which allows sequential logic to be implemented.

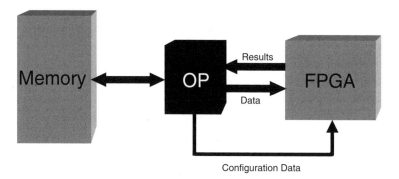

Figure 15.6
FPGAs are usually used as accelerators. The master processor (microprocessor and memory) programs the slave processor (FPGA) to perform the most computationally intense tasks.

can program the FPGA to perform that task much faster than if it was executed by the main processor. The configuration data of the FPGA, which specify the values in the LUTs and the interconnection pattern, are stored in an external memory, in most cases an electrically programmable read-only memory (EPROM), and downloaded into the FPGA chip on demand. The microprocessor just feeds the data into the FPGA and waits for the results; all the cumbersome computation has been hard wired inside the FPGA.

Although the size of these devices, in logic gates, can vary among different models and manufacturers, they can easily contain on the order of 10^5 gates, and the trend is to keep increasing the logic density to go beyond the million-gate FPGA. This means that the configuration data page for a medium-sized FPGA can be as large as 1 Mbit. Despite the fact that the FPGA can be reprogrammed multiple times, the user typically does not take advantage of this feature. In most cases, the FPGA is configured only once and this configuration is downloaded into the FPGA offline, before the execution is started. The main reason for not dynamically reconfiguring the device, that is, changing its internal configuration once the execution has started and some data are already flowing into it, has been the small communication bandwidth between the external configuration memory and the FPGA chip itself. The configuration bandwidth of the FPGA has not scaled well enough to keep up with the enormous data throughput.

Upon programming, the configuration data are downloaded serially by shifting a long bitstream into the FPGA. The data transfer rate between memory and the FPGA is only in the range of 100 megabits per second (Mbps), which results in configuration times of tens or even hundreds of milliseconds. These long reconfiguration times, if compared with clock cycles of just tens of nanoseconds and input-output throughputs reaching 100 Gbps, become an important overhead. Some attempts to decrease the reconfiguration times have been proposed, such as providing a dedicated parallel bus to increase the bandwidth with the configuration memory, or having fast-access cache memory built into the chip (Trimberger et al., 1997; Motomura et al., 1998). Both solutions only further increase the already high power dissipation of the FPGAs, which although application dependent, can easily be in the range of 1 to 10 W.

Holographic Memories
Holographic memories offer a potential solution to this demand for high-capacity memory. Holography was invented by Gabor in 1948 (Gabor, 1948, 1949a,b) and volume data storage was proposed already in the early 1960s (van Heerden, 1963; Leith et al., 1966), but it was not until the early 1990s that advances in optoelectronic devices and materials made holographic memories viable (Psaltis and Mok, 1995; Mok, 1993). In a holographic memory, the information is recorded by the inter-

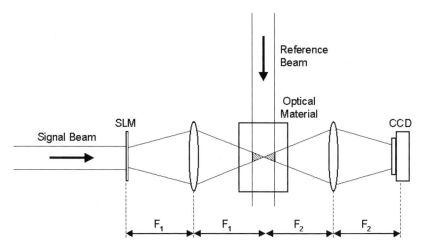

Figure 15.7
Typical holographic setup: Two beams of coherent light are crossed inside an optical material. The spatial light modulator (SLM) transfers a page of digital data into the signal beam, while the reference beam carries no information. The pattern displayed on the SLM is imaged onto the detector [a charge-coupled device (CCD) camera] using two lenses with focal lengths F_1 and F_2.

ference of two coherent beams of light inside an optical medium (figure 15.7). One of the beams (signal beam) is encoded using a spatial light modulator (SLM) or a mask containing the data formatted as a page of pixels, while the other beam (reference beam) is usually a plane wave. The unique interference pattern created between the two beams is then recorded as a hologram inside the optical material. During readout, when the original reference beam illuminates the material, the hologram causes the light to be diffracted and to reconstruct the recorded signal beam.

Owing to the Bragg effect, it is possible to superimpose several holograms on the same location without cross-talk, achieving densities as high as 100 bits/μm^2 (Pu, 1997). Several multiplexing techniques have been developed and they involve some change in a property of the reference beam [angle (Mok, 1993; Curtis et al., 1994), wavelength (Rakuljic et al., 1992; Yin et al., 1993), or shift (Psaltis et al., 1995; Barbastathis et al., 1996) multiplexing] or in its wavefront [phase-code (Denz et al., 1991) or speckle (Markov et al., 1999) multiplexing]. The number of holograms that can be stored on a single location depends on the recording geometry and the dynamic range of the material. Further pages of data can be stored by recording in multiple locations (spatial multiplexing), for example, on a spinning holographic disk (Pu and Psaltis, 1996).

Another unique feature of holographic memories is that the data are written to and retrieved from the memory in a page-oriented way. Pages can contain from just several kilobits to a few megabits encoded as pixels whose size can be as small as

1×1 µm or even in the submicrometer range (Liu and Psaltis, 1999). This parallelism provides the optical memory with gigantic data transfer rates in the range of terabits per second.

Besides high storage capacity and fast transfer rates, it is important that holographic memories be compact in order to be able to compete with other technologies, such as magnetic storage. Even though a typical holographic system may involve very few optical components, the space constraints imposed by the optics result in bulky setups. One way of minimizing the volume of the system is by using phase-conjugated readout (Feng and Sayano, 1996). Instead of reconstructing the hologram with the same reference beam as the one used for recording, the counterpropagating beam is used to read out the hologram. As a result, the reconstructed signal backpropagates as well, and self-focuses on the input plane, which now becomes the output plane and can be separated from the former by a beam splitter (figure 15.8). Since no lens is required for the readout, the holographic module becomes very compact (Drolet et al., 1997).

An important aspect of the memory concerns the selection of the optical material. For read-only (or write-once-read-many, WORM) applications, polymer-based materials can be used. In these media, readout of the stored data does not result in erasure, so the lifetime of the holograms is limited only by the aging of the polymer

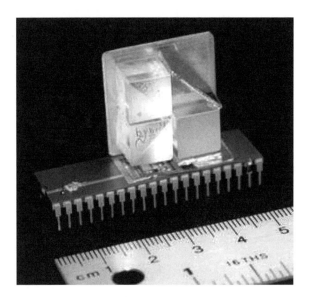

Figure 15.8
Holographic random access memory (RAM) module that makes use of the phase-conjugated readout technique. Two beam splitters (one on top of the other in the picture) direct the laser beam into the photorefractive crystal (on the back under the 45-degree mirror) during the write-read cycles.

itself. The recording of successive holograms bleaches the material's absorption spectrum until eventually it reaches saturation, which means that the material has used up its dynamic range and is insensitive to further illumination.

One important metric that is commonly used to characterize optical materials is the M/No. (Mok et al., 1996), which measures their dynamic range and is defined as the sum of the strengths of the recorded holograms. Rewritable holographic memories are usually implemented on photorefractive materials, typically lithium niobate ($LiNbO_3$) crystals. They have traditionally suffered from the fact that the information stored in them is volatile during readout, even in the dark; however, recent research has successfully developed nonvolatile rewritable memories using doubly doped crystals (Buse et al., 1998). In this class of materials, the M/No. is directly related to the asymmetry between the recording and erasure rates.

Optically Programmable Gate Array
Optical memory modules inherently possess a high degree of parallelism, since the data are handled in the format of pages. Such parallelism results in a large communication bandwidth between the memory and the array of photodetectors during a readout cycle, or the SLM upon recording. The use of optical memories in information-processing systems makes it necessary to consider the interface between the holographic module and the silicon circuitry that processes the data retrieved from the memory and stores computational results.

Traditionally, holographic systems have not addressed this issue, so even though the information can be transferred very quickly to and from the optical memory, this parallelism is lost in the communication between the optoelectronic chips and the processor, becoming a bottleneck. Therefore, a direct interface between memory and processor would be much more effective since the parallelism would always be preserved, as suggested in figure 15.9. The direct interface avoids the slow interchip communication by simply integrating the logic circuitry and an array of photodetectors on the same silicon die. However, the question now is to identify which computing devices have enough hardware parallelism to exchange data efficiently with the optical memory. It is here that the distributed hardware resources of the FPGA marry the parallelism of the optical memory.

Based on the FPGA architecture, the optically programmable gate array (OPGA) (Mumbru et al., 1999) is a device in which the computation is still performed by programmable logic blocks and interconnects as in the conventional FPGA, but the configuration data are brought into the chip optically. This optical reconfiguration capability results from interfacing an optical memory with a silicon chip in which, in addition to the logic resources, an array of photodetectors has been incorporated, as illustrated by figure 15.9. The holographic memory can store a large number of configuration templates that can be transferred down to the FPGA chip as a single

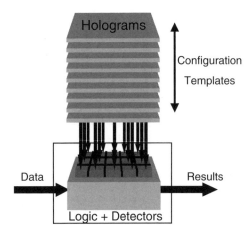

Figure 15.9
Direct interface between the optical memory and the silicon chip carrying photodetectors and logic circuitry. The configuration templates stored as holograms (depicted as slices) can be downloaded to the chip in parallel.

page. By taking the reconfiguration circuitry out of the FPGA chip, the OPGA can achieve a larger logic density, that is, more CLBs can be implemented than in the conventional device.

In its initial implementation, the OPGA module is intended to operate as a holographic read-only memory (HROM), where a priori and for a given application, the user will decide on the library of configuration templates that needs to be stored in the memory. This frees the OPGA module from all the optics and optoelectronics required to write in the memory, like the SLM, and makes it very compact. However, later OPGA designs will encompass both read and write capabilities, which will provide an increased computational flexibility.

The OPGA is basically the integration of three main components or technologies: an array of vertical cavity surface-emitting lasers (VCSELs) used to retrieve the templates stored in the memory; the optical memory, which contains a large set of configuration contexts; and the VLSI chip, which combines complementary metal-oxide semiconductor (CMOS) logic and photodetectors. Each of these components presents a number of issues that are discussed in this section.

VCSELs operating in the infrared wavelengths are widely used in fiber optics data links, optical interconnects, and storage applications. In contrast to conventional laser diodes, which emit light from the edge of the chip, VCSELs emit light vertically from the wafer surface. Therefore, instead of having to cleave the wafer into single elements, they can be packaged as large arrays (Krishnamoorthy, 2000). The first VCSELs emitting in the red wavelengths were reported in 1993 (Schneider and Lott, 1993). The shift toward shorter wavelengths has presented the possibility of using

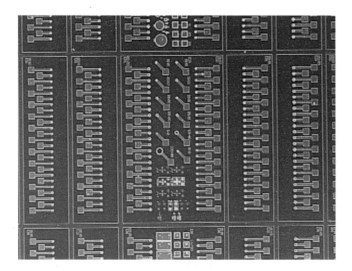

Figure 15.10
Photograph of the die containing several 25×1 arrays of red wavelength vertical cavity surface-emitting lasers (VCSELs), arranged in columns. The size of each device, the small circles at the end of the square pads, is 20 μm. The VCSELs operate at a wavelength of 680 nm (photo provided by Honeywell Corp.).

such devices in holography, since most optical materials are sensitive in the visible range of the spectrum.

An array of VCSELs is used as a light source for the OPGA module to selectively retrieve one data page of the optical memory at a time. Arrays of different sizes provided by Honeywell Corporation (figure 5.10) have been tested and characterized. Their very good power and wavelength stability over time have revealed that this type of laser diode is suitable for holographic recording (figure 15.11). The two most important parameters for the VCSELs, if they are to be used in the OPGA module, are their output power and wavelength uniformity across the array. The improvements in newer arrays have been able to meet such requirements; however, the consistency from die to die seems to require further research in the fabrication process.

The technique used to store and multiplex the holograms in the optical memory determines the architecture of the entire module. For this reason it is not possible to discuss the holographic memory without giving a more global view of the system that encompasses both the VCSEL array and the array of photodetectors in the chip.

Owing to the limited output of optical power available from each VCSEL, we have developed a novel technique to multiplex the holograms in which we still achieve short reconfiguration times, in the range of tens of microseconds, but without a demanding requirement on the power per VCSEL. This technique combines both spatial and shift multiplexing. Upon recording (figure 15.12), a lens focuses the

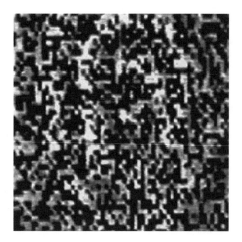

Figure 15.11
Reconstruction of a hologram using VCSELs. The digital data, the 1s and 0s, are encoded as bright and dark square pixels in the hologram. In this case, the hologram corresponds to a 34-μm pixel size mask.

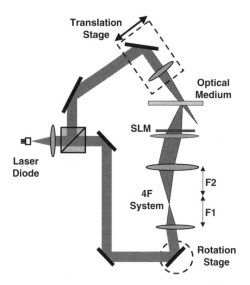

Figure 15.12
Optically programmable gate array (OPGA) recorder setup. The linear translation stage in the reference arm, combined with the rotation stage and the lenses in the 4F system in the signal arm, is used for the shift-multiplexing of the holograms.

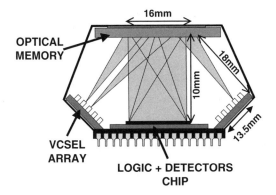

Figure 15.13
OPGA reader module. The light emitted by each VCSEL is used to read out a different hologram that self-focuses, owing to phase-conjugation, on the array of photodetectors in the chip.

beam that impinges the SLM onto a small spot on the recording medium. By changing the angle of incidence of the beam on the lens, the signal spot can be made to focus on a different location in the material, which partially overlaps the previous ones. The pages of data are recorded in these partially overlapping circles, which span a stripe on the optical material. To achieve Bragg mismatch among holograms, a converging reference beam needs to be shifted accordingly to illuminate the corresponding signal spot.

In the recording setup (figure 15.12), a laser diode with enough coherence length can be used instead of the VCSEL array. The beam emitted by the diode is collimated and split into the signal and reference arm. The angle of the signal beam is adjusted with a rotation stage before it illuminates the SLM. The reference beam is focused by a lens mounted on a mechanical scanner used to translate the beam beyond the shift selectivity of the optical medium.

During readout, the system becomes very compact (figure 15.13), for two reasons. First, we use reflection geometry for recording, so upon readout, the reading beam from the VCSEL and the array of photodetectors are both located on the same side of the material. Second, phase-conjugated readout makes the use of any extra components unnecessary. The VCSEL array is placed at the plane where the converging reference beams used for recording focus. Upon read out each VCSEL illuminates one of the spots in the memory, and all the reconstructed images backpropagate to the plane of the SLM, where the photodetector array is located.

As a benefit of this architecture, we obtain larger values in the diffraction efficiency per hologram, which scales, not as the total number of stored holograms, but as the number of overlapping ones at any location. A simple system design calculation helps to illustrate the fact that the power required per VCSEL is compatible with the levels that we have in our VCSEL arrays. Assume that we design the memory to store 100 configuration pages; each page is 10^6 pixels with a pitch of 5 μm, and we use an optical material 200-μm thick with M/5. If the number of overlapping holograms is set to 20, then the diffraction efficiency per hologram is as high as 6.25%. Therefore if we consider the photon budget at the photodetectors and choose 1000 photons to be detected in order to have an acceptable signal-to-noise ratio (SNR), we can parameterize the power per VCSEL as a function of the integration time of the detectors. If the integration time is set to be just 1 μs, each VCSEL must output 6.4 mW. If a longer integration time is allowed, the power required per VCSEL falls into the range of values of the present VCSEL array.

Another advantage of this architecture is the small area used on the recording medium to store all the holograms. If the lens that focuses the signal beam has a focal length of 10 mm, the signal spot size on the material is only 2.7 mm in diameter, and 100 holograms can be stored on a stripe 2.7 mm wide by 16 mm long. Given the small dimensions of the area where the pages are recorded, the holograms are much less sensitive to any nonuniformity on the medium and, consequently the quality of the reconstructed images is higher.

Once the mechanism to store the configuration templates in the optical memory is chosen, we need to consider which optical media are appropriate for the OPGA system. Holographic polymers are interesting because they present good dynamic range and have high sensitivity. However, polymers like DuPont or methylene blue (MB)-doped polyvinyl alcohol (PVA) (Blaya et al., 1998) suffer from shrinkage and poor optical quality that is due to nonuniformity in the material, which distorts the reconstructed images. This problem becomes more important as the pixel size is reduced, even if phase-conjugated readout is used.

The possibility of using phenanthrenequinone (PQ)-doped polymethylmethacrylate (PMMA) (Steckman et al., 1998) has also been explored. This material shows good optical quality and M/No. (Steckman et al., 1998). However, the material has extremely poor absorption in the red. This means that the material is not useful for the OPGA unless we use green light sources, which does not seem a plausible solution at present. The most solid choice seems to be Aprilis film (Waldman et al., 1998), which enjoys both good recording dynamics and high optical quality.

Another alternative is iron-doped lithium niobate crystals. Experiments have revealed that their performance in the red wavelengths for reflection geometry is fairly good in terms of dynamic range. Although there is a drop in their sensitivity compared with polymers, this is relatively unimportant for this application. The excellent optical quality (figure 15.14), combined with the fact that LiNbO3 has very low scattering, makes it a good alternative to be used in this project.

The development of active pixel sensors (APS) (Mendis et al., 1994) using standard CMOS technology, the same that is used for most microprocessors and memory

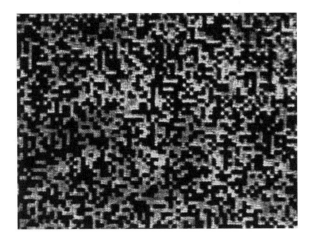

Figure 15.14
Phase-conjugated reconstruction of a random-pixel hologram stored in a lithium niobate crystal with traces of iron. The reconstruction exhibits very good quality despite the small pixel size (4 μm) used in the experiment.

modules, enables the integration of photodetectors with on-chip processing circuitry and has resulted in the expression "camera-on-a-chip" (Fossum, 1997). The OPGA chip makes use of this idea and integrates an array of pixels to detect the reconstructed hologram as well as the logic circuit of a conventional FPGA on the same die, as shown in figure 15.15. The detectors must have a very small pitch to result in a low area overhead and enough sensitivity to guarantee a reconfiguration time in the range of 1 to 100 μs.

There are two competing topologies for the spatial layout of the detectors and the logic. We could sparsely distribute the detectors with the logic, as shown in figure 15.15a, so the optical bits are detected exactly where they are used to program the logic, or conversely, concentrate all the detectors on a single array and distribute the detected signals across the chip, as in figure 15.15b. The second topology makes the optics simpler because the quality of the hologram needs to be more uniform over a smaller area than in the first case. However, the first case greatly simplifies the mesh of metal buses used to deliver the detected signals to the logic blocks.

The light detected by each APS needs to be converted into a logic value of 1 or 0 by comparing this signal with some threshold. The simplest way to perform such a conversion is to set the same threshold for all the photodetectors in the chip. However, a global threshold cannot compensate for spatial variations in intensity across the entire data page. An alternative is to use different threshold levels across the area of the chip. This is not a perfect solution either, even assuming that generating many different bias voltages for the thresholds is not an issue, because the spatial

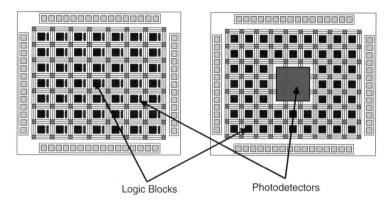

Logic Blocks   Photodetectors

Figure 15.15
Detector distribution on the OPGA chip: (*a*) sparse, where the photodetectors are interleaved with the logic or (*b*) concentrated, where all the photodetectors are implemented as an array and the detected signals need to be delivered to the programmable elements.

nonuniformity in the reconstructed hologram can change from one holographic page to another.

An efficient way to be more robust to this nonuniformity of intensity is differential encoding (Heanue et al., 1994; Psaltis and Burr, 1998). In this case, a pair of pixels in the hologram represents each single bit of information required to program the chip. The differential photodetector must have two photosensitive areas, referred to as left and right pixels, which need to be matched to the pixel pair in the hologram. The logic 1 is then represented by left pixel on and right pixel off and logic 0 by left pixel off and right pixel on. This coding scheme makes it unnecessary to set any threshold for the photodetectors. Since the global variation of the incident illumination is reduced, the signal-to-noise ratio is increased and therefore the bit error rate (BER) is improved. From the optics point of view, this type of data representation is simple and does not increase the system's cost.

The OPGA chip (Mumbru, 2000) (figure 15.16) mimics a small-scale FPGA. The chip combines a 64×32 array of differential APS sensors (the large big block at the left center in figure 15.16); the logic array (the small block on the right) containing four logic blocks, based on five-input LUTs; and switching matrices to fully interconnect the logic blocks among them and with the input-output buses, as sketched in figure 15.17. In the full OPGA chip, the strategy adopted has been to concentrate all the photodetectors in one block separated from the logic array.

The last issue concerns the integration of the three major components—VCSELs, optical memory, and CMOS chip—in a single package. The main goal is to make the OPGA module small enough to be mounted on a board in a computer, or to be easily worn in a neural prosthetic context. The main constraint is the height of the module, and this depends only on the focal length of the lens used before the SLM.

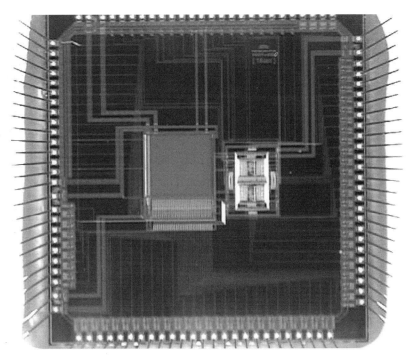

Figure 15.16
The full OPGA chip, designed by Photobit in a 0.35-μm standard complementary metal-oxide semiconductor (CMOS) process, integrates a 64 × 32 array of differential photodetectors (the large block at the left center) and fully connected logic array (the small block on the right center).

As already discussed, this distance can be made as small as 1 cm. The module is very compact, owing to the lensless readout and to the small area of recording medium used to store the holograms. The package shown in figure 15.18 houses the optical memory on the top rectangular window. The VCSEL arrays, integrated on both sides, retrieve the holograms detected on the chip located on the bottom of the package. The package also needs to be robust to ensure alignment between all the components. It is important to preserve the one-to-one correspondence between the pixels in the hologram and the photodetectors on the chip and also to avoid any change in the areas illuminated by the VCSELs on the optical material.

A first prototype has been successfully developed to demonstrate that it is possible to integrate all three elements in a compact module (figure 15.19). The module uses a 5 × 1 array of VCSELs to read out the holograms that have been stored in the holographic memory, a 100-μm-thick layer of DuPont photopolymer. For this demonstration module, instead of the OPGA chip, a simple charge-coupled device (CCD) chip was interfaced to the optical memory to detect the reconstructed holograms. During recording, a laser diode stores two shift-multiplexed holograms in the

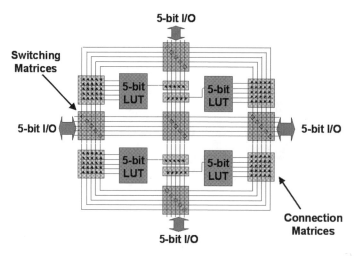

Figure 15.17
Schematic of the programmable logic array. The logic circuitry consists of a 2 × 2 array of five-input LUTs
with one buffered output each. The LUTs are fully interconnected by five switching matrices located in the
center, left, right, top, and bottom of the array.

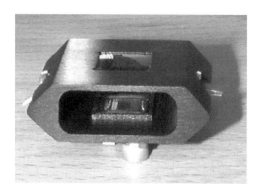

Figure 15.18
Mechanical design of the OPGA module integrating in a compact package the optical memory (window
on the top), VCSEL arrays (one on each side) and the chip (bottom).

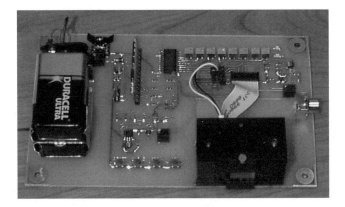

Figure 15.19
First-generation OPGA prototype mounted on the board that carries the circuitry to drive single VCSELs in the array and to power up the module.

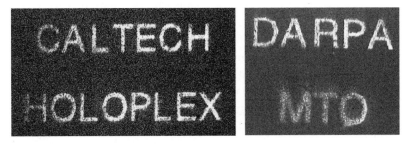

Figure 15.20
Reconstruction of the two holograms stored in the optical memory of the OPGA prototype. Two different VCSELs are used to retrieve one hologram at a time.

memory at the two locations that match the position of the two VCSELs at each end of the array. Once the recording operation is finished, the VCSELs are assembled into the OPGA reader module and the module is removed from the setup of the recorder. The OPGA module is mounted on a demonstration board (figure 15.19) that contains the additional circuitry to drive the VCSELs and select which element in the array is active, and the interface to the monitor where the holograms are displayed as they are read out by the VCSELs (figure 15.20).

Reconfigurable Processors Applied to Neural Prosthetic Systems

As we saw in the last section, reconfigurable processors possess a powerful blend of speed and flexibility. Speed is achieved through optimized and often parallel circuits, akin to those found in ASICs, while flexibility results from the ability to perform a wide range of computations, approaching the breadth found in microprocessors. Even greater speed and flexibility is possible by reconfiguring and optimizing the hardware for each class of computation, with faster reconfiguration times leading to greater optimization and total processing power. Unfortunately the traditional, all-electronic reconfigurable processors available today (e.g., FPGAs) have relatively slow reconfiguration times (1–10 ms). These slow rates are due largely to low-bandwidth buses retrieving from serially addressable electronic memory. We introduced an OPGA system that overcomes this reconfiguration bottleneck by pairing a high-bandwidth optical bus with a page-addressable optical memory. OPGAs achieve very fast reconfiguration times (1–10 μs) by simultaneously reading an entire page of reconfiguration data from the holographic memory onto an FPGA circuit, which we modified to include an array of photodetectors. The resulting increase in speed and flexibility has important consequences for a wide range of computational systems, including those envisioned to power emerging neural prosthetic systems.

How could reconfigurable processors in general, and OPGAs in particular, be applied to neural prosthetic systems? To be a bit more specific, we return to the prosthetic arm example introduced in the first section. The goal of the discussion in the following two subsections is simply to point out a few of the central architectural principles relevant when considering reconfigurable processors in the context of neural prosthetic systems. It is beyond the scope of this chapter to present a detailed design, and any such design would necessarily depend on the particular reconfigurable hardware used and the specific neural prosthetic computations to be performed.

A Prosthetic Arm System Revisited
Figure 15.21 is identical to figure 15.1, except that several elements have been grouped according to how they could be implemented. There are three of these groups, which we refer to as subsystems. The first subsystem is the front end, which consists of amplifiers, filters, and analog-to-digital (A/D) converter(s) needed to transform the continuous-time and continuous-voltage neural wave form from each electrode into discrete-time and discrete-voltage (digitized) signals. Since these functions require highly specialized and optimized circuits (e.g., low-noise amplifiers, fast high-precision A/D converters), they are best implemented in an ASIC. As we will discuss later, it is also possible that additional front-end functions such as signal buffering, which is straightforward to include on an ASIC, could simplify overall system design.

The second subsystem is the neural prosthetic processor (NPP), which we suggest could be implemented in a reconfigurable processor with a fast reconfiguration time (i.e., OPGA). The reconfigurable NPP (RNPP) as drawn in figure 15.22 would handle four major functions described previously: (1) spike sorting and spectral anal-

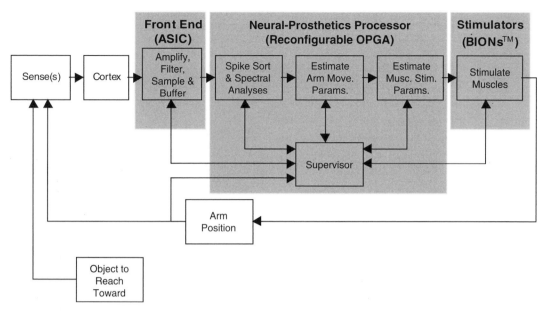

Figure 15.21
Block diagram of the example prosthetic arm system with elements grouped according to their possible implementation. The front end requires specialized circuitry that may best be implemented as an application-specific integrated circuit. The reconfigurable neural prosthetic processor (RNPP), which could be implemented with a reconfigurable processor like the OPGA, performs many of the block element operations. Muscle stimulation could be performed with BION-like stimulators injected into muscles.

yses, (2) estimating (decoding) arm-movement parameters from the neural data, (3) estimating (inverse kinematics) appropriate muscle stimulation parameters given the estimated arm-movement parameters, and (4) supervising performance and adjusting the system's parameters accordingly. The RNPP could also perform two additional functions that are needed in the system architecture envisioned for this example. First, when a block of neural data is needed, the RNPP requests these data from the front-end subsystem that temporarily buffers data for each electrode channel. Second, when stimulation parameters have been estimated, the RNPP sends these parameters on to the stimulation subsystem. Both of these communications would most likely proceed via telemetry, which is transparent in this discussion because we assume that a transmit-receive subsystem handles all error correction. The RNPP is described in more detail later in this chapter.

The final subsystem illustrated in figure 15.21 consists of the muscle stimulators. Current state-of-the-art muscle stimulators, such as the BION (Loeb and Richmond, 2000), are capable of being injected into muscle with a hypodermic needle, powered wirelessly, and receiving a wireless digital transmission, including a stimulator-specific identifier and stimulation parameters. Thus to move the arm, the RNPP

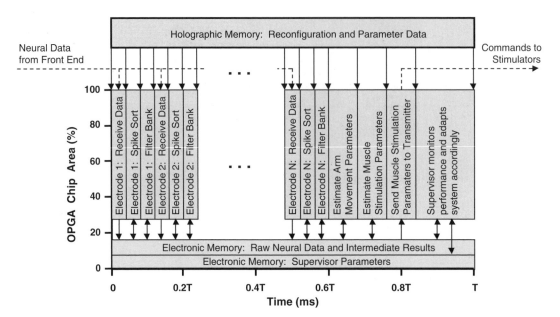

Figure 15.22
Possible RNPP architecture employing an OPGA. Neural signals from the front-end ASIC enter from the left (dashed lines) and muscle-stimulation parameters exit on the right (dashed lines). The OPGA is represented in two main parts, both of which are shaded gray. The electronic portion is represented as an OPGA chip area versus time plot, which illustrates how the OPGA electronics are allocated and reconfigured through time. The RNPP operates in cycles, with a period of T (ms). The holographic memory is depicted at the top of the figure. Lines indicate information flow, with arrows indicating the direction of this flow. See text for a complete description of all elements.

need only encode the muscle stimulation parameters appropriately and issue the data packets.

Reconfigurable Processor Subsystem

This example applies an OPGA to the prosthetic arm system described earlier and is intended to suggest a general architecture, not a fully functional design. Neural data flow in from the left, through the RNPP (depicted in gray), and muscle-stimulator commands flow out on the right. Figure 15.22 shows an OPGA chip area versus time plot, which suggests how OPGA electronics could be reconfigured through time, as well as the OPGA holographic memory (at the top of the figure).

When operation begins, the front-end ASIC starts storing neural data samples in an on-chip buffer. This buffer can be thought of as a memory page, with rows corresponding to sample number (time) and columns corresponding to electrode number. The number of rows equals the sampling rate termed R (e.g., 40 kHz or 40 samples/ms) multiplied by the period of time required to service all data in the buffer, which we term T (ms). We term the number of columns (electrodes) N, which could be on the order of 10 to 100 s. Each memory element is B bytes, which is typically two (e.g., 12–16-bit samples). From time $0–T$, the first buffer is filled and from time $T–2T$ a second buffer is filled. This allows the RNPP T ms ($T–2T$ in real time) to service the neural data stored in the first buffer. The first buffer is overwritten from $2T$ to $3T$, while the RNPP services the second buffer, and so on. This architecture allows the ASIC to implement most of the data memory (e.g., 2 buffers $\times$ RT samples $\times$ N electrodes $\times$ B bytes/sample = $2RTNB$ bytes) freeing the RNPP to store only a small amount of neural data at any time (e.g., RT samples $\times$ 1 electrode $\times$ B bytes/sample = RTB bytes). For example, if a 10×10 electrode array were implanted, and the electrical signals sampled at 40 kHz for a 20-ms time frame and afterwards digitized with 12-bit precision, a 120-kbyte RAM memory for each page would be enough to store all the neural data in the ASIC. The OPGA would require $1/N$ as much on-chip memory, 1.2 kbytes.

As shown in figure 15.22, the RNPP must complete all of its operations within one period (T ms). This period is bounded by the maximum allowable time between muscle-stimulator updates, which could range from hundreds of milliseconds for coarse motor control to just a few milliseconds for fine motor control. While T may be made as small as current technology will allow, the ultimate limit rests with the time scale of neural representations and the information transmission rate achieved by the front-end sensors. An important point is that while T ms pass between muscle-stimulator updates, the absolute latency of the system (i.e., time from neural event until muscle stimulation) is $2T$ ms because T ms is consumed in the front end and T ms is consumed in the RNPP. Therefore, the maximum allowable period T must also take into consideration the maximum allowable latency in the closed-feedback prosthetic system.

The first RNPP operation in this example architecture is to configure the OPGA to request, receive, and store neural data. The OPGA is configured by reading a page of configuration data from the holographic memory (the downward-directed arrow from holographic memory at the far left of figure 15.22) and is fast enough (1–10 µs) that we do not allocate any appreciable time to this operation in the figure. The second OPGA operation is to request T ms of electrode 1 data from the front-end ASIC, receive these data, and place them in OPGA memory. This operation consumes some finite amount of time, illustrated as the width of the "Electrode 1: Receive Data" bar, and occupies some fraction of the total OPGA electronics area, illustrated by the height of the bar. Again, this figure is meant simply to be suggestive of architectural principles. A certain fraction of the OPGA electronics area is configured as memory, with raw neural data and intermediate results and supervisor parameters each having their own reserved regions.

The next RNPP operations are to configure the OPGA for spike sorting, spike sort T ms of electrode 1 data, and place the results in OPGA memory. Spike sorting requires the OPGA electronics to be configured as an efficient DSP-like processor in order to correlate the neural data with neural wave form templates (Wheeler, 1999). Electrodes typically sense action potentials originating from many neurons, with 1–4 of these neurons being identifiable by their voltage-time wave form shapes. Statistical neural templates appropriate for each electrode can be learned offline, stored in the holographic memory, and then retrieved just before spike sorting data from a given electrode. Cross-correlating these neural wave form templates (1–4 templates, roughly 2–3 ms in duration) with the neural data from electrode 1 (T ms in duration) requires shift (delay), multiplication, and addition operations that are straightforward to implement in FPGAs-OPGAs.

Let us consider a hypothetical, although not unrealistic, OPGA device containing 3500 CLBs and a 30-kbyte bank of on-chip RAM memory. In such a device, four template-matching filters for a 2-ms-long sequence each could be simultaneously implemented using slightly less than 1000 CLBs, assuming that we take advantage of efficient distributed computing algorithms, such as the ones described in Andraka and Berkun (1999). This low CLB count would even allow multiple electrodes to be processed in parallel. The identity and time of each action potential in the T ms of electrode 1 data are stored for later analysis. This does not consume large amounts of memory since spike rates are relatively low (e.g., <100 spikes/s on average) and identity and time information can be compact. Just 80 bytes per electrode are used, for example, if 10 matches are found on average in each one of the filters and each match is encoded as 2 bytes.

The final RNPP operation that must be performed on data from each electrode is spectral analysis or digital filtering. Digital filters appropriate for estimating the power in a given frequency band, for example, can be designed offline, given offline data from each electrode. These filter coefficients are most likely specific to each electrode. Since the power in multiple frequency bands may be of interest, the OPGA could be configured as a DSP filter bank, which again requires delays, multiplication, and addition operations. A 256-tap filter, using 12-bit precision complex coefficients, can be implemented in the OPGA using just 715 CLBs (Andraka and Berkun, 1999). Therefore there is enough hardware available to implement a bandpass filter bank to obtain the spectral information for the neuronal signals in three different regions of the spectrum simultaneously. This suggests that even fast Fourier transform (FFT) analyses are possible. Filter coefficients for each electrode's digital filters and the electronics configuration data for the filter bank are stored in the holographic memory and downloaded just before data from a given electrode are analyzed. After analysis, the relatively compact spectral estimates, perhaps just 16 bytes per electrode, are stored for later use.

This sequence of operations—receive T ms of buffered neural data, spike sort, and filter—repeats until all N channels of electrode data have been processed. Together all such operations must consume less than T ms (shown as $0.6T$ ms in figure 15.22) to allow sufficient time to complete the remaining RNPP operations (shown as $0.4T$ ms). Continuing with the example, if the OPGA could be clocked at 166 MHz, the time required to compute the spike sorting and the spectral analysis could be as low as 116 μs, which with the reconfiguration overhead of 2 μs for the two reconfigurations, becomes 118 μs per electrode. Therefore the array of 100 electrodes could be processed in 13 ms (within 60% of 20 ms).

We can already see the key reconfigurable processing architectural principles at work. First, the diverse neural prosthetic computations are rapidly accommodated by the OPGA rewiring to efficiently perform a range of calculations. Second, the OPGA meets the real-time demands by being "wired" nearly optimally for any given task, which includes parallel-processing topologies. Finally, the OPGA is able to scale well with the number of electrodes (sensors) delivering neural data by time-multiplexing its operations. The number of electrodes this OPGA can handle is set by the speed of the processor, not by the number of parallel circuits that will fit within the area of the chip. This ability to time-multiplex the processing of data from increasing numbers of electrodes, as opposed to adding more physically parallel circuits that consume more chip area, is afforded by the relatively slower biological time scale and by the fast and parallel circuits possible in FPGAs-OPGAs.

The next RNPP operation is to estimate the arm-movement parameters. The goal is to estimate how the arm should move (e.g., new x, y, z location in space) given the new neural observations extracted from the preceding T ms in time (e.g., spike times and spectral power density). Although the best way to perform this estimation is a matter of current research, all methods require a database for how each neuron or electrode responds for real or intended reaches in numerous directions. This database can be constructed offline, stored in the holographic memory, and retrieved when the RNPP needs to estimate arm movements. The OPGA should also be configured to perform any of a number of estimation algorithms (e.g., maximum likelihood, Bayesian analysis, neural network) and, again, these configuration data are stored in the holographic memory. As before, these algorithms reduce to multiplications and additions, and the FPGA can perform millions of those per millisecond (Andraka and Berkun, 1999). The results of this estimation are quite compact, potentially as small as the new x, y, z arm location; for example, 6 bytes. It is important to note that estimation of arm movement scales well as the number of neurons and electrodes increases.

After estimating and storing the new arm location, for example, the RNPP must estimate how each of several (S) muscle stimulators should be activated to direct the arm to this desired location. Estimates of this sort require a model for where each muscle stimulator is implanted, how muscle stimulation leads to muscle contraction, and how this contraction moves the arm. These models are then run in reverse to arrive at stimulation parameters, given the desired arm location. These reverse models, and the OPGA electronics needed to run them efficiently, are stored in the holographic memory. Upon completion, each stimulator's identity (1 byte) and its stimulation current level (1 byte) and duration (1 byte) are stored in the on-chip memory for delivery to BION-like stimulators (Loeb and Richmond, 2000).

The last RNPP operation before the arm starts moving is to send these muscle-stimulation parameters to the transmitter. As with the front-end ASIC-to-RNPP connection, the RNPP-to-muscle-stimulator connection is envisioned to contain a wireless link. Therefore the RNPP must send the wireless transmitter each muscle-stimulator's identity and stimulation parameters, perhaps in an appropriately en-coded packet, and the transmitter will broadcast the instructions. Each muscle stimulator will activate accordingly.

The final RNPP operation is to perform the supervisory duties described in the first section of this chapter. In brief, many signals and conditions are expected to change throughout the lifetime of such a neural prosthetic system. While the system can be initially calibrated using offline analyses, as we have seen, continual adjust-ments are almost certainly needed for adequate performance over months or years. At the front end, electrodes may drift or become encapsulated, thereby changing the recording characteristics. The RNPP should adjust the spike-sorting and spectral-analysis algorithms accordingly, or even actively move the electrode tips to track neurons when this capability is available. At the arm-movement estimation stage, neural plasticity can change the response characteristics of neurons, and the response database and/or estimation algorithms must learn or adapt accordingly. System per-formance should actually benefit from such neural plasticity.

Finally, at the back end, it is likely that over time muscle stimulation will even-tually lead to slightly different arm movements. Again, the supervisor should adapt the model's parameters appropriately. While the basic supervisory logic circuitry can be stored in, and retrieved from, the holographic memory, much of the infor-mation needed by the supervisor must be stored in OPGA electronic memory (see "Electronic Memory: Supervisor Parameters" in figure 15.22). The supervisor must analyze past neural signals and system performance, store intermediate assessments, and store numerous adjusted parameter values to be accessed by the other RNPP operations (e.g., new spike-sort parameters). At present this information is best stored in electronic memory because OPGA holographic memory is read-only, al-though this is expected to change.

Here we have attempted to illustrate how a reconfigurable processor, the OPGA, might be used in an example neural prosthetics system, the prosthetic arm system. This so-called reconfigurable neural prosthetic processor subsystem performs most, if not all, of the signal processing, estimation, and control essential for a prosthetic arm system. The OPGA-based RNPP is able to achieve this level of performance by virtue of its inherent (optical) reconfiguration speed, parallel and optimized circuitry, and the use of a time-multiplexing scheme. By our estimates, a single OPGA built in current FPGA technology would be able to perform all RNPP tasks for approximately 100 electrodes. As semiconductor and optical technologies continue to advance, we expect a single OPGA to be capable of processing neural signals from more electrodes, perform more complex computations and control, or both. We also envision that OPGAs could contribute meaningfully to sensory prosthetic systems (e.g., transforming images into electrical-stimulation patterns) since FPGAs have already made an important impact on image processing.

Discussion

In this chapter we have attempted to convey the unique processing demands of neural prosthetic systems, the powerful and flexible nature of reconfigurable processors, and the potential of applying novel reconfigurable processor technologies to the emerging field of neural prosthetics. To address the current bottleneck in field-programmable gate arrays, namely, long reconfiguration times, we reviewed our recent efforts to develop optically programmable gate arrays. These devices derive their extremely short reconfiguration times from the enormous memory bandwidth afforded by parallel optical interconnections between a page-readable holographic memory and the reconfigurable electronics. Finally, we suggested a potential architecture for how OPGAs might be applied to a representative neural prosthetic system, the prosthetic arm system.

According to our stated assumptions and approximations regarding current technology, it should be possible to process neural data from roughly 100 electrodes (spike-sort and estimate spectral power densities) and estimate arm movements and muscle-stimulation parameters on a single OPGA. Clearly, the next step toward realizing reconfigurable neural prosthetic processors would be to implement these functions in current FPGA technology and verify processing speed. Processing signals from even a few electrodes would considerably increase our understanding of how neural processing, including online learning, should be mapped onto reconfigurable processor architectures. The FPGA reconfiguration times are much longer than those assumed for OPGAs, but the FPGA experiments could take this into consideration when projecting more accurate OPGA performance metrics. With these performance benchmarks in hand, an appropriate OPGA-based RNPP could be designed and tested. Again, our suggestion is that the power and flexibility of reconfigurable processors, which can behave like an efficient (e.g., parallel) DSP or microprocessor at different times, may outperform other processors on neural prosthetic computations. Moreover, reconfigurable processors may scale better than other processors as the number of sensors increases or the number of estimates grows, for similar reasons.

Finally, we would like to again emphasize the broad range of neural prosthetic systems that can be envisioned, and for which reconfigurable processors seem applicable. Although we have chosen to focus on a particular motor prosthetic system to more easily discuss the role of reconfigurable processors, we believe that FPGAs-OPGAs may be well suited for many neural prosthetic functions. Returning to the idea of an artificial vision system, a reconfigurable processor could, in some sense, substitute for the retinal and thalamic neural processing that is circumvented when the striate cortex is stimulated directly. Since these functions are related to other image-processing tasks currently implemented in FPGAs, it seems plausible for FPGAs-OPGAs to play an important role in transforming scenes derived from digital imaging into stimulation patterns appropriate for delivery to the brain.

Acknowledgments

The authors want to acknowledge the experimental research done by Chris Moser and Wenhai Liu on the advanced package for the OPGA, and to thank Eric Fossum and Sandor Barna from Photobit Corporation for their contribution to the design and testing of the OPGA chip, and David Waldman from Aprilis Inc. and Arrigo Benedetti for helpful discussions on the FPGA in computation. This research is funded by the Defense Advanced Research Projects Agency through contract F30601-98-1-0199, a Burroughs Wellcome Fund Career Award in the Biomedical Sciences, and by a National Science Foundation Engineering Research Center grant to California Institute of Technology.

References

Andraka, R., and Berkun, A. (1999) FPGAs make a radar signal processor on a chip a reality. In *Proceedings of the 33rd Asilomar Conference on Signals, Systems and Computers*, IEEE, Vol. 1, pp. 559–563.

Barbastathis, G., Levene, M., and Psaltis, D. (1996) Shift multiplexing with spherical reference waves. *Appl. Opt.* 35(14): 2403–2417.

Barinaga, M. (1999) Turning thoughts into actions. *Science* 286: 888–890.

Benabid, A. L., Pollak, P., Gao, D., Hoffmann, D., Limousin, P., Gay, E., Payen, I., and Benazzouz, A. (1996) Chronic electrical stimulation of the ventralis intermedius nucleus of the thalamus as a treatment of movement disorders. *J. Neurosurgery* 84: 203–214.

Benedetti, A., and Perona, P. (1998) Real-time 2-D feature detection on a reconfigurable computer. In *Proceedings of the 1998 IEEE Conference on Computer Vision and Pattern Recognition*. New York: Institute of Electrical and Electronics Engineer, pp. 586–593.

Blaya, S., Carretero, L., Mallavia, R., Fimia, A., Madrigal, F., Ulibarrena, M., and Levy, D. (1998). Optimization of an acrylamide-based dry film used for holographic recording. *Appl. Opt.* 37(32): 7604–7610.

Brown, S. D., Francis, R. J., Rose, J., and Vranesic, Z. G. (1992) *Field-Programmable Gate Arrays*. Norwell, Mass.: Kluwer.

Buse, K., Adibi, A., and Psaltis, D. (1998) Non-volatile holographic storage in doubly doped lithium niobate crystals. *Nature* 393(6686): 665–668.

Chapin, J. R., Moxon, K. A., Markowitz, R. S., and Nicolelis, M. A. L. (1999) Real-time control of a robot arm using simultaneously recorded neurons in the motor cortex. *Nature Neurosci.* 2(7): 664–670.

Curtis, K., Pu, A., and Psaltis, D. (1994) Method for holographic storage using peristrophic multiplexing. *Opt. Lett.* 19(13): 993–994.

Denz, C., Pauliat, G., Roosen, G., and Tschudi, T. (1991) Volume hologram multiplexing using a deterministic phase encoding method. *Opt. Comm.* 85(2–3): 171–176.

Drolet, J.-J. P., Chuang, E., Barbastathis, G., and Psaltis, D. (1997) Compact integrated dynamic holographic memory with refreshed holograms. *Opt. Lett.* 22(8): 552–554.

Feng, Z. O., and Sayano, K. (1996). Compact read-only memory with lensless phase-conjugate holograms. *Opt. Lett.* 21(16): 1295–1297.

Fetz, E. B. (1999) Real-time control of a robotic arm by neuronal ensembles. *Nature Neurosci.* 2(7): 583–584.

Fossum, E. R. (1997) CMOS image sensors: Electronic camera-on-a-chip. *IEEE Trans. Electron. Dev.* 44(10): 1689–1698.

Gabor, D. (1948) A new microscopic principle. *Nature* 161: 777.

Gabor, D. (1949a) Microscopy by reconstructed wavefronts: II. *Proc. Physics Soc.* B64: 449.

Gabor, D. (1949b) Microscopy by reconstructed wavefronts. *Proc. R. Soc.* A197: 454.

Hatsopoulos, N. G., Ojakangas, C. L., Maynard, E. M., and Donoghue, J. P. (1998) Detection and identification of ensemble codes in motor cortex. In H. B. Eichenbaum and J. L. Davis, eds., *Neuronal Ensembles Strategies for Recording and Decoding.* New York: Wiley-Liss, pp. 161–175.

Heanue, J. F., Bashaw, M. C., and Hesselink, L. (1994) Volume holographic storage and retrieval of digital data. *Science* 265(5173): 749–752.

Isaacs, R. E., Weber, D. J., and Schwartz, A. B. (2000) Work toward real-time control of a cortical neural prosthesis. *IEEE Trans. Rehabil. Eng.* 8(2): 196–198.

Jean, J., Liang, X. J., Drozd, B., Tomko, K., and Wang, Y. (2000) Automatic target recognition with dynamic reconfiguration. *J. VLSI Sig. Proc. Syst. Sig. Image Video Technol.* 25(1): 39–53.

Kaps, J. P., and Paar, C. (1999) Fast DES implementations for FPGAs and its application to a universal key-search machine. *Selec. Areas Cryptography, Lecture Notes in Comp. Sci.* 1556: 234–247.

Kennedy, P. R., Bakay, R. A. E., Moore, M. M., Adams, K., and Goldwaithe, J. (2000) Direct control of a computer from the human central nervous system. *IEEE Trans. Rehabil. Eng.* 8(2): 198–202.

Krishnamoorthy, A. V., Goossen, K. W., Chirovsky, L. M. F., Rozier, R. G., Chandramani, P., Hobson, W. S., Hui, S. P., Lopata, J., Walker, J. A., and D'Asaro, L. A. (2000) 16×16 VCSEL array flip-chip bonded to CMOS VLSI circuit. *IEEE Photon. Technol. Lett.* 12(8): 1073–1075.

Lauer, R. T., Peckham, P. H., Kilgore, K. L., and Heetderks, W. J. (2000) Applications of cortical signals to neuroprosthetic control: A critical review. *IEEE Trans. Rehabil. Eng.* 8(2): 205–208.

Lee, D., Port, N. L., Kruse, W., and Georgopoulos, A. P. (1998) Neural population coding: Multielectrode recordings in primate cerebral cortex. In H. B. Eichenbaum and J. L. Davis, eds., *Neuronal Ensembles Strategies for Recording and Decoding.* New York: Wiley-Liss, pp. 117–136.

Leith, E. N., Kozma, A., Upatnieks, J., Marks, J., and Massey, N. (1966) Holographic data storage in three-dimensional media. *Appl. Opt.* 5(8): 1303–1311.

Liu, W., and Psaltis, D. (1999) Pixel size limit in holographic memories. *Opt. Lett.* 24(19): 1340–1342.

Loeb, G. E., and Richmond, F. J. R. (2000) BION™ implants for therapeutic and functional electrical stimulation. In J. K. Chapin, K. A. Moxon, and G. Gaal, eds., *Neural Prostheses for Restoration of Sensory and Motor Function.* Boca Raton, Fla.: CRC Press, pp. 75–99.

Markov, V., Millerd, J., Trolinger, J., Norrie, M., Downie, J., and Timucin, D. (1999) Multilayer volume holographic optical memory. *Opt. Lett.* 24(4): 265–267.

Mendis, S., Kemeny, S. E., and Fossum, E. R. (1994) CMOS active pixel image sensor. *IEEE Trans. Electron. Dev.* 41(3): 452–453.

Mok, F. H. (1993) Angle-multiplexed storage of 5000 holograms in lithium niobate. *Opt. Lett.* 18(11): 915–917.

Mok, F., Burr, G. W., and Psaltis, D. (1996) A system metric for holographic memory systems. *Opt. Lett.* 21(12): 896–898.

Motomura, M., Aimoto, Y., Shibayama, A., Yabe, Y., and Yamashina, M. (1998) An embedded DRAM-FPGA chip with instantaneous logic reconfiguration. In *Proceedings of the IEEE Symposium on FPGAs for Custom Computing Machines*. Los Alamitos, Calif.: IEEE Computer Society, pp. 264–266.

Mumbru, J., Panotopoulos, G., Psaltis, D., An, X., Mok, F., Ay, S., Barna, S., and Fossum, E. (2000) Optically programmable gate array. *Proc. SPIE* 4089: 763–771.

Mumbru, J., Zhou, G., Ay, S., An, X., Panotopoulos, G., Mok, F., and Psaltis, D. (1999) Optically reconfigurable processors. *SPIE Critical Review 1999 Euro-American Workshop on Optoelectronic Information Processing*, 74: 265–288.

Psaltis, D., and Burr, G. W. (1998) Holographic data storage. *Computer* 31: 52–60.

Psaltis, D., and Mok, F. (1995) Holographic memories. *Sci. Amer.* 273(5): 70–76.

Psaltis, D., Levene, M., Pu, A., Barbastathis, G., and Curtis, K. (1995) Holographic storage using shift multiplexing. *Opt. Lett.* 20(7): 782–784.

Pu, A. (1997) Holographic 3-D disks and optical correlators using photopolymer materials. Ph.D. thesis, California Institute of Technology, Pasadena.

Pu, A., and Psaltis, D. (1996) High density recording in photopolymer-based holographic 3D disks. *Appl. Opt.* 35(14): 2389–2398.

Rakuljic, G. A., Leyva, V., and Yariv, A. (1992) Optical data storage by using orthogonal wavelength-multiplexed volume holograms. *Opt. Lett.* 17(20): 1471–1473.

Schmidt, E. M. (1999) Electrodes for many single neuron recordings. In M. A. L. Nicolelis, ed., *Methods for Neural Ensemble Recordings*. Boca Raton, Fla.: CRC Press, pp. 1–23.

Schneider Jr., R. P., and Lott, J. A. (1993) Cavity design for improved electrical injection in InAlGaP/AlGaAs visible (639–661 nm) vertical-cavity surface-emitting laser diodes. *Appl. Phys. Lett.* 63(7): 917–919.

Shenoy, K. V., Kureshi, S. A., Meeker, D., Gillikin, B. L., Dubowitz, D. J., Batista, A. P., Buneo, C. A., Cao, S., Burdick, J. W., and Andersen, R. A. (1999) Toward prosthetic systems controlled by parietal cortex. *Neuroscience* 25: 152.19.

Si, J., Lin, S., Kipke, D. R., Perepelkin, P. D., and Schwartz, A. B. (1998) Motor cortical information processing. In H. B. Eichenbaum and J. L. Davis, eds., *Neuronal Ensembles Strategies for Recording and Decoding*. New York: Wiley-Liss, pp. 137–159.

Steckman, G. J., Solomatine, I., Zhou, G., and Psaltis, D. (1998) Characterization of phenanthrenequinone-doped poly(methyl methacrylate) for holographic memory. *Opt. Lett.* 23(16): 1310–1312.

Stogiannos, P., Dollas, A., and Digalakis, V. (2000) A configurable logic-based architecture for real-time continuous speech recognition using hidden Markov models. *J. VLSI Sig. Proc. Systems Sig. Image Video Technol.* 24(2–3): 223–240.

Trimberger, S., Carberry, D., Johnson, A., and Wong, J. (1997) A time-multiplexed FPGA. In *Proceedings of the IEEE Symposium on FPGA-Based Custom Computing Machines (FCCM '97)*. Los Alamitos, Calif.: IEEE Computer Society, pp. 34–40.

van Heerden, P. J. (1963) Theory of optical information storage in solids. *Appl. Opt.* 2(4): 393–400.

Waldman, D. A., Li, H.-Y. S., and Cetin, E. A. (1998) Holographic recording properties in thick films of ULSH-500 photopolymer. *Proc. SPIE* 3291: 89–103.

Wheeler, B. C. (1999) Automatic discrimination of single units. In M. A. L. Nicolelis, ed., *Methods for Neural Ensemble Recordings*. Boca Raton, Fla.: CRC Press, pp. 61–77.

Wolpaw, J. R., Nirbaumer, N., Heetderks, W. J., McFarland, D. J., Peckham, P. H., Schalk, G., Donchin, E., Quatrano, L. A., Robinson, C. J., and Vaughan, T. M. (2000) Brain-computer interface technology: A review of the First International Meeting. *IEEE Trans. Rehabil. Eng.* 8(2): 164–173.

Yin, S., Zhou, H., Zhao, F., Wen, M., Zang, Y., Zhang, J., and Yu, F. T. S. (1993) Wavelength-multiplexed holographic storage in a sensitive photorefractive crystal using a visible-light tunable laser-diode. *Opt. Comm.* 101(5–6): 317–321.

16 The Coming Revolution: The Merging of Computational Neural Science and Semiconductor Engineering

Dan Hammerstrom

There is a large class of problems in merging computational engineering with neural applications that are still only poorly solved. These involve the transformation of data across the boundary between the real world and the digital world. They occur whenever a computer is sampling and/or acting on real-world data. Examples of these "boundary transformation" problems include computer recognition of human speech, computer vision, textual and image content recognition, robotic control, optical character recognition (OCR), and automatic target recognition. These are difficult problems to solve on a computer, since they require the computer to find complex structures and relationships in massive quantities of low-precision, ambiguous, noisy data. "Boundary transformations" are important. Our inability to adequately solve these problems constitutes a significant barrier to computer usage:

I claim that if you take anything that's a human skill—speech, listening, hand-writing, touch—it's totally predictable that those are key technologies ... that people should invest millions and millions of dollars in. (Bill Gates, *Upside Magazine*, May 1992)

We have made much progress in front-end processing (such as in the digital signal processing of one and two-dimensional signals), but the solutions to complex recognition problems still elude us. Neither artificial intelligence, artificial neural networks (ANN), or fuzzy logic has given us effective and robust solutions to these problems.

This chapter discusses an approach that has the potential to move us closer to solving these problems. I first begin with a discussion of intelligent signal processing (ISP), which attempts to solve complex problems in recognition and control. I then look at biological computing models, which offer insight into new techniques for doing intelligent signal processing. However, these biological models are radically different and require radically different implementations.

In parallel with these revolutionary advances in computational neurobiology, silicon technology has been advancing at a phenomenal pace. Although previous attempts at combining them were premature, silicon technology and computational neurobiology are beginning to merge to create a powerful and radically new form of computation. This synthesis will result in a large, new market in neuromorphic silicon for solving a number of important problems ranging from genetic sequencing and Internet routing and content recognition to robotic control and speech processing.

Intelligent Signal Processing

A new research area, intelligent signal processing, is now emerging that is devoted to consolidating and refining existing solutions, and finding better solutions to transformation problems. The term *intelligent signal processing* is being used to describe algorithms and techniques that involve the creation, efficient representation, and effective utilization of complex models of semantic and syntactic relationships. It uses learning and other "smart" techniques to extract as much information as possible from signal and noise data (Haykin and Kosko, 1998). In other words, ISP augments and enhances existing digital signal processing (DSP) by incorporating contextual and higher-level knowledge of the application domain into the data transformation process. ISP techniques, in essence, enhance boundary transformations. One of the most common ISP techniques in use today is the hidden Markov model (HMM) (Rabiner, 1989). In an HMM, the states in the model are discrete activations, with transition and symbol emission probabilities obtained by training on real-world data. HMMs do not approach human capabilities. The representation of higher-level structure is limited to keep model sizes under control. Only moderate parallelism is used, further limiting model size.

Researchers believe that what makes human beings so good at pattern recognition is that:

- We generate numerous hypotheses based on incomplete and noisy data.
- We select the "best" hypothesis based on previously observed data from the process in question, which is remembered as a "model" that has evolved from repeated encounters with a particular context.
- We make efficient use of historical statistical information in the selection process.
- We do all this in real time.

When attempting to recreate humanlike intelligence in a computer, an open question is how accurately must one model the way humans perform these computations? For many years, the symbolic, modestly parallel, approach (which has little biological relevance) was used and has not achieved great success. Many researchers, even in the artificial intelligence community, are beginning to agree that a key component of human intelligence is its ability to effectively use massive parallelism and statistical, fuzzy processing.

An experiment that demonstrates the significant differences between how computers currently perform boundary transformations and how real neural circuitry works is Feldman's "100 step rule." Take a simple cognitive task that involves briefly exposing a human subject to the image of an alphanumeric character on a screen. The subject is to push a button if the character is a numeral, but do nothing if it is a letter. For humans, the time for processing such a task, after practice, is typically about half a second (500 ms). Given that the typical switching time for neurons is on the order of a few milliseconds, the brain performs this complex task in roughly a couple of hundred sequential steps, which implies massive parallelism. Looking at biological computing systems, this is an obvious conclusion, since the human cerebral cortex is estimated to consist of about 10 billion relatively slow neurons. A computer program designed to accomplish the same task would be mostly sequential; it could easily require up to a billion steps and can best be described as "massively sequential."

The first attempt to create more brainlike models for knowledge representation problems consisted of the connectionist models (Feldman et al., 1996). They are a first step to more neural-like solutions. These models are often highly structured and problem specific. Each node generally implies a specific meaning, each connection a relationship. Sparsely connected and activated, computation was generally done in parallel using constraint relaxation (for example, by energy minimization). Other related models are spreading activation semantic networks and Bayesian networks (Heckerman, 1996).

Computers are getting faster and can execute larger and more complex versions of existing ISP techniques. However, we need to do more than just rely on higher clock rates and larger memories to move to the next level in recognition capability—we need new solutions. We know that biological computing solves complex ISP problems. Perhaps we should turn there for inspiration.

Biological Computing Models

Even the most primitive biological systems are capable of performing complex ISP. In addition, biological computing is robust in the presence of faulty and failing systems and requires no intrinsic synchronization.[1] It is energy efficient, consists of networks of sparsely connected and sparsely activated nodes, and requires only moderate levels of precision (often binary).

Other current hypotheses about neurobiological computation include the following:

• Communication is expensive (mostly in energy), so biological systems tend to trade off local computation for nonlocal communication.

• It is most likely that data representation is partially distributed or "vector encoded," with each node participating in a number of representations; this enhances fault tolerance and response time, and allows more efficient representation of knowledge.

• There seems to be high-level linkage (hierarchical and bidirectional) between large subnetworks.

• They tend to be dynamic, with multiple feedback loops.

If these models are so promising, why haven't our current batch of artificial neural network algorithms been more successful at performing ISP? ANN models create a powerful set of tools for solving a number of interesting problems, but most of the models have little biological relevance. Among other things, they are too small and not dynamic enough. In addition, they are limited to moderate levels of parallelism, unlike biological networks that are massively parallel. For all these reasons, biologically inspired models have great potential for providing us with new, scalable ISP algorithms.

Before we can be inspired by computational neurobiology, there have to be abstract functional representations of these systems. What may actually be the most important result from the recent resurgence in neural network research, is a major shift in perspective in the neuroscience community. In the past 10–15 years, many neuroscientists have been looking at functional models ("what does it compute?") and not just structural models ("what is it connected to?"). As researchers attempt to model ever more complex, higher-order functionality, computational models are emerging from neuroscience laboratories all over the world. Such models will be the primary inspiration for the next generation of ISP algorithms.

There are a number of excellent examples of the reverse engineering of biological computing systems. These models are abstracted from the original biology and are scalable to large configurations.

An important model is the cortronic network, which has been developed under the leadership of Robert Hecht-Nielsen (1999). These networks are abstract models of the cerebral cortex that create associations. They are sparsely connected and scalable to extremely large networks. The basic computation is straightforward and the models are stable. They are now being used to perform complex language-processing tasks.

Another important set of models consists of those developed by Lynch and Granger (Coultrip and Granger, 1994). They and their co-workers have "reverse engineered" the olfactory pyriform cortex and hippocampus. Their hippocampus model performs Bayesian classification with Parzen windows using a network of a nonobvious and amazingly efficient design. It is sparsely connected and activated, and data are represented in a partially distributed manner in which the network design uses the statistical aspects of neuron connectivity. The models are now being used to solve many real-world pattern recognition problems.

The third set of models includes cortical models from Douglas and Martin's group (Douglas and Martin, 1992). In addition to computational models, they have created silicon implementations, and are now applying these implementations to a number of real-world applications in areas such as robotic control and computer vision.

Other interesting and relevant models include those of Berger (Berger et al., 1994) and von der Malsburg (Wiscott et al., 1997), as well as those of Lansner and his group (Lansner and Holst, 1996). The latter are doing some interesting work in reinforcement-based learning (Barto and Sutton, 1998).

Implementation Issues

It appears that one of the problems with current ANN models is a lack of sufficient parallelism; therefore it is most likely that successful, biologically inspired ISP will utilize large numbers of nodes. The ability to execute such models in real time requires radically new silicon architectures—even the fastest projected microprocessors will be insufficient. For example, emulating a network of 1 million nodes and 1 billion connections (each node is connected to 1000 other nodes) in real time, where the network is updated once every 100 μs, requires more than 10 tera-ops/s.[2] In addition, many of the envisioned applications require this performance in low power and inexpensive implementations.

Many neural network chips have been built, but none have been commercial successes. These early efforts were either analog (Faggin and Mead, 1995) and suffered from design and technology limitations, or they were digital (Hammerstrom, 1995), with moderately parallel models and limited input-output (I/O) and transistor counts. Thus they found themselves competing directly with mainstream microprocessor and DSP technologies, where they lost.

In addition to the need to provide more powerful ISP, another reason for looking to biological systems for inspiration for future very large-scale integrated (VLSI) structures is Moore's law, which the semiconductor industry has been following for almost 30 years (i.e., the number of transistors that can be manufactured cost-effectively doubles every 18–24 months). It has been said that this is not really a physical law, but an article of faith, and now there is increasing pressure on our faith. As gate lengths shrink:

· Quantum effects become more common.

· Transistors are increasingly leaky, noisy, and unreliable.

· Metal interconnects appear as long, slow transmission lines.

· Communication becomes expensive relative to computation.

· It is increasingly difficult to synchronize an entire chip at multiple gigahertz clock rates.

- It is almost impossible to perform design verification and validation of a 100 million transistor design.

Another threat to Moore's law is fabrication cost. Intel Corporation is building a $2.3 billion chip fabricator in Oregon; —a lot of chips need to be sold to amortize this kind of investment.

Looking at this problem differently, much of the pressure on Moore's law results from existing computational models, which:

- are fault intolerant,
- require high precision,
- are globally synchronized, and
- perform extensive global communication, which is required, for example, in high-precision, parallel multiplication and score-boarding and conditional execution.

These characteristics are quite different from the capabilities that deep submicron transistors offer. In short, there is an increasing discrepancy between what these tiny, transistors can do and what we want them to do.

The Opportunity

Biological systems have figured out how to use loosely coupled, globally asynchronous, distributed computing with unreliable (and occasionally failing) components. Furthermore, even simple biological systems perform highly sophisticated ISP.

The models being derived from work in computational neurobiology, the awesome capabilities of silicon, and the fact that transistors are starting to behave like neurons creates a unique opportunity for radical new architectural models. These technologies, coupled with the significant need for more powerful ISP solutions, are creating what has been referred to as a strategic inflection point. The fundamental premise of our research project is that computational neurobiology will inspire new ISP models, and that these models will be massively parallel and require massively parallel silicon architectures for efficient execution.

The implication is not that Moore's law will end for traditional computing structures, since it will continue for some time. In the next 5 years (SIA, 1997) we will have the ability to place tens of thousands of simple processors on a single piece of silicon (table 16.1), although many engineers now acknowledge that there will be a slowing down as the fabrication of deep submicron circuits becomes ever more complex and expensive, and the behavior of the transistors themselves becomes more problematic. The main point of the discussion here is that biological computing offers models that will allow more rapid scaling because they are fundamentally tol-

Table 16.1
The relationship of transistors number and feature size over time

Year of First Product	1999	2003	2009
Feature size (nanometers)	180	130	70
Dynamic random access memory total bits	1.1 billion	4.3 billion	68.7 billion
Microprocessor transistors	21 million	76 million	520 million

erant of many of the deleterious effects of extreme scaling. These models will also lead to significantly cheaper implementations, providing massively parallel computation using small, low-power, fault-tolerant processors.

Just as it is clear that Moore's law will continue to hold (more or less) for traditional computational structures, so too, the biologically inspired systems discussed here are not being considered as a replacement for current computing models. Rather, they will augment and enhance what we currently do now with computers, acting as ISP co-processors.

The Impact on VLSI Architecture

To create silicon structures to emulate biologically inspired computing, we need a better understanding of biological computing models, and we need VLSI design techniques that emulate these models efficiently. We also need to identify which aspects of computational neurobiology are necessary and which are not. For example, analog computation has advantage in low-precision computations and low-power applications, and impressive computational density. However, analog computation also has disadvantages in stability, temperature sensitivity, communication, and ease of design. And it is not clear that analog's computational density is an advantage in sparsely activated, sparsely connected networks.

Digital technology is less area efficient, especially for certain types of functionality (e.g., leaky integration). It is also power intensive, and the representation of time tends to be more complicated (events are typically synchronized to a global clock). However, digital technology allows efficient multiplexing of scarce computational and communication resources.

One of our research tasks is to determine the combination of implementation techniques that is best for this architecture's space. We suspect that hybrid, analog-digital or "mixed-signal," techniques may well constitute the optimum design.

There are numerous other implementation issues in the adaptation of biological models for a vastly different implementation technology:

· capturing high-order and temporal information efficiently,

· stability,

• robustness in the face of faulty hardware—silicon also has different failure modes than biological structures, and

• connectivity—silicon does not have the same storage and connectivity capabilities as biological systems, which could ultimately limit silicon-based ISP.

Of these, connectivity is one of the most important characteristics of biological neural structures. As Mead expressed so eloquently in his ground-breaking book on neural-inspired VLSI:

Computation is always done in the context of neighboring information. For a neighborhood to be meaningful, nearby areas in the neural structure must represent information that is more closely related than that represented by areas further away. Visual areas in the cortex that begin the processing sequence are mapped retinotopically. Higher-level areas represent more abstract information, but areas that are close together still represent similar information. It is this map property that organizes the cortex such that most wires can be short and highly shared; it is *perhaps the single most important architectural principle* in the brain. (Mead, 1989)

Unfortunately, connectivity is perhaps the one area where silicon is significantly less robust than biological systems. Communication in silicon is generally limited to a two-dimensional plane (although with several levels—six to eight with today's semiconductor technologies). It is still one of the most important problems as we consider scaling to very large models. The following theorem (Bailey and Hammerstrom, 1988) demonstrates why.

Theorem: Assume an unbounded or very large rectangular array of silicon neurons in which each neuron receives input from its N nearest neighbors—that is, the fanout (divergence) and fan-in (convergence) is N. Each such connection consists of a single metal line, and the number of two-dimensional metal layers is much less than N. Then the area required by the metal interconnect is $O(N^3)$.

This result has profound implications for the general emulation of biological computation in silicon. If, for example, we double the fan-in from 100 to 200, the silicon area required for the metal interconnect increases by a factor proportional to $8\times$.

This unfortunate result means that for even moderate connectivity, the silicon area[3] devoted to the metal interconnect will dominate. Research at Oregon Graduate Institute (Bailey and Hammerstrom, 1988) has indicated that even moderate multiplexing of communication resources would greatly decrease the silicon area requirements without any real loss in performance. Means (1991) studied the implementation of the Lynch-Granger pyriform cortex model with multiplexed and nonmultiplexed communication and obtained a similar result.

Concurrently, Mead's group at California Institute of Technology and others developed "address-event representation" or AER communication (Mahowald, 1992; Mortara and Vittoz, 1994). The address-event technique has also been expanded into a hierarchical structure by Lazzaro and Wawrznyk (1995). When analog computation is used, signals can be represented by action potential-like "spikes" (generally a neuron unit exceeding its threshold). These signal "packets" or "pulses" are transmitted asynchronously at the moment they occur by sending the originating unit's address on a single multiplexed bus. This "pseudodigital" representation allows multiplexing of the bus and retention of temporal information, if competition for the units sharing the bus is minimal.

The issue of synchronization and clocking is related to multiplexing. If significant multiplexing is used, then it becomes more difficult to operate in real time, and a simulated virtual clock is required. There are already some interesting techniques that have been developed for synchronizing large-scale single-instruction multiple-data systems that may be of use here (Bengtsson and Svensson, 1998; Söderstam et al., 1998).

In studying potential implementations of cortical structures, we have developed an efficient multiplexing architecture in which data transfer occurs via overlapping, hierarchical buses (Bailey, 1988; Hammerstrom, 1991; Hammerstrom and Bailey, 1991; Bailey et al., 1990). This structure, the broadcast hierarchy (TBH) allows simultaneous high-bandwidth local connectivity and long-range connectivity, thereby providing a reasonable match to many biological connectivity patterns.

Braitenberg (Braitenberg and Schüz, 1998) postulates two general connectivity systems in cortex: "metric" (high-density connections to physically local cells, based on an actual two-dimensional layout), and "ametric" (low-density point-to-point connections to all large groups of densely connected cells). Connectivity is significantly denser in the metric system, but with limited extent, whereas connectivity in the ametric system is very sparse and random. There are actually many other reasons for such bimodal connectivity schemes (Anderson, 1999). One hypothesis that we will be investigating is that these localized connectivity patterns actually enable certain kinds of advanced cognitive processing, such as abstraction and hierarchical representations. So it is possible that in solving the scaling problem, biological computation created a structure of great power and flexibility.

Assume the network discussed earlier with 1 million nodes and 1000 connections per node, which is 1 billion connections. If we have a simple analog processor per neuron, then we can compute all 1000 connections simultaneously. If we are using micropower techniques, each processor could take a few microseconds; assume 100 μs. So we are computing 1 billion connections in 100 μs, which gives us a computation rate of 10 trillion connections computed per second. Assume that 10% of the neurons are active (i.e., they produce output pulses) and that each active neuron communicates 10 pulses[4] on average during a single network update. This is about 100,000 pulses per second per active neuron. The entire communication network then must handle 1 million × 10% × 100,000, or 10 billion pulses per second.

Figure 16.1 shows a simple, two-level broadcast hierarchy with four "nodes" (digital or analog processors) in each low-level region. A node can broadcast to any other node in its low-level region or any node in the high-level region.

Assume we have a two-level broadcast hierarchy, and that 95% of the messages from each node are to other nodes that can be reached by broadcasting the pulses on the lower layer. In addition, assume that each lower level broadcast region is connected to 1000 neurons; that means that each low-level broadcast region needs to handle about 9.5 million pulses per second, which is not a terribly large bandwidth. Recall that there are 1000 of these lower layers, so the accumulated bandwidth is 9.5 billion pulses per second.

The top broadcast region, which will cover all 1 million neurons, needs to handle 5% or 500 million pulses per second, which is certainly achievable in today's semiconductor technology. Messages can be "pipelined" through buffers and routers, since even in neural circuitry there is often a fair amount of signal delay—although it is important that the delay be reasonably consistent and predictable.

This example is quite simple; a real implementation would probably have several broadcast layers and possibly even some point-to-point connectivity. We believe that we can meet the connectivity requirements of large neural network models with current silicon techniques. However, it is necessary that the networks being emulated exhibit reasonably localized interconnections, which has been shown to be the case in cortical structures (Braitenberg and Schüz, 1998; Anderson, 1999; Abeles, 1991).

When implementing neural-like structures in silicon, an important issue concerns how the synapse is represented, in particular, how information is stored in the synapse. For digital systems, such information storage is straightforward. Single bits can be stored in dynamic, static, or floating-gate devices, since even in a noisy environment, signal restoration to a 1 or 0 is reasonably straightforward. However, storing analog values is more error prone and complex. There has been much work in creating floating-gate structures for analog learning systems (Diorio et al., 1997). We intend to exploit this technology to the degree that we use mixed-signal (analog-digital) data representations. It should be pointed out that the models we are considering here use either a single bit or at most a few bits to represent information at each synapse. It is possible that multilevel logic would provide the best representation compromise and the most efficient utilization of scarce communication resources.

Another important issue affecting VLSI architecture is fault tolerance. Research at Oregon Graduate Center (May, 1988) has shown that even with all-digital implementations, massively parallel hardware that emulates neural network models has a reasonable degree of fault tolerance. This is because most of the silicon area contains circuitry whose failure has a local functional impact. Another interesting question concerns whether there is some degree of design fault tolerance. The Adaptive

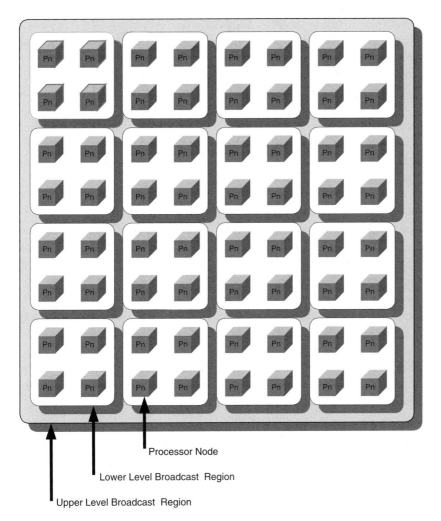

Figure 16.1
A two-level broadcast hierarchy for efficient emulation of cortical-like connectivity.

Solutions connected network of adoptive processors (CNAPS) chip had two design errors in the processor nodes arithmetic unit that were not discovered for several years. This problem was invisible mainly because most applications did not need precise arithmetic results. More work is needed in this area as these architectures evolve.

Then there is the need to test the manufactured chip. It is not clear exactly how one tests a faulty, mixed-signal chip like this, so the development of test methodologies optimized for this kind of architecture is important. Although the efficient testing of such chips is challenging, we do not view this as an impediment to the long-range success of the technology. However, we do foresee a fair amount of work required to create the necessary testing techniques.

Commercial Realization

The goal of our project is to create a family of commercial integrated circuits for use in a range of ISP solutions. Tentatively we expect the first commercial chip to be derived from this work to be the associative data processor (ADP).[5] The ADP will implement high-speed, high-capacity, best-match, associative memory. Because of algorithm and application dependencies, it is difficult to estimate at this time the implementation parameters of the resulting chip. However, Palm (Palm et al., 1997) has shown that these networks operate best with a very large number of nodes. Our goal will be tens of thousands of nodes for preliminary implementation.

In addition to large numbers of nodes, associative memory operation is highly dependent on having a sparse data representation. Since few natural data representations are sparse, we will need input and output pre- and postprocessing to "sparsify" and then "desparsify" input and output. Fields (1999) has shown that sparse representations may be a more suitable representation for preprocessed data. Small networks with a moderate number of inputs and a large number of outputs can be trained to efficiently map application-specific external representations to the distributed internal representations used by the network. A similar technique would be used for system output. Also, the input-output networks can be used to convert temporal to spatial information and vice versa.

For the first generation of ADPs we envision that the basic functionality will be "best-match" associative processing. For the most part, the "content-addressable" memory function that has been implemented to date is considered an "exact" match. Examples include cache and virtual page addressing in modern microprocessors, and domain name to internet protocol address look-up in Internet domain servers where a portion of a record is used as input and the memory returns the rest of the record. In contrast, with best-match processing, an arbitrary subset of a record is input, which may not match any record in the memory. In this case then, the memory returns the closest match (or matches) according to some metric. Incidentally, a best-match memory will always return the exact match first if such a match exists.

Best-match is significantly more powerful and more difficult to implement using traditional computing structures (it generally requires a complete search of the data in the memory). However, it can gracefully deal with errors and missing data and perform reasonable "generalization."

The metric used to determine how "close" an input vector is to a stored vector is generally an emergent property of the interconnection structure and the methods used in setting the connection or "synaptic" weights between nodes. For many applications, the metric can be a simple measure of vector distance. However, for more complex applications, the metric becomes a function of the higher-order internal data representation.

For the algorithms we are considering, the resulting weights tend to create a "distance-likelihood" metric that approximates Bayesian[6] classification. That is, the ADP will return the match (or set of matches) that is the most likely according to Bayesian rules.

A common operation in the applications being developed in other groups at Oregon Graduate Institute is that of finding complex higher-order structures in data (sound waves, image pixels, Internet text). Although limited in capability, and computation intensive, hidden markov models (Rabiner, 1989) are currently the best ISP technique for this task. One possibility we are considering is using a temporal version of best-match to approximate HMM functionality. Most of the neural models we are considering are capable of some form of this type of processing. For example, one of the Lynch-Granger models has already been used in simple speech applications (Aleksandrovsky et al., 1996). Just demonstrating superior results emulating HMMs would be a powerful proof of existence for this technology, and implementing HMMs on an ADP would provide marketable functionality since HMMs have a ready set of applications in speech recognition, OCR, handwriting recognition, and genetic sequencing.

We also intend to exploit the significant fault tolerance of these models to increase yield. All but large area faults, such as those that are due to wafer processing and power or ground shorts, should be correctable. For this reason, no chip will be exactly the same. Therefore, ADP chips will need to be trained rather than programmed. Although the training process will be nontrivial, we view this as an advantage, since it will be easier than programming a large parallel processor array. However, it will be a custom operation performed by the customer (much like burning a particular set of words into an electrically erasable–programmable read-only memory).

Conclusion

It is my belief that the convergence of high-density silicon and advanced computational models will lead to exciting new capabilities in intelligent signal processing.

In the research proposed here, our goal is to create a commercial product, based on simple models, that performs high-speed, adaptive, best-match, high-capacity associative data processing—the associative data processor.

Returning to Moore's law, Moore says there will be exponential progress and that doublings will occur every year and a half (Lucky, 1998). At first achieving exponential progress is easy, but later it becomes overwhelming—and we are starting to enter the "overwhelming" phase in semiconductors. Since the invention of the transistor, there have been about thirty-two doublings of the technology—the first half of a chessboard. The exciting question is, what overwhelming implications await us now as we begin the second half of the board?

The next 10 years will be an extraordinary time for silicon engineers and computer scientists. The challenges of Moore's law, and the search for quantitatively better ISP solutions will lead to more experimentation in new silicon architectures, fueled in part by ideas from biological computation. Understanding and mapping biological computing models to silicon, and then to real applications, will be difficult but the rewards will be great. By 2010, massively parallel, biologically inspired computational models will account for a significant portion of the global semiconductor business.

At the centenary of the Institute of Electrical and Electronics Engineers in 1984, Dr. Robert Noyce, co-founder of Intel and co-inventor of the integrated circuit, said: "Until now we have been going the other way; that is, in order to understand the brain we have used the computer as a model for it. Perhaps it is time to reverse this reasoning: to understand where we should go with the computer, we should look to the brain for some clues" (Noyce, 1984).

Notes

1. Some neuromodels exhibit synchronization, but it is generally part of the model, not a given supported by the underlying hardware.

2. It is possible that in some digital implementations, sparsely activated networks may lead to savings by having to emulate only parts of the network at any one time. However, that possibility is not considered in this simple example.

3. The cost of producing a silicon chip is directly related (in a complex, nonlinear manner) to the area of the chip.

4. In the address-event representation, each pulse is represented by the address, possibly of varying length, of the sender.

5. We intend to create a family of ADP chips that will cover a range of cost-to-performance ratios. In addition, one can envision using a variety of "intellectual property" library components such as digital signal processors and analog-to-digital converters, all integrated on a chip with the ADP circuitry.

6. Bayesian statistics guide the memory to return the stored vector most likely to have caused the input (assuming the input is a corrupted version of the returned value). Bayesian selection is optimal under certain conditions.

References

Abeles, M. (1991) *Corticonics: Neural Circuits of the Cerebral Cortex*. Cambridge: Cambridge University Press.

Aleksandrovsky, B., Whitson, J., Andes, G., Lynch, G., and Granger, R. (1996) *Novel Speech Processing Mechanism Derived from Auditory Neocortical Circuit Analysis*. New York: Institute of Electrical and Electronics Engineers.

Anderson, B. (1999) Commentary: Ringo, Doty, Demeter and Simard, Cerebral Cortex 1994; 4: 331–343: A proof of the need for the spatial clustering of interneuronal connections to enhance cortical computation. *Cerebral Cortex* 9: 2–3.

Bailey, J., and Hammerstrom, D. (1988) Why VLSI implementations of associative VLCNs require connection multiplexing. In *International Conference on Neural Network*. IEEE, vol. 2, pp. 173–180.

Bailey, J. (1988) A VISI interconnect structure for neural networks. Ph.D. dissertation. Department of Computer Science/Engineering, Oregon Graduate Center, Beaverton, Oregon.

Bailey, J., et al. (1990) Silicon association cortex. In S. F. Zornetzer, J. L. Davis, and C. Lau, eds., *An Introduction to Neural and Electronic Networks*. San Drego: Academic Press, pp. 307–316.

Barto, A. G., and Sutton, R. S. (1998) *Reinforcement Learning*. Cambridge, Mass.: MIT Press.

Bengtsson, L., and Svensson, B. (1998) A globally asynchronous, locally synchronous SIMD processor. In *5th International Conference on Massively Parallel Computing Systems—MPCS'98*. IEEE.

Berger, T. W., Chauvet, G., and Sclabassi, R. J. (1994) A biologically based model of the functional properties of the hippocampus. *Neural Networks* 7: 1031–1064.

Braitenberg, V., and Schüz, A. (1998) *Cortex: Statistics and Geometry of Neuronal Connectivity*. 2nd edition. New York: Springer-Verlag.

Coultrip, R. L., and Granger, R. H. (1994) Sparse random networks with LTP learning rules approximate Bayes classifiers via Parzen's method. *Neural Networks* 7(3): 463–476.

Diorio, C., Hasler, P., Minch, B. A., and Mead, C. A. (1997) A floating-gate MOS learning array with locally computed weight updates. *IEEE Trans. Electron. Dev.* 44(12): 2281–2289.

Douglas, R. J., and Martin, K. A. C. (1992) Exploring cortical microcircuits: A combined anatomical, physiogical, and computational approach. In T. Mckenna, J. Davis, and S. Zornetzer, eds., *Single Neuron Computing*. San Diego: Academic Press.

Faggin, F., and Mead, C. (1995) VLSI implementation of neural networks. In S. F. Zornetzer, J. L. Davis, and C. Law, eds., *An Introduction to Neural and Electronic Networks*. San Diego: Academic Press, pp. 297–314.

Feldman, J. A., and Ballard, D. (1982) Connectionist models and their properties. *Cog. Sci.* 6: 205–254.

Feldman, J., Lakoff, G., Bailey, D., Narayanan, S., Regier, T., and Stolcke, A. (1996) Lzero: The first five years. *Artificial Intell. Re.* 10.

Field, D. J. (1999) What is the goal of sensory coding? In G. Hinton and T. J. Sejnowski, eds., *Unsupervised Learning*. Cambridge, Mass.: MIT Press, pp. 101–143.

Hammerstrom, D. (1995) A digital VLSI architecture for real-world applications. In S. F. Zornetzer, J. L. Davis, and C. Law, eds., *An Introduction to Neural and Electronic Networks*. San Diego: Academic Press, pp. 335–358.

Haykin, S., and Kosko, B. (1998) Special issue on intelligent signal processing introduction. *Proc. IEEE* 86(11): 2119–2120.

Hecht-Nielsen, R. (1999) Tutorial: Cortronic neural networks. In *International Joint Conference on Neural Networks*. IEEE.

Heckerman, D. (1996) *A Tutorial on Learning with Bayesian Networks*. Redmond, Wash: Microsoft Research.

Johnson, C. (1998) Full speed ahead—Mead sees a future without boundaries. In *EE Times Special Edition—IC@40 Where We're Going*. CMP Media.

Lansner, A., and Holst, A. (1996) A higher order Bayesian neural network with spiking units. *Int. J. Neural Syst.* 7(2): 115–128.

Lansner, A., Ekeberg, Ö., Fransén, E., Hammarlund, P., and Wilhelmsson, T. (1997) Detailed simulation of large-scale neural networks. In J. M., Bower, ed., *Computational Neuroscience: Trends in Research 1997.* Boston: Plenum, pp. 931–935.

Lazzaro, J. P., and Wawrzynek, J. (1995) A multi-sender asynchronous extension to the address-event protocol. In W. J. Dally, J. W. Poulton, A. T. Ishü, eds., *16th Conference on Advanced Research in VLSI,* pp. 158–169.

Lucky, R. W., Reflections. (Sep 1998) IEEE Spectrum. 17.

Mahowald, M. A. (1992) VLSI Analogs of Neuronal Visual Processing. Ph.D. Thesis. Computation and neural systems. California Institute of Technology, Pasadena.

May, N. (1988) Fault simulation of a wafer-scale integrated neurocomputer. Department of Computer Science/Engineering, Master's Thesis. Oregon Graduate Center, Beaverton, Oregon.

Mead, C. (1989) *Analog VLSI and Neural Systems.* Reading Mass.: Addison-Wesley.

Means, E. (1991) Designs for a cortically inspired neurocomputer architecture. Department of Computer Science/Engineering, Master's Thesis. Oregon Graduate Institute, Beaverton, Oregon.

Mortara, A., and Vittoz, E. A. (1994) A communications architecture tailored for analog VLSI artificial neural networks—intrinsic performance and limitations. *IEEE J. Neural Net.* 5(3): 459–466.

Palm, G., Schwenker, F., Sommer, F. T., and Strey, A. (1997) Neural associative memories. In A. Krikelis and C. C. Weems, eds., *Associative Processing and Processors.* Los Alamitos, Calif.: IEEE Computer Society, pp. 284–306.

Rabiner, L. (1989) *A Tutorial on Hidden Markov Models and Selected Applications in Speech Recognition.* New York: Institute of Electrical and Electronics Engineers.

SIA (1997) *The National Technology Roadmap for Semiconductors.* Semiconductor Industry Association, San Jose, CA.

Söderstam, P., Taveniku, M., and Svensson, B. (1998) Adaptive beamforming on ring and torus SIMD architectures. Paper presented at *Swedish Workshop on Computer Systems Architecture.*

Wiskott, L., Fellous, J. M., Krüger, N., and Von Der Malsburg, C. (1997) Face recognition by elastic bunch graph matching. *IEEE Trans. Pattern Anal. Mach. Intell.* 19(7): 775–779.

Contributors

Xin An
Holoplex Inc.
Pasadena, California

Suat Ay
Photobit Corp
Pasadena, California

Michel Baudry
Neuroscience Program
and Department of Biology:
Neurobiology
University of Southern California
Los Angeles, California

Theodore W. Berger
Center for Neural Engineering
Department of Biomedical Engineering
University of Southern California
Los Angeles, California

Roberta Diaz Brinton
Department of Molecular
Pharmacology and Toxicology
and Neuroscience Program
University of Southern California
Los Angeles, California

Gilbert A. Chauvet
École Pratique des Hautes Études
Paris, France
and
Centre Hospitalier Universitaire d'Angers
Angers, France

P. Chauvet
Institut de Mathématiques Appliquées
Université Catholique de l'Ouest Angers
Angers, France

Ellen Covey
Department of Psychology
University of Washington
Seattle, Washington

Sam A. Deadwyler
Department of Physiology and
Pharmacology and Neuroscience
Program
Wake Forest University School of
Medicine
Winston Salem, North Carolina

Emese Dian
Department of Biological Sciences and
Center for Network Neuroscience,
University of North Texas
Denton, Texas

Howard Eichenbaum
Laboratory of Cognitive Neurobiology
Department of Psychology
Boston University
Boston, Massachusetts

Kah-Guan Au Eong
Wilmer Eye Institute
Johns Hopkins University
Baltimore, Maryland

J. Finch
Raytheon RIO Corporation
Goleta, California

Shahram Ghandeharizadeh
Department of Computer Science
University of Southern California
Los Angeles, California

Dennis L. Glanzman
Theoretical and Computational
Neuroscience
National Institute of Mental Health
Bethesda, Maryland

R. Graham
Raytheon RIO Corporation
Goleta, California

Alexandra Gramowski
Institute for Cell Technology
University of Rostock
Rostock, Germany

Richard Granger
Brain Engineering Laboratory
Computer Science Department
University of California
Irvine, California

Guenter W. Gross
Department of Biological Sciences and
Center for Network Neuroscience,
University of North Texas
Denton, Texas

Dan Hammerstrom
Electrical and Computer Engineering
Department
Portland State University
Portland, Oregon

Robert Hampson
Department of Physiology and
Pharmacology and Neuroscience
Program
Wake Forest University School of
Medicine
Winston Salem, North Carolina

James J. Hickman
Director, Nanoscience Technology
Center
Burnett College of Biomedical Sciences
University of Central Florida
Orlando, Florida

J. G. Howard
U.S. Naval Research Laboratory
Washington, D.C.

M. Humayun
U.S. Naval Research Laboratory
Washington, D.C.

B. Keith Jenkins
Department of Electrical Engineering
University of Southern California
Los Angeles, California

E. de Juan, Jr.
Wilmer Eye Institute
Johns Hopkins University
Baltimore, Maryland

Brian Justus
U.S. Naval Research Laboratory
Washington, D.C.

Edward G. Keefer
Department of Biological Sciences and
Center for Network Neuroscience,
University of North Texas
Denton, Texas

R. Klein
U.S. Naval Research Laboratory
Washington, D.C.

Alexei Koulakov
Department of Physics
University of Utah
Salt Lake City, Utah

Gerald E. Loeb
Biomedical Engineering
University of Southern California
and
Medical Device Development Facility
A.E. Mann Institute for Biomedical
Engineering
Los Angeles, California

E. Margalit
Wilmer Eye Institute
Johns Hopkins University
Baltimore, Maryland

Vasilis Z. Marmarelis
Department of Biomedical Engineering
University of Southern California
Los Angeles, California

Charles Merritt
U.S. Naval Research Laboratory
Washington, D.C.

Fai Mok
Holoplex Inc.
Pasadena, California

Jose Mumbru
Department of Electrical Engineering
California Institute of Technology
Pasadena, California

Richard A. Normann
The Center for Neural Interfaces
University of Utah
Salt Lake City, Utah

George Panotopoulos
Department of Electrical Engineering
California Institute of Technology
Pasadena, California

M. Peckerar
U.S. Naval Research Laboratory
Washington, D.C.

F. K. Perkins
U.S. Naval Research Laboratory
Washington, D.C.

Demetri Psaltis
Department of Electrical Engineering
California Institute of Technology
Pasadena, California

Dean Scribner
U.S. Naval Research Laboratory
Washington, D.C.

Krishna V. Shenoy
Divison of Biology
California Institute of Technology
Pasadena, California

Bing J. Sheu
Nassda Corporation
Santa Clara, California

John Simeral
Department of Physiology and
Pharmacology and Neuroscience
Program
Wake Forest University School of
Medicine
Winston Salem, North Carolina

Walid Sousou
Department of Biology Neurobiology
University of Southern California
Los Angeles, California

Simone Stuewe
Institute for Cell Technology
University of Rostock
Rostock, Germany

Armand R. Tanguay, Jr.
Departments of Electrical Engineering,
Materials Science and Biomedical
Engineering
University of Southern California
Los Angeles, California

S. Taylor
Raytheon RIO Corporation
Goleta, California

Mark Thompson
Department of Chemistry
University of Southern California
Los Angeles, California

C. Trautfield
Raytheon RIO Corporation
Goleta, California

David J. Warren
The Center for Neural Interfaces
University of Utah
Salt Lake City, Utah

J. Weiland
Wilmer Eye Institute
Johns Hopkins University
Baltimore, Maryland

Index

Abdelrazzaq, F. B., 223
Abeles, M., 59, 378
Aboitiz, F., 286
Acetylcholinesterase (AChE), 197
Acoustics, 4–7
Action potentials. *See* Synapses
Active pixel sensor (APS) arrays, 307, 352–354
Adaptive Solutions network, 378, 380
Adhesion
 CAMs and, 180, 221–225
 decapeptide and, 235
 electrode coatings and, 221–233
 microelectrode array/electrode coupling and, 186–188
 RGDS and, 235
 strength of, 181–182
 surface preparation and, 178–181
Age-related macular degeneration (AMD), 16, 19, 23, 29–30
Agnew, W. F., 15
Ahmed, B., 281
Aiple, F., 43–44
Aizawa, M., 206
Alataris, K., 249
Albus, K., 55
Aleksandrovsky, B., 279, 284, 286, 291, 381
Alfred E. Mann Institute for Biomedical Engineering, vii
Algorithms, 37–38, 278
 dynamic learning, 250, 252
 fast Fourier transforms, 362
 intelligent signal processing, 369–382
 K-Means, 169–170
 K Nearest Neighbor (KNN), 170
 multichip modules and, 309–311
 query processing, 168–170
 shuffling, 46
 striatal complex and, 286–291
 thalamocortical circuits and, 280–286, 290–291
Allen, J. F., 164, 165
Alzheimer's disease, 241, 290
Amacrine cells, 16

Amaral, D. G., 244
Ambros-Ingerson, J., 279, 283–284, 291
Amnesia, 92
Amyotrophic lateral sclerosis (ALS), 335
An, Xin, 335–368, 385
Analog-digital design, 243, 252–256
 dynamic synapse network, 261–263
 high-density hippocampal processor, 259–261
 multichip modules and, 323–326 (*see also* Multichip modules)
 second-order nonlinear models, 257–259
Analogical approach, 129–130
Analog-to-digital converters, 358
Anandamide, 199
Andersen, P., 244
Anderson, B., 377–378
Anderson, C. M., 234
Anderson, D. J., 28
AND gates, 261
Andraka, R., 362
Angel dust, 217
Anterior neocortex, 286
Anton, P. S., 212, 291
Aplysia, 180
Application-specific integrated circuit (ASIC), 340–341
Arbib, M. A., 328
Arginine, 235
Arieli, A., 59
Arm system, 336–338, 358–359, 362–365
Arrhythmic bursting, 281–282
Artificial neural networks
 conventional, 249–250
 defined, 131
 dynamic synapse, 250–252, 261–263
 hierarchical representation and, 133–136
 high-precision computation and, 277–291
 hippocampus and, 249–257, 261–263
 intelligent signal processing and, 369–382
 mathematical modeling of, 129–157
 speech recognition and, 252–257
Aschner, M., 234